Physicians' Pathways to Non-Traditional Careers and Leadership Opportunities

Richard D. Urman · Jesse M. Ehrenfeld
Editors

Physicians' Pathways to Non-Traditional Careers and Leadership Opportunities

Editor, "Leaders in the Successful Pursuit of Non-Traditional Careers in Medicine"

N. Stephen Ober, M.D., M.B.A.
Executive Director, Business Incubation
Boston University Technology Development
Faculty Director, MD/MBA Dual Degree Program
Boston University School of Medicine
Boston, MA, USA

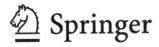 Springer

Editors

Richard D. Urman, M.D., M.B.A.
Assistant Professor of Anesthesia
Harvard Medical School
Director, Hospital Procedural Sedation
Management and Safety
Co-Director, Center for Perioperative
Management and Medical Informatics
Brigham and Women's Hospital
Boston, MA 02115, USA

Jesse M. Ehrenfeld, M.D., M.P.H.
Assistant Professor of Anesthesiology
Assistant Professor of Biomedical
Informatics
Director, Center for Evidence-Based
Anesthesia
Director, Perioperative Data Systems
Research
Medical Director, Perioperative Quality
Vanderbilt, University Medical Center
Nashville, TN 37232, USA

ISBN 978-1-4614-0550-4   e-ISBN 978-1-4614-0551-1
DOI 10.1007/978-1-4614-0551-1
Springer New York Dordrecht Heidelberg London

Library of Congress Control Number: 2011940804

Cover Illustration: © Joachim Wendler

Printed on acid-free paper

Springer is part of Springer Science+Business Media (www.springer.com)

*I would like to thank all my colleagues
for helping me learn from their aspirations
and experiences, my mentors for their
support and encouragement,
my students for asking insightful questions
and for providing inspiration to write this
book, and my family for their love
and patience. Very special thanks to my
parents, Dennis and Tanya Urman,
and to my wife, Dr. Zina Matlyuk-Urman,
for her editorial input.*

RDU

*I would like to dedicate this book
to my mentors, who have given of themselves
selflessly, and tirelessly, in order that
others may succeed. To all of you,
I am forever indebted.
Special thanks to Warren Sandberg,
Katharine Nicodemus, David Ehrenfeld,
Joshua Ehrenfeld and all of my family and
friends without whose support none of my
achievements would have been possible.*

JME

Foreword

Medicine has changed dramatically over the past several decades. State-of-the-art imaging technologies, minimally invasive surgery, and targeted cancer diagnostics and therapeutics are now standard. Individual private practices have given way to large group practice models. The changes in the practice and outcomes of medicine are breathtaking.

Many forces that shape medicine (and the healthcare of the American public) now are driven from outside of our profession. Insurance reform, research funding, medical student debt, medical malpractice insurance, drug prices, and access to primary care are just a few of the current challenges. Although traditional medical education does not formally train physicians in economics, management, or organizational behavior, the structure of residency education and practice does provide physicians with leadership, teaching, and supervision skills. Many physicians also informally learn basic accounting skills over time in the management of their clinical practice or academic department.

The input of physicians with their practical understanding of the current impediments to effective healthcare delivery into the medical policy debate is critical. Increasingly physicians need to leverage their medical expertise with business skills to remain leaders in the healthcare industry.

Over my career, and especially as my last 7 years as dean of the Boston University School of Medicine, I have met with hundreds of medical students, resident physicians, and practicing clinicians who share the vision of wanting to make the world a better place and specifically to fix healthcare. Although physicians are well grounded in clinical medicine and in the practical aspects of healthcare delivery, they have less experience in reaching these goals politically on a macro level.

In this book, Dr. Richard Urman, his coauthors, and more than 30 physicians have documented their careers and outlined opportunities for physicians in addition to those in clinical medicine. Their experiences considerably broaden career options and leadership opportunities for physicians and provide a wider framework for physicians to take leadership roles in health policy and delivery. Whatever career trajectory chosen by a physician to improve our healthcare system, those in administration, research, financial services, consulting, industry, or managed care still adhere to one of the most sacrosanct phrases in the original translation of the Hippocratic Oath: "In every house where I come, I will enter only for the good of my patients."

I hope you enjoy this book and that you will think broadly about the impact you can make in reshaping the future of medicine.

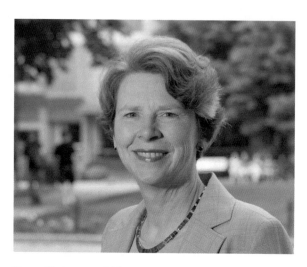

Karen H. Antman, MD
Provost, Boston University Medical Campus
Dean, School of Medicine

Preface

Many physicians are in search of opportunities to enrich their professional lives by obtaining additional experiences and education outside of their area of practice as a way to help their patients, provide leadership in healthcare, advance their careers, or perhaps pursue excellence in a new area or field. Some physicians will choose to pursue another degree, while others will seek to expand their horizons in non-academic settings such as public service, business, education, and organized medicine.

This book fulfills an unmet need by serving as a practical guide and offering advice on how to make sense of one's career goals, what questions to ask, and how to position oneself for success. Many medical students, residents, fellows, and physicians in practice want to continue their clinical work and provide direct care for patients, while pursuing other interests. This book discusses how mentorship, formal and informal educational opportunities, volunteer and public service can enrich your professional life. We begin with an overview of healthcare today and a discussion of the relationship between personality type and job satisfaction.

Our goal is to guide you through the process of formulating concrete questions, which can then help you devise a short- and long-term career plan. A practicing physician might ask herself, "I would like to work more closely toward improving the overall health of my community – should I get an MPH degree?" A resident-physician might be wondering what the best way would be to get involved with organized medicine, and how to find good mentors. A medical student might wonder, "What kind of meaningful volunteer work should I pursue to enrich and guide my educational experiences and help me choose a specialty?" Others with an interest in business or consulting might want to know the utility of pursuing an MBA degree. This book offers advice to individuals seeking to pursue a variety of professional endeavors both within and outside of medicine.

We include a few first-hand accounts of those physicians who have distinguished themselves in a variety of career pursuits outside of traditional career paths. They tell their stories and discuss their paths toward success. We believe that there is currently no other source that addresses these important issues, and hope that you and other medical students, residents, fellows, and practicing physicians find this book a useful tool in pursuing your dreams – wherever they may take you.

Boston, MA, USA   Richard D. Urman, MD, MBA
Nashville, TN, USA   Jesse M. Ehrenfeld, MD, MPH

Contents

Contributors

Rebecca Aft, MD, PhD Department of Surgery, Washington University, St. Louis, MO, USA

Edward L. Amaral, MD, FACS Department of Surgery, University of Massachusetts School of Medicine, Shrewsbury, MA, USA

Alexander F. Arriaga, MD, MPH Department of Health Policy and Management, Harvard School of Public Health, Brigham and Women's Hospital, Boston, MA, USA

Michael S. Axley, MD, MA Department of Anesthesia and Perioperative Medicine, Oregon Health and Science University, Portland, OR, USA

Christopher W. Baugh, MD, MBA Department of Emergency Medicine, Brigham and Women's Hospital, Harvard Medical School, Boston, MA, USA

Paul D. Biddinger, MD, FACEP Department of Emergency Medicine, Massachusetts General Hospital, Boston, MA, USA

Mark A. Bloomberg, MD, MBA HealthNEXT, Sudbury, MA, USA

Richard Bohmer, MBChB, MPH Harvard Business School, Soldiers Field Road, Boston, MA, USA

Spencer Borden IV, MD, MBA, FACR, FAAP, FACPE Concord, MA, USA

Sheng F. Cai, MD, PhD Medical Scientist Training Program, Washington University in St. Louis School of Medicine, Sunnyside, NY, USA

David M. Center, MD Department of Medicine, Boston University Clinical and Translational Science Institute, Boston University Medical Campus

Pulmonary, Allergy, Sleep and Critical Care Medicine, Boston Medical Center, Boston, MA, USA

Maria Young Chandler, MD, MBA University of California, Irvine, USA

The Children's Clinic, Long Beach, CA, USA

Association of MD/MBA Programs, Inc., Sunset Beach, CA, USA

Alexander Ding, MD, MS Department of Radiology, Massachusetts General Hospital/Harvard Medical School, Boston, MA, USA

Lena Ebba Dohlman, MD, MPH Department of Anesthesiology, Critical Care & Pain Medicine, Massachusetts General Hospital/Cambridge Health Alliance, Brookline, MA, USA

Gregory Dolin, MD, JD University of Baltimore School of Law/Johns Hopkins University School of Medicine, Baltimore, MD, USA

Joseph S. Fastow, MD, MPH, FACEP Physician Management, Ltd., Bethesda, MD, USA

Department of Health Policy & Management, Johns Hopkins Bloomberg School of Public Health, Baltimore, MD, USA

Stan N. Finkelstein, MD MIT Engineering Systems Division and Harvard-MIT, Division of Health Sciences & Technology, Harvard Medical School, Cambridge, MA, USA

Kathleen Franco, MD, MS Cleveland Clinic Lerner College of Medicine of Case Western Reserve University, Cleveland, OH, USA

Ingrid Ganske, MD, MPA Department of Plastic and Reconstructive Surgery, Massachusetts General Hospital, Boston, MA, USA

Deeona Gaskin Student at Harvard Law and Harvard School of Public Health, Boston, MA, USA

Jonathan P. Gertler, MD, MPH, FACEP Back Bay Life Science Advisors, Boston, MA, USA

Annekathryn Goodman, MS, MD Department of Obstetrics and Gynecology, Gillette Center for Women's Cancers, Harvard Medical School, Boston, MA, USA

Jean Hess, MS Harvard Medical School, Boston, MA, USA

Jeremy M. Huff, DO, CAPT, USAF Medical Corps Department of Anesthesia, Wright-Patterson Medical Center, Wright-Patterson AFB, OH, USA

Steve Alan Hyman, MD, MM Department of Anesthesiology, Vanderbilt University School of Medicine, Nashville, TN, USA

Richard Kalish, MD, MS, MPH Medical Director, Boston Medical Center, HealthNet Plan and Boston HealthNet

Assistant Professor, Departments of Medicine and Family Medicine, Boston University School of Medicine

Director of Community Engagement, Boston University Clinical and Translational Science Institute, Boston, MA, USA

Mary Kraft, MD, MPA Department of Anesthesia, Baystate Medical Center, Springfield, MA, USA

Lisa Soleymani Lehmann, MD, PhD, MSc Division of General Medicine, Brigham and Women's Hospital, Harvard Medical School, Boston, MA, USA

Lisa Bard Levine, MD, MBA Associate Director, Navigant Consulting, Inc., Needham, MA, USA

Melvin C. Makhni, MD, MBA Candidate Harvard Medical School, Harvard Business School

Richard Marshall, MD Department of Pediatrics, Harvard Vanguard Medical Associates, Boston, MA, USA

Darshan Mehta, MD, MPH Benson-Henry Institute for Mind Body Medicine, Massachusetts General Hospital, Boston, MA, USA

D. Kiley Mortensen, DO, CAPT, USAF Medical Corps Department of Anesthesia, Wilford Hall Medical Center, Lackland AFB, TX, USA

Katharine M. Nicodemus, PsyD, MA Clinical Neuropsychologist, Greenville, DE, USA

N. Stephen Ober, BA, MD, MBA Executive Director, Business Incubation, Boston University Technology Development

Faculty Director, MD/MBA Dual Degree Program, Boston University School of Medicine, Boston, MA, USA

Shalini Reddy, MD Department of Internal Medicine, University of Chicago, Pritzker School of Medicine, Chicago, IL, USA

David A. Rosman, MD, MBA Instructor in Radiology, Harvard Medical School, Assistant Radiologist, Associate Director Business Development, Department of Imaging, Massachusetts General Hospital, Boston, MA, USA

Samantha Rosman, MD Department of Pediatrics, Division of Emergency Medicine, Harvard Medical School, Children's Hospital Boston, Boston, MA, USA

Peter R. Russo, MBA Boston University School of Management, Boston University, Boston, MA, USA

Rahul Sakhuja, MD, MPP, MSc Department of Cardiology, Massachusetts General Hospital, Boston, MA, USA

Jason Sanders, MD, MBA Consultant McKinsey & Company, Boston, MA, USA

Palak Shah, MPP Harvard Kennedy School of Government, Boston, MA, USA

Simona F. Shaitelman, MD, EdM Department of Radiation Oncology, Division of Radiation Oncology, The University of Texas MD Anderson Cancer Center, Houston, TX, USA

Erica Seiguer Shenoy, MD, PhD Division of Infectious Diseases,
Department of Medicine, Massachusetts General Hospital, Boston, MA, USA

Peter L. Slavin, MD President, Massachusetts General Hospital, Boston,
MA, USA

Mary E. Thorndike, MD, MPA Division of General Medicine,
Department of Medicine, Hospitalist Service, Brigham and Women's Hospital,
Brigham and Women's Hospital, Jamaica Plain, MA, USA

Jack T. Watters, MD Pfizer Medical Department, Pfizer Inc.,
New York, NY, USA

Part I
How to Choose a Balanced Career Path

Chapter 1
Changing Landscape of Career Opportunities in Medicine in the 21st Century: A Brave New World

David M. Center

Key Points
- The importance of the Bayh-Dole Act in creating opportunities for university-based physician-scientists to become entrepreneurs.
- New opportunities for physicians with computational mathematical skills in electronic clinical data management.
- New opportunities in health-law, ethics, and informatics.

Introduction

For most of the history of formal training in medicine, individuals sought a post graduate degree (MD) to devote themselves to care for the sick. The many specialties of medicine and surgery evolved out of need and were maintained by highly structured apprenticeships and rites of passage. As types of treatments grew, medical practice expanded in both hospital and office settings and by the first third of the twentieth century practices in specialties of medicine and surgery became popular. By the mid 1960s there was deemed to be a major shortage of physicians, and medical schools were mandated to increase their enrollments to meet these needs. Forty years later we stand in the shadow of that expansion with a wide variation of

D.M. Center, MD (✉)
Department of Medicine, Boston University Clinical and Translational Science Institute,
Boston University Medical Campus, Boston, MA, USA

Pulmonary, Allergy, Sleep and Critical Care Medicine, Boston Medical Center,
72 East Concord Street, Boston, MA 02118, USA
e-amil: dcenter@bu.edu

R.D. Urman and J.M. Ehrenfeld (eds.), *Physicians' Pathways to Non-Traditional Careers and Leadership Opportunities*, DOI 10.1007/978-1-4614-0551-1_1,
© Springer Science+Business Media, LLC 2012

interpretation of its impact. One of the mandates for that expansion was the shortage of what we now call primary care physicians (either Family Practitioners with skills in multiple disciplines or Internal Medicine trained generalists who do not practice a medical subspecialty). At one extreme, it is clear that the expansion of medical school classes markedly increased the number of specialists in all fields and with very unique skills. Many of these specialists are more highly compensated than general practitioners. Specialty skills have driven many fields to levels of sophistication of care not possible if medical care delivery was completely entrusted to generalists. It is unfair to generalize and state that specialties and subspecialties are now oversubscribed, as it is clear that some still have huge work forces shortages (e.g., critical care medicine). On the other extreme, the need for primary care physicians went unmet and as a corollary it has been suggested that the costs of medical care have been driven up by the presence of specialists intent on discovering and inventing new, more sophisticated and more expensive technologies to care for patients. The trend in medical care away from private practices to hospital-based employment is an indication that the priorities of practicing physicians have changed. As such, this is an opportune time to consider new (non-traditional) career opportunities in medicine.

As you will read in the chapters of this book, physicians have expanded their career horizons from full time clinical medicine to careers as diverse as law, politics, entrepreneurship, research, consulting, financial services, public health, administration, journalism, and business (to name just a few), all the while leveraging their clinical knowledge and experience to make an impact on the healthcare system in their own unique way. How did we get here and what are some of the innovations we can expect from not only traditional clinicians, but from those pursuing some of the non-traditional career tracks mentioned above? It is clear that the discoveries of the past few decades will need both more entrepreneurial MDs to drive the science of medicine and practitioners to deliver traditional and new treatments. This chapter will briefly highlight some historical events that have opened a Pandora's Box of new directions, fields and applications of science in medicine with a diversity of exciting opportunities for those with medical degrees to make local, regional, national and international impact on the health of individuals and global populations.

Historical Perspective

We can attribute a vast majority of new MD career opportunities to discoveries and inventions in three fields (engineering, computer science, and genetics) and an extraordinary Act of Congress (Bayh-Dole Act). The remarkable giants of clinical medicine, like Osler and Freud created the modern approaches to the diagnosis and practice of medicine in what we now know as its traditional form of care for the sick. These hypothesis-driven approaches are based on careful observation. Physiology, anatomy and natural history generated the focus of training in medicine and therefore shaped MD career opportunities well into the latter half of the twentieth century. Almost all of primary and specialty care careers are derived from their approaches to applying new knowledge of pathophysiology of organ-specific diseases. At the same time, careers in medical research and the pharmaceutical industry were derived from a parallel group of physicians from the nineteenth century whose careers and impact were devoted to disease prevention. The impacts on health of providing uncontaminated drinking water and milk; the concept of vaccination to protect against infectious diseases (e.g., smallpox), and vector (mosquito) control to prevent spread of other infectious diseases (malaria and yellow fever) still resonate as the most important concepts in medicine in the twenty-first century.

Once it became clear that natural or synthetic products could prevent disease or affect health the pharmaceutical industry became a part of daily life. Because these corporations produced healthcare products, the input from physicians at all stages of drug and device development became essential. Among the first, and persistent alternate career opportunities for physicians were in industry. Product ideas and development and regulatory requirements defined by the FDA generated the need for input in design and implementation of clinical trials in patients. As more new products become available, the need for physician input will continue to grow in order to recruit subjects and provide insights into study design. As new targets for drugs are discovered, the need for physicians with knowledge of clinical disease genotypes and phenotypes, disease processes, and desirable disease outcomes will continue to grow. The opportunities range from development of new vaccines to better drugs with fewer side effects. These are not new opportunities, but they are examples of a few of the ones that will continue to grow in need.

However, the research and initial development stage of tomorrow's medical breakthroughs do not guarantee an innovation's success, regardless of whether the product is fundamentally sound. As these technologies advance, there are important issues that must be addressed to assure their success. Critical matters such as pricing, reimbursement policy, regulatory approvals, product development, product sales, marketing, financing, training, and ethical impact are a few of the areas that can make a new innovation a block buster or a total commercial failure. While these matters have traditionally been the domain of non-physicians, more and more medical professions are realizing that careers in these areas can be personally rewarding. In addition, by combining these new skill sets with their clinical expertise, many physicians realize that they can truly excel in these careers, often resulting in an expedited track to leadership positions in their chosen fields.

The Changing Complexion of Medicine

Is there a "Brave New World" of career opportunities? As noted above, discoveries in three fields, two non-medical have been a driving force behind providing new opportunities for careers in medicine. The non-medical fields, engineering and computer science are intimately related and one could argue the former spawned the latter. Biomedical engineering can claim its modern roots in the Curies' discovery of the diagnostic and therapeutic effects of X-rays. Those discoveries required design and manufacture of an ever more sophisticated series of machines capable of imaging and X-ray delivery. Biomedical engineering has prospered from an ever increasing array of variations on this theme in imaging, improving our understanding of disease process and chronology, staging, therapy, drug delivery, disease tracking, and so on. From devices to sutures to implantable materials and artificial organs, advances in engineering have been rapidly incorporated into daily patient care. Whether it is faster more reliable in vitro testing devices or diagnostic equipment (e.g., fiberoptics), technology becomes available and used more rapidly than new drugs and other therapies.

New areas in engineering which offer potential career opportunities to provide medical expertise, direction, and testing include microfluidics for point of care diagnostics using extremely small amounts of body fluids, design and development of new synthetic organs or devices that assume the functions of diseased organs (e.g., artificial pancreas, hearts, miniaturized implantable kidneys to avoid bulky inconvenient dialysis machines and overcome the transplant shortage), sophisticated nanotechnology and particle design for localization of areas of disease, polymer design for use in delivery of drugs and as scaffolding for repair of surface structures, new techniques for low scatter radiation therapy, and many others.

More and more sophisticated engineering like robotics and better miniaturization of testing and delivery devices will continue to drive whole fields of new job opportunities for MDs trained in various specialties. These techniques are not only essential for progress in medical care delivery, but one also expects that they will eventually drive the costs of care down as monitoring-free modalities for earlier detection and prevention become available, and costly medical therapies like dialysis are eliminated.

Perhaps even more important for the future is the revolutionary impact that computer science has and will have on medicine. The blending of computers into healthcare is now so complete, it is hard to imagine a time when computer technology was not available. Computer science will continue to open new career opportunities at an ever increasing pace far outstripping the opportunities generated by other engineering and human genetics (see below). The need for more sophisticated and useful software is the current major career opportunity and is expected to expand with time. It is expected that the use of electronic records will become ubiquitous and with it a need for MD sophistication in tools and applications (e.g., voice recognition programs). The Brave New World of computer diagnosis is already here in programs like IBM's Watson technology recently showcased on the game show Jeopardy. There are now voice recognition systems that completely scan the entire world's literature (including the newest publications) for diagnostic searches and then rank-order treatment options. Newer

Table 1. Examples of alternate career paths for physicians

Engineering	Information Technology	Genetics/Genomics	Entrepreneurship
New Biomedical diagnostics and treatments	Development of electronic medical records	Development of individual genome sequencing	MD-Scientist (e.g., drug discovery)
Artificial organs	New tools for storing and access of clinical and research data	Personalized medicine	MD-MBA (e.g., company CEO)
New point of contact diagnostics	High speed, point of contact (voice recognition) diagnostics	Environmental medicine	MD-JD (e.g., patent law)
Individualized disease-specific monitoring devices	Computer-based monitoring and self-therapy	Genetic/genomic diagnostic and prognostic tools	

computer-assisted physiologic monitoring equipment is also on the horizon. Perhaps the most important impact of computers on medicine has been the ability to store huge amounts of clinical and scientific data and then to analyze it. This made possible the sequencing of the human genome and now the sequencing of any individual's genome at a low cost. Without computational mathematics and new algorithms genetics, systems biology (genomics, proteomics etc) and personalized medicine would be science fiction. The opportunities are limitless and will enable MDs with sophisticated mathematics skills to develop unique careers.

The third field which will continue to have an increasingly greater role in providing new non-traditional careers in medicine is genetics. By this I mean all the fields related to human genes and their expression. The fields of population, group, family and personalized medicine have developed from the various components of the human genome research. These fields combine essential computing power with genetic, epigenetic and gene-environment interactions. The new career opportunities are limitless as pharmaceutical industry-government partnerships are formed to identify targets for new diagnostics and therapies. Table 1.1 summarizes various career opportunities available for physicians. These include MD expertise in new drug and device development, conceptualization of techniques for surrogate physiologic ex vivo high throughput screening, and means for proof of concept before human testing. In this regard, the field of regenerative medicine has already begun to provide organ-specific cells with the mature disease phenotype from skin of affected individuals from autologous iPS cells. These ex vivo systems will someday be used for screening for efficacy and side effects of new agents before testing in whole human beings.

Careers in Business

December 12, 2010 marked the thirtieth anniversary of the single most important piece of legislation in scientific entrepreneurship. In addition to its many consequences, it paved the way for numerous new opportunities in business careers in medicine. This is the Bayh-Dole Act [1]. Co-sponsored by Birch Bayh of Indiana and Robert Dole of Kansas, it is generally considered the most important piece of biotechnology legislation ever passed by Congress. Known as the Patent and Trademarks Amendment of 1980, it granted the ability of non-profit institutions, in particular universities, to file for patents based on discoveries that arose from federally funded research. The importance of this piece of legislation on expanding the types of career options for MDs and scientists cannot be overstated. It had six major provisions:

1. Non-profits, universities, or small businesses could elect to retain rights to inventions made with federally funded research.
2. It specifically encouraged universities to file patents on these discoveries.
3. It explicitly encouraged non-profits to make collaborations with other entities for the development of related products from their IP (e.g., licensure of patents to pharmaceutical companies to develop drugs).

But it retained some caveats:

4. Universities were supposed to give preference to licensing agreements with small businesses (an unenforceable provision).
5. The government retained the non-exclusive right to practice any patents generated from federally funded research anywhere in the world.
6. The government retained "march in" rights.

This required formal reporting of inventions and technology derived from government grants as part of the continuing non-competitive renewal reports and in the final grant summary at the conclusion of funding. From this act a number of alternate career opportunities for MDs emerged:

1. The MD Scientist as Reimbursed Discoverer. First, it created a concrete basis for MD (and PhD) scientists to become entrepreneurs based upon their science. In many ways, it helped give birth to the translational science movement. In addition to traditional biomedical science, funded by National Institutes of Health (NIH), National Science Foundation (NSF), Veteran Affairs (VA), Department of Defense (DoD) or private institutions, it gave universities the incentive to encourage filing for patents on intellectual property (IP) developed by their scientists. The hope is that these discoveries would someday return a profit, and in fact in a growing number of instances this has been accurate and true. Large profits have been garnered by universities and the scientists for inventions that are now everyday drugs. In addition, after Bayh-Dole Act, tools, reagents, and similar byproducts of research were licensed to small and large businesses that made biologicals for research purposes. Some of these products, like monoclonal antibodies developed by basic scientists for uses in experiments were licensed to reagent companies

for a wide variety of uses (e.g., immunocytochemistry, western blotting, ELISAs, neutralization in vitro or in vivo) and then became drugs for human use. Similarly, vectors, recombinant proteins, and other reagents first licensed for research uses subsequently found their way into clinical therapeutics. MDs could now derive opportunities to fund their research with program income, even if the discoveries were made from federal funding, in addition to trading reagents for collaborations. By and large, Bayh-Dole Act was a huge success.

Second, Bayh-Dole Act opened the opportunity for MD discoverers to start create their own biotechnology companies, seek further NIH support in the form of SBIR development grants to convert their own basic discoveries to diagnostics and therapeutics on their own terms, rather than as licensers of technology. In the early days of Bayh-Dole Act, many of these companies were able to identify Wall Street interest in marketing the companies' expertise and became public offerings. As these offerings dried up, the model shifted to driving products past proof of concept and towards investigator initiated investigational new drugs (INDs) to the FDA to a point of interest for venture capitalists to invest or big pharmaceutical companies to license the technology or buy the companies outright.

Thus, Bayh-Dole Act revolutionized the universities' outlook on basic science (T1 type) research when they realized this research could be translated to profit. The opportunities for the classical MD scientist followed, including leaving academia for full time devotion to their biotechnology interests, or shared private sector-university employment. The role this has played in education of young scientists is unclear. As the primary goal of scholarly academic careers shifts from creation of new knowledge to successful product development from pressure by the universities and the NIH, training and education are certainly to suffer in some ways. MDs will have less time to teach. And if their basic research is to be funded, the newest NIH mandate is drug and device development.

The sequencing of the human genome was mentioned above; and its consequences on Bayh-Dole type entrepreneurship are as yet unknown. Many university-based patents have as their IP a cloned gene and its products. If the public publication of the human genome creates prior art for patenting the gene structure, the field will shift to use patents. Whatever the future holds, there are certainly many new opportunities for a physician scientist entrepreneur who drives the development of her/his own discoveries.

2. Bayh-Dole Act also opened the floodgates to biotech law. More patents, more companies generate a seemingly bottomless need for highly trained biological scientists with secondary law degrees specializing in IP. These opportunities range from becoming in-house counsel in biotech companies to becoming associates/partners in private law firms specializing in patent and corporate law. The opportunities include expert advice on filing for IP and management of IP portfolios, including refinement of claims, extensions of concepts, and filing for complementary claims. MD-law expertise is now needed for the interpretation of value of filings in all the separate countries of the EU, Canada, and Asian countries based on international practice of medicine and specific markets. Finally, MD expertise is needed for patent infringement law for both sides of potential litigation as expert witnesses and as litigators with sufficient background

knowledge of the medical implications of the law. Many of these scientist-law positions have been filled by PhD scientists, expert in various areas of science (in particular molecular biology following the surge in patents related to cloned genes), but the need for MD-JDs has markedly expanded because of the need for expertise on the medical applicability of products.

3. A completely different type of MD entrepreneur evolved from Bayh-Dole Act, the MD-MBA CEO. These are individuals who enter MD-MBA programs, then do post-doctoral training in specific areas directed at providing expertise in an area of business medicine (e.g., clinical pathology), and then market themselves as CEOs for startup biotechnology companies. They use their business skills to create marketing plans and approaches that help drive the companies' portfolio to raise capital. The MD degree is essential as it provides the framework for understanding the potential value of discoveries for clinical practice in ways that MBAs without this background cannot. These CEOs work for salary and receive stock in lieu of additional compensation. When capital is raised, they are either retained to direct the companies interests, or move on to similar opportunities.

Summary

To summarize, there are too many fields with broad implications to discuss in this brief introduction to future opportunities in medicine. Careers associated with bioengineering, computer science, genetics (including gene therapy), regenerative medicine, unique and effective ways for healthcare delivery, drug, device and vaccine development and delivery, entrepreneurial science, health law and ethics, patent law, and the business of medicine are evolving. Aldous Huxley set his futuristic satire, *Brave New World* in the twenty-sixth century where genetic manipulations, cloning, universal vaccination and other "far out" medical advances were commonplace [2]. It has taken only 70 years to get to the point where these concepts are part of everyday medical science, not science fiction, and are ready for practical application. These new fields will require totally unique skill sets for physicians of the future. The hope is that the following chapters in this book will provide some guidance in how to pursue these careers while advancing innovation and directly or indirectly continuing our clinical mission of improving ways to care for the sick.

References

1. Bayh-Dole Act: patents and contracts amendment of 1980. Sponsored by senators Birch Bayh, Indiana; Robert Dole, Kansas. (Pub. L. No. 96–517).
2. Huxley A. Brave new world. London: Chatto and Windus; 1932.

Chapter 2
Personality Type and Job Satisfaction

Katharine M. Nicodemus

Key Points

- Dispositional factors (how you think, feel, and act) are important determinants of job satisfaction.
- Personality and the employment environment have a reciprocal relationship.
- The quality of the match between your work environment and personality will dramatically impact your overall job satisfaction.

Introduction

The vocational choices in our society are amazing, but the process of choosing can be ambiguous at best. Throughout this chapter three points will be discussed in varying ways, and deserve mention at the start, because of their impact on the successful attainment of job satisfaction by much of the information reviewed: [1] Dispositional factors; how you think , feel, and act, are important in determining job satisfaction; [2] there is significant data indicating that a reciprocal relationship between your personality and the employment environment exists; and [3] the quality of the match between your personality and the work environment you chose will dramatically impact your chances for job satisfaction. Keep these three points in mind as we briefly explore the traditional ways that we choose professions, and then examine a combination of resources, structures, and strategies to make the process less chaotic and more productive.

K.M. Nicodemus, PsyD, MA (✉)
Clinical Neuropsychologist, 4011 Springfield Lane, Greenville, DE 19807, USA
e-mail: drnicpsyd@comcast.net

R.D. Urman and J.M. Ehrenfeld (eds.), *Physicians' Pathways to Non-Traditional Careers and Leadership Opportunities*, DOI 10.1007/978-1-4614-0551-1_2, © Springer Science+Business Media, LLC 2012

11

When you ask people why they chose to go into medicine or dentistry, or any other discipline you will find an astounding array of answers. Influence can range from strong familial input, to varying degrees of school influence, to the effect of a positive relationship in the community, to no advice at all. Of course we do know that a great deal of self-selection goes on in this process. We may start out adopting mom's view of us as a surgeon, until we have difficulty with anatomy. We tend to follow paths supported by things we excel in. How do we choose something that will make us happy? And even more problematic, how do we know that a particular job, or specialty will be a good fit with our talents and or, temperament, and is that necessary anyway? The caveat is that past methods of choice can be improved upon, and this chapter's purpose is to delineate some of the resources that are available to make the process less confusing.

You are probably wondering why is this important to me now? I'm an adult and I've made my vocational choice. Why the historical backdrop? Here's the reason. Sometimes we get it completely right the first time and feel 100% satisfied with what we are doing with our lives. Other times we need to find more to challenge ourselves as we garner greater competence in our respective fields. In some cases, we start on a career track and discover half way down the path it isn't what we expected, like the second year surgical resident who thought to himself "oh my God what have I done, and what am I going to do now!" Confusion can be a problem, especially when you begin a rigorous stair-step training program like most medical schools provide, and are expected to have some idea of where your interests will lie in the future. Yes I want to help people, but how? Under what parameters? Pathology is very different from general medicine! How am I suppose to know what will fit my personality? On the other hand, we may find we need completely different outlets to balance what we do professionally. We may have a passion that only an avocational pursuit can accommodate. Like the Internist, who enjoyed the practice of medicine, but found hospital politics difficult to manage. He discovered painting landscapes helped him to dissipate some of the tension and relax; or the Orthopedic Surgeon who wanted to have more involvement with his community, and ran for political office. A newly developed passion can nurture our sense of purpose on multiple levels, making us more satisfied and hence more present in our daily routines, as well as satisfy a need for stretching ourselves beyond our current limits. Adding a new skill set can benefit a person in a way that was dreamed of (I always wanted to be part of Speakers Bureau), or of ultimately fulfilling dreams that they didn't know they had, or were going to have. This is especially true in adults who want to transition from one field to another, but don't know specifically what to look for, just that something is missing. Like the Psychiatrist who said "I love treating my patients, and I'm happy working with them, but I just feel itchy. There must be more!" "How do I figure out what that more might be?" A great starting point is knowing your strengths and weaknesses. Not just in a concrete way, like I loved calculus but hated neuroanatomy. But instead knowing yourself in a global sense, your personality and its unique features. To do this you need to look at ways of formulating personality, and then discover how your particular personality profile might intersect with job satisfaction, and some facts related to increasing its optimal occurrence.

The purpose of this chapter is to begin to address some of these issues. We will look at two different personality type systems, and some of the most cogent ideas available about what makes job satisfaction likely. We will end by giving you several references so that if you are interested, you can obtain more information on your own. Let's get started!

Personality Type, Just What is That?

To some degree personality type will depend on the system that is being used. A traditional way to frame personality is that it is both "ingrained and habitual ways of psychological functioning that emerge from the individuals entire developmental history" [1]. There are many personality measures that have been used historically. We will look at two systems that are still being used a great deal, and that might be useful in a practical way, to help you understand your individual personality type, and how it relates to job satisfaction. The Myers-Briggs Type Indicator and the work of Dr. John L. Holland. It is important to note that both of these systems are complex and rich in detail, and the breadth and depth of this chapter does not allow for a critical analysis, but is meant to give you the essence of each as a starting point.

The Myers-Briggs Type Indicator

The Myers-Briggs Type Indicator (MBTI) is a personality theory that was developed by Isabel Briggs Myers and Katharine Briggs, and has been in use for over 60 years [2]. It has received a resurgence of interest, due in part, to its widespread use in the competitive world of business. The MBTI was an outgrowth of the initial work of C.G. Jung's theory of personality, most particularly his theory about introversion and extraversion. The concept is a dichotomy revolving around how individuals deal with energy in their world. The extravert engages the world in direct ways and takes pleasure in doing so; their energy comes from those interactions. The introvert is more reserved, taking pleasure in the world of ideas, the interior of the self is their favored domain, and it is the joy of this world that provides the source of most of their energy. The Myers-Briggs family expanded on Jung's theory of introversion-extroversion, and found a way to practically apply this theory [3]. Unlike many personality theories, the MBTI is based on the assumption that people prefer a certain way of being. It is about preferences, not pathology. During development each individual acquires a preference for certain styles of thinking or relating to others that affects their interpersonal relationships, both in the workplace and privately. The major focus of the theory is the interaction of four basic preferences, making each personality dynamic in nature [2]. A good way to explain these may be to list them and then describe each with an example. These include the dichotomies listed in Table 2.1.

Each of these dichotomies represents a preferred style that the individual has adopted over the course of their development. Some people are more introverted or extraverted than others. There is always a continuum. When taken together, these dichotomies represent 16 personality types. The goal of the MBTI is to identify

Table 2.1 The four basic dichotomies of Myers-Briggs

Introversion-Extraversion (I or E)	Sensing-Intuition (S or N)
Where is the energy coming from, interior or exterior?	*How is information gathered?*
Introversion = focus on the world of ideas	Sensing = need for exact information
Extraversion = focus on the exterior world in an active manner	Intuition = casual approach to information
Thinking-Feeling (T or F)	**Judging-Perceiving (J or P)**
How decisions are made	*How do you deal with daily life?*
Thinking = objectively	Judging = need to plan carefully
Feeling = subjectively	Perceiving = spontaneous approach

which of the opposing dichotomies each person prefers on each of the four categories. A label is assigned, like INTJ, once the person's preferences are known. This is an indication of their "habitual choice," [2] but because there is inherent flexibility in the system, a person may choose the opposing pole choice on occasion. There is a dominant process that is usually in charge, and there is the auxiliary process that compliments, and takes care of issues that must be dealt with, but are not necessarily favored. Let's use an introverted librarian as an example. Most of the time his dominant process (I) is utilized, but on occasion, when the need arises, (say some unruly people burst into his library), he will raise his voice and let the auxiliary process of extraversion (E) take over. A great deal of work has been done to compile data on what different combinations mean in terms of personality style, and how they are represented in different fields in the workforce. [2] This is fascinating reading, and interesting data is available. For example, most dentists, cross culturally, have very similar dominant personality types on the MBTI [4]. It is important to keep in mind that each combination represents a different set of strengths and no one combination is viewed as superior over another.

The Holland Personality Assessment

Dr. John L. Holland developed several assessment measures helpful for a wide range of client populations; from the high school, college or graduate student, to adults in transition. His instruments are designed to assist in decision-making about personality type, as well as how an individual's unique qualities might best fit into the workforce. There is a significant body of research indicating that people do best at work, and are happiest when there is a "good fit between their personality type and the characteristics of the environment." [5] He developed a personality type system called the Holland Codes. It is in fact a theory revolving around career and vocations, and is represented by six personality and work environment types. I'll list them with an example: (see Table 2.2).

Each of these is called a sub-type, and a person's unique profile can be made up of some of them or all of them, to varying degrees. The system is frequently referred

Table 2.2 Holland code sub-types – RIASEC

Realistic (R) = practical	Social (S) = cooperative/nurturing
Investigative (I) = analytical	Enterprising (E) = leadership
Artistic (A) = creative	Conventional (C) = organized

to as RIASEC. Holland thought that an individual could utilize more than one type, and the idea was to prioritize the person's preferences numerically to ascertain which were strongest. Usually the highest three codes were used for assessment purposes. People with comparable codes have similar profiles of vocational preferences and seem to do well in the same sort of occupational environments [6]. Like the MBTI, one code or type was not seen as superior to another. Holland believed that occupational choice made a very strong statement about an individual's personality, and for optimal job satisfaction, the individual's code profile must be congruent with their work environment. For example, if your top three codes were AES (artistic, enterprising, social), you wouldn't be a good candidate for a work environment that was too conventional and restricting, so anything resembling the environment of a research lab probably wouldn't be a good fit for you. Holland stated that vocational identity, the adoption of a consistent ideal of one's self in the vocational world, was critical to job satisfaction, and had been demonstrated to be highly correlated ($r=0.70$) with it as well [7]. He reasoned that an individual with vocational identity had a clear sense of what their skills were, what reasonable career goals might be, as well as occupations that might be compatible. That sort of self-awareness coupled with knowledge of resources made it likely that they would find work that was a good fit, or congruent with their needs [5].

Holland also developed The Self-Directed Search, an assessment tool used to measure an individual's similarity to the RIASEC personality types [8]. It is made up of six scales, and is one of the most widely used interest inventories available. It is designed to be user friendly, and the test can be taken and scored without assistance. You simply fill in the answers in the booklet, score it, take your three highest codes, which comprise your code profile, and compare that with the one that most closely approximates it on the occupation finder. In addition, the dictionary of Holland occupational codes [9], which lists over 12,000 occupations, is a tremendous resource guide. Both of these instruments have been invaluable in the career guidance of thousands of people in this country. A plethora of research has documented the capacity of Holland's instruments to be both appropriate and useful in academic and vocational settings.

The Relationship Between Job Satisfaction and Personality

One thing seems clear; our jobs are never done in a vacuum. There is always a relationship between the holding environment that supports us, and the dispositional factors we bring to bear as individuals. You might ask, what about those dispositional factors? They are the way we think, feel and behave [10], and have the capacity to influence most everything we do. Research by Watson and Slack concurred that dispositional issues can influence job satisfaction [11]. Recently, a study of Dutch Nurse Anesthetists was done with the MBTI to study personality dimensions and job satisfaction in an effort to predict factors that might help aid nurse retention. The author's reported two factors, "easy going, $(r=0.18)$" and "orderly, $(r=0.11)$," as both correlating positively with job satisfaction [12], but predictive value using the MBTI was reported as minimal.

In a meta-analysis article focusing on the five factor model of personality and job satisfaction, Judge and his collaborators found that Neuroticism $(\rho=-0.29)$ Conscientiousness $(\rho=0.26)$ and Extraversion $(\rho=0.25)$ were most strongly corre-lated with job satisfaction[1] [13]. By definition, if you are high on the Neuroticism scale, you are likely to carry a rather negative world view that permeates most everything you do, making you less likely to be happy in general, and more specifi-cally in the workforce. Conversely, the higher you were on the Conscientiousness and Extraversion scales the more likely you were to be satisfied in your work. Anecdotally, it follows that if you are engaged in an active way (Extraversion), and put great effort into your work product (Conscientiousness), your chances of suc-cess and satisfaction go up.

Studies on the relationship between job and life satisfaction have found support for the Spillover Hypothesis [14], which states that the affective valence from both sides of the equation, job and life, are equally important and affect each other. *If your personal life is going well, the positive affect attached to that experience will follow you into the workplace, creating a similar impact.* You can see there is quite a bit of data suggesting a reciprocal relationship between your personal life and your job [15]. This clearly ties in with what we know about Holland's work regarding the critical need for congruence between our work environment and personality type for job satisfaction. Equally important is Holland's concept of vocational identity, which we defined previously, and which we know is highly correlated with job satisfaction [7], and when well developed, is relatively consistent and stable across time.

Summary

We've seen that there are many dispositional factors that potentially influence our interpretation of our employment settings, and can therefore affect job satisfaction. It also seems clear that a reciprocal relationship exists between the personality of an individual and the job setting, so that how well they are matched becomes critical for job satisfaction. Equally important is the concept of vocational identity, because it can serve as a guide to aid you in your search, whether you are a student or a seasoned profes-sional looking for an outside interest or to make an important professional transition.

---

[1] ρ=estimated true score correlation.

Lastly, what seems crucial to the success of anyone searching for a new beginning is that they know where to start, with themselves. You may not know exactly which job or volunteer position you want, but you know your strengths; capitalize on them. Understanding your uniqueness through personality type, if it resonates, or therapy, or any way you choose, is a good place to begin. Then use the resources that are available to create some structure, and a plan. Remember, if you can visualize a plan, you can likely achieve it as well.

References

1. Millon T, Davis RD. Disorders of personality: DSM-IV and beyond. New York, NY: John Wiley & Sons, Inc.; 1996.
2. Myers IB, Mc Caulley MH, Quenk MH, Hammer AL. Manual: a guide to the development and use of the Myers-Briggs type indicator instrument. 3rd ed. Mountain View, USA: CCP, Inc; 2009.
3. Myers IB, Myers PB. Gifts differing: understanding personality type. Mountain View, USA: CCP, Inc.; 1995.
4. Jessee SA, O'Neill PN, Dosch RO. Matching student personality types and learning preferences to teaching methodologies. J Dent Educ. 2006;70:644–51.
5. Holland JL. Exploring careers with typology: what we have learned and some new directions. Am Psychol. 1996;51:397–406.
6. Brown SD, Lent RW. Career development and counseling: putting theory and research to work. Hoboken, USA: John Wiley & Sons, Inc.; 2005.
7. Holland JL, Daiger DC, Power PG. Some diagnostic scales for research in decision-making and personality: identity, information, and barriers. J Pers Soc Psychol. 1980;39:1191–200.
8. Holland JL, Fritzsche BA, Powell AB. The self-directed search technical manual-1994 edition. Odessa, USA: Psychological Assessment Resources; 1994.
9. Gottfredson GD, Holland JL. Dictionary of Holland occupational codes. 2nd ed. Odessa, USA: Psychological Assessment Resources; 1989.
10. Eagly AH, Chaiken S. The psychology of attitudes. Forth Worth, USA: Harcourt Brace Jovanovich; 1993.
11. Watson D, Slack AK. General factors of affective temperament and their relation to job satisfaction over time. Organ Behav Hum Decis Process. 1993;54:181–202.
12. Meeusen VCH, Brown-Mahoney C, van Dam K, van Zundert AAJ, Knape JTA. Personality dimensions and their relationship with job satisfaction amongst dutch nurse anaesthetists. J Nurs Manag. 2010;18:573–81.
13. Judge TA, Heller D, Mount MK. Five-factor model of personality and job satisfaction: a meta-analysis. J Appl Psychol. 2002;87:530–41.
14. Rain JS, Lane IM, Steiner DD. A current look at the job satisfaction/life satisfaction relationship: review and future considerations. Hum Relat. 1991;44:287–307.
15. Judge TA, Locke EA. Effect of dysfunctional thought processes on subjective well-being and job satisfaction. J Appl Psychol. 1993;78:475–90.

Chapter 3
Career Decision-Making in Medicine: Practical Approaches

Shalini Reddy

Key Points

- Consider both traditional (rational) and non-traditional (emotional, life) factors when making a career decision.
- Obtain an objective assessment of your abilities and ask yourself "Do these abilities match the skills necessary for the job I am considering?"
- Realize that ambivalence and ambiguity are always a part of any major decision.

Introduction to Career Planning

In years past, the career trajectory of a physician has been linear. In more recent years, however, the progression of an individual through their medical career is better characterized as meandering with physicians leaving and entering clinical practice and pursuing a variety of non-traditional careers. The reasons for the change in this trajectory are many-fold. The options available to one entering the medical profession have expanded; there are more opportunities for enhanced interaction between physicians and those outside the practice of medicine; and the rapid and constant changes in our healthcare system are forcing a new need for adaptation. There is also some speculation that current generations ("Gen X" and "Gen Y") are more apt to change careers to fit their changing life contexts. Overall, the paradigm has shifted from a desire to find the "one best fit" to a state in which physicians now ask "how can I adapt to change?"

S. Reddy, MD (✉)
Department of Internal Medicine, University of Chicago, Pritzker School of Medicine,
924 E 57th Street, Suite 104, Chicago, IL 60637, USA
e-mail: sreddy@uchicago.edu

R.D. Urman and J.M. Ehrenfeld (eds.), *Physicians' Pathways to Non-Traditional Careers and Leadership Opportunities*, DOI 10.1007/978-1-4614-0551-1_3,
© Springer Science+Business Media, LLC 2012

Career decision making has its theoretical roots in the work of Plato and Eastern philosophy. Platonic theory postulates that the brain is governed by rationality and emotionality and that ideal decision-making should rely heavily on the former rather than the latter [1]. The Tao de Ch'ing advises that "in work, do what you enjoy [2]." Modern vocational theory embraces the notion that rational and "alternative-to-rational" thinking are both valid and necessary for arriving at mature decisions. This chapter describes ways in which one can make "rational" decisions while incorporating emotional and contextual underpinnings.

Considerations for Choosing an Ideal Vocation

The majority of individuals reading this book have likely utilized traditional, rational approaches in their decision-making. A traditional list-based approach to rationally quantifying career parameters is delineated in Table 3.1. When developing a list of characteristics for an ideal vocation, consider traditional and non-traditional factors. Factors that are traditionally considered include the daily tasks involved in the job, interest in the intellectual aspects of the work, monetary rewards and a match between the individual's abilities and the type of work performed. When constructing a list of properties of the "ideal job," aspects that are less frequently considered include the ability to balance work with interests outside of work and with family, the ability to be creative in the job, and the ability to serve others. Both of these traditional and non-traditional factors are summarized in Table 3.2.

Table 3.1 List-based approach to rational decision-making

Characteristics of the ideal vocation
Skills possessed by the individual
Jobs that match the individual's interests and skills
Skills necessary for proficiency in the ideal vocation

Table 3.2 Characteristics of the ideal vocation

Characteristic	Category of consideration
Daily tasks associated with job	Traditional
Interest in the work	Traditional
Intellectual challenge of the work	Traditional
Monetary rewards	Traditional
Work-life balance	Nontraditional
Creativity	Nontraditional
Service to others	Nontraditional
Flow	Nontraditional

Assessment of Personal Qualities

In addition to delineating aspects of a career which may interest an individual, it is also necessary to recognize one's own qualities as they relate to the career being considered in order to determine if there is opportunity for overlap between one's abilities and the qualifications necessary to be successful in a particular career. Constructing this list requires a clear assessment of one's own skills and interests. The ability to objectively assess one's strengths can often be difficult and can frequently be best done by those who are closest to the individual. Co-workers, supervisors, friends, and family can be invaluable in helping to define areas of strength and weakness. Along with skills, a list of interests is necessary when choosing a career or deciding to switch careers. Such a list should encompass both intellectual and outside of work interests.

Predicting Career Fit

Once the skills necessary to perform a job and one's own abilities have been delineated a true assessment of the fit between the career and the individual can be made. A construct that is helpful in assessing whether a particular career may be a good "fit" is the concept of Flow. This construct was developed by psychologist Mihály Csíksentmihályi who described flow as a mental state during which an individual is fully absorbed in the task at hand [3]. In this state, perceived ability is matched to the perceived level of challenge, and an individual is in a state of full engagement. When an individual's perceived ability exceeds the level of challenge, a state of boredom ensues and when the level of challenge exceeds ability, one is likely to experience anxiety or frustration. This concept is illustrated in Fig. 3.1.

Skills: Assessment and Development

It is uncommon for an individual's skills to perfectly match the level of challenge of a particular career at the onset of that career. This is especially true for fields such as medicine that require direct apprenticeship or practice in order to gain proficiency. Many skills necessary for a profession can be obtained through practice or study. The overall goal of professional development is to develop the necessary skills, throughout the course of one's career, in order to successfully progress from Novice to Master, as illustrated in Fig. 3.2. However, a baseline level of ability is necessary in order to avoid frustration. A practical example is an individual who wishes to perform population-based research involving complex statistical analysis. If that individual's area of weakness is mathematics, pursuing additional statistical training may become an exercise in frustration.

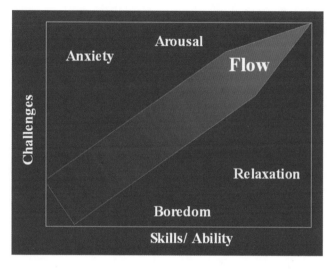

Fig. 3.1 Flow (used with permission from Vivek Prachand, MD.)

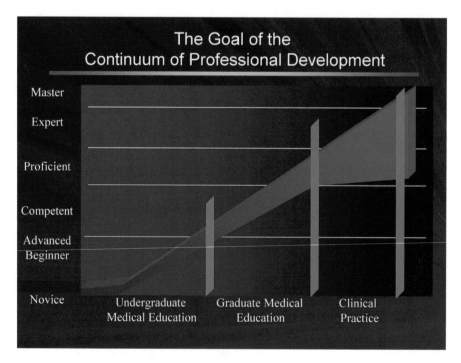

Fig. 3.2 The goal of the continuum of professional development

Once the level of baseline skills and interest is established, one can begin assessing what additional skills may be necessary to pursue a career or to change careers. If individuals who are already working in the areas of interest can be identified, they can be immensely helpful in outlining the skills necessary to succeed in a particular career. This is particularly useful when considering careers that are "off the beaten path." It is easy to find role models in traditional medical careers but finding such role models in alternate medical careers often requires non-traditional search strategies. Social media internet-based resources and professional school alumni offices can also be good starting points for finding individuals who are involved in alternate careers in medicine.

Conclusions and Other Factors to Consider

Decision-making which considers rational factors in the context of a person's life (i.e., "alternate to rational") may result in more satisfying career decisions. The context of an individual's life includes factors such as one's worldview, culture, and family considerations. Gut instinct should not be undervalued as a source of input into a decision as life and work experience may contribute subconsciously to the development of instincts.

There are some important caveats to consider when making any major decisions. Depression can make even the most ideal situation appear gloomy and individuals must thoughtfully examine whether they are making decisions because of their current emotional state. Secondly, even a carefully made decision that takes emotional and rational factors into account is often accompanied by ambivalence. This is particularly true when one is leaving a job that they enjoy to pursue a career path that may be even more fulfilling. Leaving one situation for another, less well-known position can naturally create uncertainty and some level of anxiety. A familiar situation, even when suboptimal, may often feel more comfortable than making a major life change. Allowing that these feelings of ambivalence are normal can help to mitigate "buyer's remorse" that may accompany the decision to change career paths. The ability to remain flexible and open to change is essential to success in today's society and is certainly true when choosing a non-traditional career in medicine. The last pitfall to be wary of is the decision to pursue an opportunity solely because it is available. Opportunities present themselves on a daily basis; however, it may not be the right thing for an *individual* to avail themselves of that opportunity. Are the skills, time and energy needed to pursue this option at this time the right thing for you?

Deciding what career to pursue is one of the major choices that one makes during their life. Considering both rational and emotion points in the decision-making process can help to mitigate some of the ambivalence and anxiety that commonly accompany big decisions. Because there is little that is written about alternate career choice, the chapters which follow will provide information designed to help you in your decision-making process.

Case Example

Bob is a second year medical student who is interested in international travel. Because of this interest, he pursued an international medicine experience in Somalia in the summer between his first and second years of medical school. During this time, he worked with an international medical relief organization and found that he was excited at the prospect of working with a similar non-profit organization when he finished residency. At the end of his third year of medical school, Bob found himself struggling to decide which specialty to pursue. His ideal job would be to serve as the medical director for an international medical relief organization and he feels that being in this position would allow him to serve others, work internationally, and have an intellectually challenging and satisfying career. Given that there are few individuals in these positions, he identified some individuals within the institution who worked with international medical relief organization in the past and interviewed them about what skills and qualities might be necessary to pursue such a career. In the course of these discussions, Bob discovered that what he was truly passionate about was the business of non-profits and managing volunteers, funds and administrative staff. Although he took undergraduate courses in business management, he determined that he needed more skills in order to serve as an effective leader for an international medical relief organization. He reviewed this plan with his advisor and researched various MBA programs in the country and ultimately decided to obtain his MBA between his third and fourth year of medical school at a business school that offers a specialized healthcare MBA.

References

1. Irwin T. Plato's ethics. New York: Oxford University Press; 1995.
2. Cleary TF, Lao-tzu Tao tc, Chuang-tzu. Nan-hua ching. 1991. The essential tao: An initiation into the heart of taoism through the authentic tao te ching and the inner teachings of chuang-tzu. 1st ed. San Francisco: Harper San Francisco.
3. Csikszentmihalyi M. Flow: the psychology of optimal experience. Harper perennial modern classics. New York: Harper Perennial Modern Classics; 2008.

Chapter 4
Work–Life Balance

Annekathryn Goodman

Key Points

- Work–life balance will change over the course of one's medical career as life goals change.
- To achieve work–life balance, one must identify personal and career goals and constantly re-evaluate them.
- Happiness and satisfaction will impact both one's work and home environment.

Engrossed late and soon in professional cares, getting and spending, you may so lay waste your powers that you may find, too late, with hearts given away, that there is no place in your habit-stricken souls for those gentler influences that make life worth living [1].

Sir William Osler (1849–1919)

Love and work are the cornerstones of our humanness [2].

Introduction

Fifty days into her hospitalization after a pelvic exenteration for recurrent cervical cancer, the 41-year-old woman looked up at me from her bed and said, "Doctor! You just don't know what is going to happen to you in life."

A. Goodman, MS, MD (✉)
Department of Obstetrics and Gynecology, Gillette Center for Women's Cancers,
Harvard Medical School, Yawkey 9, 55 Fruit Street, Boston, MA 02114, USA
e-mail: agoodman@partners.org

R.D. Urman and J.M. Ehrenfeld (eds.), *Physicians' Pathways to Non-Traditional Careers and Leadership Opportunities*, DOI 10.1007/978-1-4614-0551-1_4,
© Springer Science+Business Media, LLC 2012

When asked at a recent medical school seminar when they knew they wanted to be doctors, the student responses ranged from before kindergarten to after college. At some point in a person's life at both rational and emotional beckoning brings them to pursue a career in medicine. My call came as a toddler. My first acts of charity and healing included rescuing stray cats and wrapping my mother in ace bandages. By adolescence, I was wheeling elderly women to their physiotherapy appointments and visiting devastatingly ill children at a long-term care facility.

When at age 14, I read the physician novelist, AJ Cronin's book "Keys of the Kingdom" about a priest tending to plague victims during an epidemic in China; I was smitten [3]. He captured my goal and dream to devote my whole heart and soul to caring for the desperate and dying.

However, midway through my Obstetrics and Gynecology residency training, I realized that there was a personal price to constant work and altruism with no thought to my own welfare. My 8-year personal relationship ended and five residents in our 20-resident program developed significant illness. As residents, we were covering three hospitals and working 120 hours a week.

External forces have led to improvements in work hours [4]. But the challenge to harness the inspiration and intensity of patient care with both self-care and self-realization must come from each individual physician's internal forces. Work–life balance is part of our challenge. This balance will be different for each person and will change through different periods of one's life. The power of a medical career with both its pressures and rewards makes our work also very intimately the essence of our lives.

I have spent my whole professional life learning how to respond to the call to heal and care and at the same time to continue to grow and develop as a human being. I have learned that my personal evolution is directly linked to my effectiveness as a physician, family member, and friend.

This chapter examines the various components and realizations of balance in life. The literature on physician work satisfaction is reviewed. Different dimensions of life balance are examined and linked to the importance of continued spiritual and intellectual growth through one's career. Twenty students and doctors at various stages of their careers graciously agreed to be interviewed for this chapter. Their personal journeys and insights about life balance are included.

Work-life balance will change as life goals develop and mature during the phases of one's medical training and career (Table 4.1). The field of medicine offers diverse career options. Individual physicians come to medicine at different stages in their life development.

Why Pursue Work–Life Balance?

After completing my fellowship, I joined a busy academic practice in gynecologic oncology. I found the work infinite. It was not possible to finish all the dictations, lab reviews, and telephone calls each day. My husband decided to set limits and at 8 pm each night, he drove over to the hospital to rescue me and bring me home.

Table 4.1 Life goals and challenges in a medical career

Medical school
Goals
  Medical knowledge
  Learning how to be a doctor
Challenges
  Huge work load
  Existential challenge of developing a new identity
  Losing a previous life identity
  Lack of autonomy

Residency
Goals
  Development of specialty expertise
  Finding a life partner
  Starting a family
Challenges
  Long hours
  Lack of autonomy
  Learning how to teach and mentor medical students
  Balancing work commitment with social engagement

Subspecialty training
Life goals
  Subspecialty expertise
  Choosing an academic track
  Finding a life partner
  Starting a family
Challenges
  Long hours
  Learning how to teach and mentor medical students and residents
  Balancing work commitment with social engagement

First job
Life goals
  Becoming boarded in specialty
  Continued education and training in specialty
  Negotiating a work schedule
  Balancing work commitment with social engagement
Challenges
  Finding a work mentor
  Learning how to teach and mentor medical students and house staff
  Learning how to multitask work commitments and home commitments

First decade
Life goals
  Developing a professional reputation
  Developing an academic or private practice niche
  Learning how to teach
  Learning how to write grants
  Learning how to balance clinical medicine and research

(continued)

Table 4.1 (continued)

Learning management and business skills in managing private practice
Learning how to manage office staff (secretaries, nurses, office managers)
Raising a family
Nurturing hobbies and play time
Challenges
Finding a work mentor
Finding time for life care
Taking emotional care of one's partner and children
Second decade
Life goals
Retraining and learning new skills relevant to specialty
Development of leadership skills
Learning how to mentor junior faculty and colleagues
Deepening relationships with friends and family
Challenges
Deciding appropriate career goals (administrative versus teaching versus clinical)
Promotions in academic career tracks
Deciding on career changes (relocating to a new city, retraining in a new field)
Taking care of friends and family in times of crisis and illness

Balance can be defined as "a state of equilibrium or equipoise, something used to produce equilibrium, counterpoise, mental steadiness or emotional stability, habit of calm behavior, judgment" [5]. The 31 definitions in *dictionary.com* for balance highlight the importance of this concept in our society. Balance can be a subjective concept. To address this concept, one needs to identify personal and career goals. These goals will shift and change and need to be reviewed frequently.

Balance in a life as a physician requires work satisfaction and personal well-being. The stresses of intensive medical training and patient care were discussed in several focus groups at Massachusetts General Hospital. Table 4.2 summarizes examples of personal solutions that were identified at all levels of training and career paths.

Mayo Clinic examined the negative effects of overwork and burn-out to identify interventions to improve physician satisfaction [6]. Seven factors identified as important for physician well-being are summarized in Table 4.3. Three of these focused on the work that physicians do: meaningful work, having challenges appropriate for the skills and interests of the physicians, and opportunities for professional development. Two factors involved the atmosphere at work: a culture of professionalism and physician autonomy. The final two areas addressed the need to support and encourage outside interests and to affirm the importance of self-care.

A survey of 895 surgeons looked at the risks associated with career dissatisfaction and the inability to achieve work–life balance [7]. While most surgeons were satisfied with their careers, 33.5% did not achieve work–life balance. Surgeons felt that their lives could be improved by limiting emergency call, diminishing litigation, and improving reimbursement.

Work–family balance is one important challenge. A survey from Switzerland evaluated the impact of gender and parenthood on physicians' careers. They found

Table 4.2 Personal solutions to work stress

Third year medical student: "I have daily telephone conversations with my sister."

Fourth year medical student: "Knowing that the rotation will be over after a month, helps me cope with today's stress."

Intern in Obstetrics and Gynecology: "I set my goal to do one personal thing each day such as running, calling family, reading a few pages of a book."

Third year resident in Obstetrics and Gynecology: "My husband and I see one movie a week."

Senior surgical resident: "I blog about patient care related stories."

Second year fellow in Gynecologic Oncology, recently married: "I am still in my honeymoon phase. I am happy every day."

Faculty member in the Cancer Center, first year out of training with one child: "My wife completely understands my work and supports me. I could not do this without her."

Faculty member in Primary Care 5 years out of training with two children. "I work 50 % time and I can only do this because of my full time nanny."

Faculty member in Surgery, 7 years out of training with one child. "My mother moved in and takes care of my son. I schedule my work and my surgical cases to be out of the hospital by 5 pm every day."

Faculty member in Obstetrics and Gynecology 10 years out of training with two children. "I work 4 days a week. I have one personal day a week where I read and do yoga while the kids are in day care."

Faculty member in Gynecologic Oncology, 20 years out of training. "I sit in the kitchen and watch my husband cook. We each share the events of our day with each other."

Table 4.3 Factors for workplace well-being

Meaningful work

Challenges appropriate to skill set

Opportunities for professional development

Culture of professionalism

Physician autonomy

Support for outside interests

Importance of self-care

that there was less career-orientation and more part-time work among women physicians with children. Compared to male physicians, women had fewer mentors, fewer academic positions, and more private practice work. However, women in this survey had higher levels of overall life satisfaction [8]. Interestingly, our world and social norms keep changing. A growing proportion of women are becoming physicians. A growing proportion of men are taking more child care responsibilities. Another challenge of the workplace in life balance is to overcome gender stereotypes [9].

Part-time careers in medicine allow work–family balance. The Association of Specialty Professors formed a task force to establish guidelines for incorporating part-time faculty into departments of internal medicine. They concluded that part-time faculty could benefit departments and provide cost-effective patient care, research, and education [10].

Personal well-being is an important component to work–life balance. A survey of general practitioners in Australia found that 10% of respondents were mild to

Table 4.4 Burnout in the workplace – contributing factors

A sense of inadequacy

A sense of guilt

Isolation

Conflicting forces and demands

Deep emotions: sorrow, fear, despair, helplessness that cannot be expressed

Repetitive or prolonged situations of stress

moderately depressed or anxious. Achieving work–life balance was an important stressor. The balance between medicine and family commitments was more of an issue for women than men in this study [11]. Stress management included talking with family, friends, peers, and having nonwork-related activities such as sports.

Physician burnout can occur when the challenges of work are overwhelming and satisfactory balances to work are lost. Work-related factors for burnout were examined in the business setting [12]. Table 4.4 summarizes key triggers for burnout.

There are several organizations that advertize training programs to help organize and control the many stressors of life. For instance, "The Life Balance Institute," a non-profit training organization, sets the goal of training individuals to develop essential life skills [13]. Websites with health advice on work balance such as the Mayo Clinic website offer structured advice on tracking work time, negotiating with superiors, and time management [14].

Equilibrium in life comes from understanding what makes life meaningful, valuing oneself, and identifying life goals. This process needs constant reassessment. It is important to get perspective from our significant relationships. There are three important categories of relationship for physicians: Family, Professional colleagues, and Patients.

Family and friends are the crucial link to the world outside of medicine. Because the pressures of workload are infinite, we need the structure and commitment of family to bring us home.

Work relationships with mentors, teachers, and peers are crucial to keep perspective. We need to identify teachers and mentors to learn new skills and to evaluate our performance. The three criteria for work balance outlined in the Mayo Clinic study, meaningful work, appropriate challenges, and professional development, require navigation through the complex hospital environment. Mentoring in academic medicine is central for growth. One review summarized the literature on this topic. It concluded that mentorship was an important influence on personal development, career guidance, and research productivity [15]. A career-success scale (CSS), an instrument to assess academic career steps, reported on items valued in academics [16]. These include lectures, publications, research collaboration, scholarship, and grants. The authors conclude that mentoring is an independent predictor of career success, and the use of an instrument such as CSS will help structure mentoring.

Patients are rich and diverse resources who help physicians grow and evolve in their careers and in life in general. Every question and dilemma about life can be found in the stories and the lives of our patients. Patients not only nourish and care

Table 4.5 Work–life balance: key concepts

Understanding personal priorites
Establishing boundaries
Acquiring specific competencies
Supportive partner and family
Professional mentors
Periodic re-evaluation of life goals

about their doctors; they give feedback and guidance to help physicians grow in their knowledge and interpersonal skills. True-patient centered learning comes from learning how to listen. David Urion writes that it is important "to avoid the great temptation to fill silences with noise and sound, instead of waiting upon meaning and sense to emerge from the quiet" [17]. Table 4.5 summarizes key concepts for work–life balance.

As a Physician, How Can I Benefit Personally?

I went to the funeral of a patient of mine who had died from a sarcoma. Her teenage children described her goodness as a mother and a teacher. She had told them to never go to bed angry at someone they love. I felt that was a direct lesson for me – to forgive and resolve problems quickly in our short, precious lives.

Intellectual balance comes from constant education and training. The journey of medical education has many layers. The goals of education are diverse and each area of learning is challenging. This constant development keeps work exciting and lessens the risk of burn out. Training also enriches life. The lessons from study and from patient interaction extrapolate to life outside of work. The areas of learning include knowledge acquisition, technical skill building, and problem-solving and synthesis. In addition, training in interpersonal skill building such as listening and conflict resolution, development of professionalism and a public persona, and inner growth and maturation are lifelong endeavors.

In medicine, there will always be the tension between wanting to be highly trained, skilled, and competent, and nourishing our personal lives. It is a reality that to become an expert, one must devote significant hours to training. Malcolm Gladwell, the author of *Outliers*, discusses the "10,000-Hour Rule," that greatness and expertise require enormous time and training [18].

Happiness at work is related to both work satisfaction and happiness outside of work.

The perfect job has been summarized as requiring three important elements: feeling competent, enjoying the work, and feeling that the work and one's moral values coincide [19]. Dissatisfaction and stress at work can challenge personal relationships. This phenomenon called "emotional spillover" must be identified and addressed. Fatigue and emotional tension can endanger personal relationships by reducing psychological availability [19]. Solutions to negative emotional spillover from work to home life are summarized in Table 4.6.

Table 4.6 Creating work – life harmony

Identify negative emotional spillover
Communicate with one's partner when work is hard
Learn to say no to jobs that are not skill set appropriate
Learn self-assessment
Check in with life partner on how your work is impacting them

How Can I Benefit My Patients?

I sat with my 16-year-old patient's mother for an hour while her daughter slept. Her daughter/my patient was dying of metastatic cancer. I listened while she shared her guilt, her anger, and her spiritual understanding of this terrible tragedy. My not being judgmental and my silence created a space for her to grieve and not be alone.

When I first completed my gynecologic oncology fellowship, I cared for a 30-year-old woman with a neglected advanced cervical cancer. She came from a different background than me and she believed that diet could treat her cancer. At that time, I was very angry with her. While I strongly recommended conventional cancer therapy, she chose a different path. Despite my frustration, she returned to see me frequently over the 2 years before her death. She taught me to listen compassionately and accept her despite my disagreement with her choices.

Each learning encounter as a result of patient teaching or continuing education influences how we understand and manage the next patient. Trained self-awareness allows one to better understand the signals that patients are sending. Trained listening helps unravel complex histories. At the same time, yearly continued education and surgical skill set training will keep one intellectually interested and engaged while benefiting our patients. Self-reflection and listening will nourish relationships with life partners, family, and friends.

Education, Other Background Needed

There are many avenues to pursue continued training, education, and get support to expand work balance while working part- or full-time. Each physician will identify over their careers areas where they want to deepen their expertise.

The following examples come from my own career development. I became interested in acupuncture because the majority of my cancer patients sought it out to alleviate cancer and treatment-related side effects. I enrolled in a Harvard-based, 300 hour-long course for physicians [20]. I have continued to train and expand my knowledge through weekend workshops at the New England School of Acupuncture [21]. Acupuncture teaches a different type of intervention for suffering. It requires sitting with patients in a nontask-based manner and just paying attention to their narratives. I have noticed that my modest acupuncture experience has increased my awareness of patients' symptoms.

I joined the federal disaster team and was deployed to several mass casualty disasters. I witnessed the depth of psychic trauma and grief in survivors and in the healthcare professionals caring for them. Witnessing grief is also a significant experience in my oncology practice. I wanted to develop a skill set to help both patients and my colleagues. I found training for this through clinical pastoral care (CPE) programs.

CPE programs focus on the practices of pastoral care and counseling and are usually located in hospitals, clinics, and community agencies [22]. CPE has a concentrated focus on pastoral care, counseling and relational skills development. While CPE can be a part of chaplaincy preparation, it is useful training for physicians who work with critically ill patients. The educational tools of narrative writing, group discussion, and verbatim exercises give a deeper inner personal understanding of illness and better patient care skills of listening and synthesis.

Listening and witnessing the suffering of patients and listening to and supporting colleagues and friends can broaden one's understanding of oneself and the world. These training experiences can be used to debrief from the challenges of work.

In conclusion, work–life balance is a highly individual journey. Regardless of the individual, creative choices doctors make about their work and home environment, happiness and satisfaction impact both settings. Self-awareness, goal setting, and constant re-evaluation are essential for this balance.

Acknowledgements I would like to thank Dr. Mary Beth Gordon and Dr. Whitfield Growdon for their invaluable comments and insights.

References

1. Osler W., "The Qualities Required of a Physician," available at http://www.oslerbooks.com/otherpages/oslerpages/thequalities.html (last accessed Sep. 18, 2011).
2. Erikson E., Childhood and Society (W. W. Norton, 1986), chap. 7 (paraphrasing Sigmund Freud).
3. Cronin AJ. Keys of the kingdom 1941. United Kingdom: Hodder and Stoughton; 2007. ISBN ISBN 0340934042.
4. Information related to the ACGME's effort to address resident duty hours and other relevant resource materials. http://www.acgme.org/DutyHours/dutyHrs_Index.asp. Accessed 22 April 2011.
5. Dictionary.com. http://dictionary.reference.com/browse/balance. Accessed 23 Sept 2010.
6. Shanafelt TD, West CP, Poland GA, LaRusso NF, Menaker R, Bahn RS. Principles to promote physician satisfaction and work-life balance. Minn Med. 2008;91(12):41–3.
7. Troppmann KM, Palis BE, Goodnight JE, Ho HS, Troppman C. Career and lifestyle satisfaction among surgeons: what really matters? The National lifestyles in surgery today survey. J Am Coll Surg. 2009;209(2):160–9.
8. Buddeberg-Fischer B, Stamm M, Buddeberg C, Bauer G, Hammig O, Knecht M, et al. The impact of gender and parenthood on physicians' careers – professional and personal situation seven years after graduation. BMC Health Serv Res. 2010;10:40.
9. Carnes M. Commentary: deconstructing gender difference. Acad Med. 2010;85(4):575–7.
10. Warde LM, Alexander RW, Demarco DM, Haupt A, Hicks L, Kutner J, et al. Part-time careers in academic internal medicine: a report from the association of specialty professors part-time careers task force on behalf of the alliance for academic internal medicine. Acad Med. 2009;84(10):1395–400.

11. Schattner P, Mazalin D, Pier C, Wainer JL, Ling MY. GP registrar well-being: a cross-sectional survey. Asia Pac Fam Med. 2010;9:2.
12. Levinson H. When executives burn out. Harvard business review on work and life balance. Boston, MA: HBS Press; 2000. p. 61–80.
13. Life balance Institute, http://www.lifebalanceinstitute.com Accessed 22 April 2011.
14. Mayo Clinic Work-Balance: tips to reclaim control. http://www.mayoclinic.com/health/work-life-balance/WL00056 Accessed 22 April 2011.
15. Sambunjak D, Straus SE, Maru A. Mentoring in academic medicine: a systematic review. J Am Med Assoc. 2006;296(9):1103–15.
16. Buddeberg-Fischer B, Stamm M, Buddeberg C, Klaghofer R. Career-success scale – a new instrument to assess young physicians' academic career steps. BMC Health Serv Res. 2008;8:120.
17. Urion DK. Compassion as a subversive activity: Illness, community, and the Gospel of Mark. Cambridge, MA: Cowley Publications; 2006.
18. Gladwell M. Outliers: the story of success. Brown and Company: Little; 2008.
19. Bartolome F, Evans PAL. "Must Success cost so much?" Harvard Business Review on Work and Life balance. Boston, MA: HBS Press; 2000. p. 31–60.
20. Structure Acupuncture for Physicians. Boston, MA. http://cme.hms.harvard.edu/cmeups/pdf/00302317.pdf Accessed 22 April 2011.
21. New England School of Acupuncture. http://www.nesa.edu Accessed 22 April 2011.
22. ACPE, Inc. Association of Clinical Pastoral Education. http://www.acpe.edu Accessed 22 April 2011.

Chapter 5
Avoiding Physician Burnout

Steve Alan Hyman

> **Key Points**
> - Burnout is likely when the job characteristics do not mesh well with personality characteristics of the individual.
> - Identify those who are risk for burnout because burnout may contribute to worsening job performance and health issues.
> - A well-lived life balances one's professional life with the personal life: personal growth and renewal are essential for maintaining this balance and may include not just time outside of work, but things like travel, family life, and other avocations or hobbies.

In the late1950s, a 4-year-old boy visited his older sister who was in nursing school (then called "nurse's training"). The visit and his sister's career choice made an indelible impression and led to his decision at that young age to become a doctor. After all, girls were nurses. If boys wanted to do the same thing, they would be doctors. Right?

The career choice was made and in a year or so, he began piano lessons. It was immediately obvious he was a gifted pianist and organist. By age 12, he was performing in many places and gained privileges other children of his age (particularly his younger twin sisters) had not. He stayed out late when others went to bed early. He identified with and acted more like an adult than most of his peers and indeed, interacted better with adults. Other kids chose teen idols like the Beatles and the Stones, but his were Van Cliburn, Vladimir Horowitz, and Arthur Rubenstein.

S.A. Hyman, MD, MM (✉)
Department of Anesthesiology, Vanderbilt University School of Medicine,
1301 Medical Center Drive 4648 TVC, Nashville, TN 37232, USA
e-mail: steve.hyman@vanderbilt.edu

R.D. Urman and J.M. Ehrenfeld (eds.), *Physicians' Pathways to Non-Traditional Careers and Leadership Opportunities*, DOI 10.1007/978-1-4614-0551-1_5,
© Springer Science+Business Media, LLC 2012

He was always a good student (not great!), but as his piano skills improved, his grades improved. As his grades improved, his piano skill improved. It was clear to everyone that he should attend a good music school – probably Julliard. However, between his junior and senior years of high school, he experienced an epiphany of epic proportion – doctors eat better than piano teachers. And statistics informed him that piano teacher was likely to be his profession with a musical education. He proposed pursing a musical education followed by medical school, but his high school guidance counselors told him that was impossible. Imagine taking counsel from people THAT ignorant! When he told his construction worker father (for whom his pianism was of the utmost importance) that he was planning to attend medical school, the Dad's reply was "You've got to be kidding!"

In college, he studied chemistry and declared himself a pre-med. He played the piano almost every night. He accompanied a choral group, taught 40 piano lessons weekly, and played at every church, wedding, funeral, and bar mitzvah he could schedule. His parents had very limited financial means, so each engagement improved his limited cash flow. He even competed in a competition with "real" musicians, because there was a cash award and he really needed the money.

College was extremely busy, but also an extremely productive period. He graduated with a high grade point average and was accepted to medical school without much difficulty. During medical school, he gave up music altogether and applied himself to his studies. He always said he wanted to give up medicine at age 50 and go to music school. He wasn't the brain of his class and didn't graduate AOA, but did well and was good at his work. He didn't LOVE medicine (as his Dad had loved the construction business), but he LIKED medicine and applied himself fully to the task at hand. He took no vacations during medical school and graduated 6 months early. During the 6 months after graduation and before residency, he worked in a research lab (remember the cash flow problem?) and was involved in music.

At this point, music was almost a "fatal attraction" and nearly derailed his medical career. While working in the research lab, he was asked to go to New England to play for Side by Side by Sondheim. *Although sorely tempted, he had made a commitment to start his internship in the summer and he intended to make good on that promise. He was not totally satisfied about this decision.*

Fast-forward 15 years. The young man is now fortyish and his residency is a decade in the past. He earned board certification in both anesthesiology and critical care and works at an academic medical center (his second job since residency) 60–90 hours weekly. He has conducted research and published papers, but was unable to create a niche for himself in the world of Academia. He went to work faithfully and put in the long hours, but was not fully engaged. He routinely brought a brief case of work home, but it almost always went back to work untouched. He dreaded the thought of another day at work, although he usually felt better after he got there. He was highly demanding of others and was often not very diplomatic in his day-to-day dealings with others.

He needed more hobbies (seriously?) so he took up tennis, bought a ski boat, and got a sports car. His marriage, while not fully satisfying, was comfortable but childless. He still worked long hours and his spouse left the workforce claiming high-stress, so he created a home-based medical billing business for the spouse, but it only received modest enthusiasm and limited success. Music, once an integral part of his life, was totally absent. He dusted his piano, and that was as close as he got to the keyboard. Once, he was asked to play something from a hymnal, and found that a challenge after not playing for such a long time.

He finally left the academic medical center for a private practice, knowing his work hours will be much better, not to mention the money. Before long, he realized that not much had changed. He still worked 60–90 hours a week, although now there was no research and no outside recognition of his efforts. He still had a full briefcase of work to accomplish each night, because someone had to do the billing and scheduling. He still dreaded going to work, but went anyway. He still had his boat and sports car, but there was no time to use them. His home-based billing business failed because he could not devote any more time to it and his spouse was not interested in the business.

One thing he did was to start playing the piano again. After so many years, he finally reached out to reclaim something that had been such an integral part of his life.

Fast-forward another 10 years. His 20 year marriage could not be salvaged, either through his own fault or that of his spouse. Depression followed this separation, but he found therapy to help deal with the issues which led to depression and failure of his marriage. After several years alone, he again married, but this time to someone with whom he shared a mutually nurturing relationship.

He decided that 60–90 hours per week didn't rise to the level of importance that they once did. He started working part-time, then on a per diem basis. At age 48, he went back to school and finally achieved his life-long dream of an advanced music degree. In fact, during this time in graduate school he didn't even work at the hospital. Talk about your "road less traveled."

Eventually, he went back to his old academic job, which is curiously stimulating this time. He works 3 days a week – no Mondays or Fridays and very few weekends. All he had to do was take a 40% pay cut and get his life back in balance! He now researches job satisfaction and burnout. He is extremely happy at work. He has some semblance of a professional music career with many concert dates in a given year worldwide. He also has an extremely happy home life with a spouse and two Schnauzers. Who could ask for anything more?

Introduction

It seems trite to say medicine is a demanding profession, but it is nonetheless true. Medical students and residents spend countless hours studying the required subjects to one day be called "Doctor." They gladly give up hobbies and outside interests, once pivotal pieces of their daily existence, with the expectation that after their training is complete and their lives are again in balance, they will resume these activities. In some cases, the resumption of life balance is achieved and these fun things resume.

Unfortunately for others, the imbalance remains and fun falls to the wayside. Time spent studying medicine is replaced by time spent practicing medicine, building a patient base, and tending the business aspects of running a practice. Personal financial requirements, marital problems, and some personality traits worsen this life imbalance and ultimately job burnout.

Although he did not give it a name, Sir William Osler noted the existence of burnout in a speech in 1899:

Engrossed late and soon in professional cares…you may so lay waste that you may find, too late, with hearts given way, that there is no place in your habit-stricken souls for those gentler influences which make life worth living [1].

The term 'burnout' was finally used in the 1970s by Dr. Herbert Freudenberger, a child psychologist and psychoanalyst. He described it thus: "to fail, wear out, or become exhausted by making excessive demands on energy, strength, or resources" [2, 3]. Burnout may occur when the demands of patient care outweigh other aspects of a physician's life. Maslach defines burnout in terms of three quantifiable terms: emotional exhaustion (EE), depersonalization (DP) or "cynicism", and a low sense of personal accomplishment (PA) [4, 5]. Spickard, Gabbe, and Christensen report that a burned out physician may also exhibit perceived clinical ineffectiveness, decreased interpersonal relationships, headaches, sleep disturbances, irritability, marital difficulties, fatigue, hypertension, anxiety, depression, and myocardial infarction [6]. Burnout is also reported to lead to alcoholism and drug dependency. Although data concerning therapy is minimal, one way of minimizing burnout may be by promoting personal and professional well-being on all levels: physical, emotional, and spiritual.

This case report clearly describes how a well-rounded, reasonably intelligent, hard-working individual achieves his goals but does not take care of his own needs. He begins to display the signs of burnout soon after his residency, but only starts to work on correcting them after a failed marriage and many years of needless unhappiness. Perhaps we can examine some of the signs of trouble and make recommendations for how to fix them.

The Physician Finds Himself

This boy first got an education. At first, it seemed his future held a musical career, but his musical education may have enhanced his ability to learn, particularly in the area of science. People have postulated that early music training could lead to improved verbal memory, more skillful abstract reasoning, greater creativity, and better performance on spatial-temporal tasks [7–9]. Rauscher et al. found significant improvements in the results of standardized spatial-temporal tests in pre-school children who studied piano compared to two other control groups [9]. Similar findings are also suggested by studies from Graziano et al. at the University of California, Irvine when they found that second graders learned proportional math skills significantly better if they also studied piano [10].

Musical study may also increase brain size. Gaser and Schlaug at the Harvard Medical School and the University of Jena (Germany) found significant differences in brain structure of professional keyboard players versus non-professional keyboard players and non-musicians [8, 11]. Using high-resolution magnetic resonance imaging (MRI), they found significant increases in the amount of musicians' gray matter in several areas including motor, parietal, and temporal regions. They also found increases in the left cerebellum (involved with coordination), left auditory cortex, and left frontal gyrus (data storage and processing). They also found the corpus callosum (the area that connects the right side of the brain to the left) to be larger in people who began music lessons before the age of 7 [11]. These brain changes were not found in non-professional musicians and non-musicians.

Raucher et al. also studied electroencephalograms in college students who listened to Mozart's Sonata in D Major for Two pianos – K448 [12–14]. Although some have doubted Rauscher's claim [15], there were significant short-term changes in waveform organization that persisted briefly while these subjects solved spatial-temporal problems [9, 12, 13].

Although it is not really provable that music had such a salutary effect on his ability to learn and become a doctor, the concept is compelling. There are no studies evaluating brain structure and function specifically in physicians, but there are studies evaluating – in the general population–some tasks that physicians likely would perform. Spatial-temporal imaging and problem-solving are important abilities for physicians, since they must visualize internal organs in the process of diagnosis. (n.b., they are also important in musicians, because they must hit the right note (the space) at the right time (tempus)). In chess players, functional MRIs show activity in the occipital and parietal lobes during the game, but not particularly in the frontal lobes, where we might assume problem-solving occurs [16]. Reukert et al. found with mental arithmetic calculations that pre-motor, parietal, and prefrontal areas were active [17]. Other researchers have found that word problems involve not only the temporal and parietal areas, but also the frontal areas [18].

One may ask "What do medicine and science have to do with music?" A historical example of the relationship between medicine and music comes from Dr. Theodore Billroth, considered the father of modern gastro-intestinal surgery. Billroth, a phenomenal pianist, often accompanied noted singers like Jennie Lind. His close friend Johannes Brahms dedicated his first two string quartets (Opus 51) to Billroth and transcribed his four symphonies into piano duet form so that he and the doctor/professor/pianist could perform them together. Joseph Attie stated in his Hayes Martin lecture to the Society of Head and Neck Surgeons in 1996: On integrating medicine and art, Billroth wrote to Brahms that "I have never known a great man in research, be it personally or from his biography, who is not essentially an artist with a rich fantasy and a childlike sensibility. Now I see it; I have again arrived at my hobby–science and art spring from the same source" [19].

The Physician Finds a Job

The vast majority of physicians have a strong work ethic. If they didn't, they probably would not have survived the rigors of medical school and residency. Nevertheless, some of us get burned out despite our willingness to work hard and forgo our own pleasure for work-related issues. When one has to give up fun things too frequently, one's life gets out of balance and places one at risk for burnout.

Burnout is likely when the job characteristics do not mesh well with personality characteristics of the individual. Job characteristics causing an increased likelihood of burnout involve workload (too much or too little), conflict, insufficient resources, insufficient social support, and lack of feedback or input into daily activities [5]. This occurs in corporations where there is downsizing – a steep organizational hierarchy exists where the same or more output is demanded of the same or fewer employees. Burned out people are often younger, well-educated adults who have never married. They are busy, have little control over daily activities, but have unrealistically high expectations for their job (sounds a little like residency, doesn't it?).

It is prudent to identify those who are at risk for burnout because burnout may contribute to worsening job performance (i.e., job turnover, decreased productivity, a negative effect on coworkers, absenteeism, and presenteeism) and health issues (i.e., substance abuse and mental and physical problems) [20]. Many of these job issues are seen in this case report. The physician had three jobs in 12 years. He didn't often accomplish what he had planned, whether it was research or simply paperwork. He was often unkind to his coworkers. Although he was fortunate not to have had physical problems or fall into substance abuse (although alcoholism was rampant in his family), he had problems with depression requiring therapy. He was not absent from work, but came to work even when he should have stayed home. This concept is called "presenteeism" [21–24] and can often be as harmful to the worker and the employer as absenteeism. One can't help but wonder what negative effects this constellation of symptoms has on the quality of patient care [25–27].

The Physician Finds a Solution

If it is not clear at this point, the case report listed above is the author, a former poster child for middle age job burnout. Although there are still moments of imbalance, I was fortunate to turn things around to experience a rewarding second act in my career.

There is no quick fix to the problem of burnout. The first step is the realization that there are job-related problems that the worker will be unable to fix by himself [5]. There are some aspects of the occupation that may never change. Workplace changes require recognition at the highest levels of the organization if there is any hope of improvement. Employers must realize that employee input is invaluable, even if not all input is implemented. In order to have faithful employees, employers will need to be faithful in return. By doing so, they encourage employees to think creatively and beyond the confines of the job.

Although the single employee cannot usually fix the workplace, he can fix his own attitudes. The following list is by no means exhaustive, but there are several important points that worked well for me:

1. Money is not the solution
2. Reclaim what is of intrinsic importance
3. Maintain goals and fulfill ambitions

Money is not the Solution

I did not come from a family of means, so when I graduated from medical school, I believed I had "made it" and assumed my financial woes were over. It didn't take me long to realize that there weren't an infinite number of zeroes after the first digit on my paycheck. Within a short time, I had spent myself into a corner and wasn't sure some months whether I would have money for groceries. I quickly got beneath, rather than above, my means. When I finally quit working full-time, it wasn't hard to get my arms around the concept of less money. For the first time in my adult life, I was going to have time to do things.

Many of my colleagues at the hospital were envious of my diminished time commitments. One surgeon said he would love to have a similar work situation. In return, I told him all he had to do was sell his Porsche, get a smaller house, and (perhaps undiplomatically) bridle his wife's uncontrolled spending habits. His response was "Oh, I couldn't sell my Porsche!" To this day I feel very sorry for him. He wanted a more balanced life, but wasn't willing to compromise to get it.

People often ask me how I can work only 3 days a week. Somewhat tongue-in-cheek I answer "All you have to do is take a 40% pay cut!" While simplistic, it is part of the answer. The other part of the answer is that you have to give your employer 110% on the days you are at work so that he feels like he gets his money's worth.

Reclaim What is of Intrinsic Importance

Personal growth and renewal are essential for maintaining this balance and may include not just time outside of work, but things like travel, family life, and other avocations or hobbies. For so many years, I didn't do what was central to my early life and what made me a well-rounded individual. For me it was music. For others it may be music, but it may be art or literature. Besides Theodore Billroth, there are many examples of physicians who are musicians. Dr. Alexander Borodin was a pioneer in the medical education of women and was the world-renowned protégé of chemist Dimitri Ivanovich Mendeleev, the creator of the periodic table of the elements. Borodin was equally world-renowned for the string quartets, symphonies, and operas written in his spare time [28, 29]. Dr. Albert Schweitzer was a physician and a famous missionary to Africa but his recordings of Bach organ works are still popular and his scholarly writings about these works are still used in music conservatories around the globe [30, 31]. Unfortunately, not all physician-musicians were successful in medicine. Dr. Hector Berlioz hated medicine so much that, against his family's will, he left the profession to compose music full-time [19, 32].

The multifaceted Thomas Jefferson once wrote that music "is the favorite passion of my soul" but music may not be the answer for some people. Dr. Arthur Conan Doyle, Dr. John Keats, and Dr. Anton Chekov practiced medicine, but were much more famous for their literary pursuits than for medicine. Gertrude Stein, who completed her medical studies but never was granted a medical degree, was also better known for her writings and bohemian lifestyle than for anything else [19].

The important thing in all these examples is that we must never let go of the things that keep us well-rounded. We must continue a commitment to the things that recharge our own batteries whether they are music, the arts, sports, or any number of other avocations. When we do, we are more likely to have extra energy to devote to our professional careers.

Maintain Goals and Fulfill Ambitions

We should all continue to have both goals and unfulfilled ambitions. By doing so, we maintain a zest for life and life-long learning. As we age and leave the workaday world, we will continue to have interests and hobbies that will keep us interested and interesting throughout our lives.

Summary

When I was a child, I sometimes got in a hurry when I played the piano. My mother called it "jet playing." This consisted of playing as fast as I could and if a composition had three counts per measure, I gave it two and a half. When I finally decided that music wasn't always fast, and measures in three-four time needed a full three counts per measure, my playing improved, my grades improved, and so on.

A well-lived life balances one's professional life with the personal. We all know what is necessary for a successful professional life, but don't always know what is important for a personal one. Balance occurs if one follows three rules described above and doesn't skimp on any one of them (i.e., give a full three counts per measure).

References

1. Osler W. Address to the students of Albany Medical College, February 1, 1899. Albany Med Ann. 1899;20:3.
2. Freudenberger HJ. The staff burn-out syndrome in alternative institutions. Psychother Theo Res Pract. 1975;12:73–82.
3. Freudenberger HJ. Burn-out: occupational hazard of the child care worker. Child Care Q. 1977;6:90–9.
4. Maslach C: MBI Manual, 3rd ed. Jackson S (ed.) Mountain View, CA: CPP, Inc., 1996.
5. Maslach C, Schaufeli WB, Leiter MP. Job burnout. Annu Rev Psychol. 2001;52:397–422.
6. Spickard Jr A, Gabbe SG, Christensen JF. Mid-career burnout in generalist and specialist physicians. J Am Med Assoc. 2002;288:1447–50.
7. Gaser C, Schlaug G. Gray matter differences between musicians and nonmusicians. Ann N Y Acad Sci. 2003;999:514–7.
8. Gaser C, Schlaug G. Brain structures differ between musicians and non-musicians. J Neurosci. 2003;23:9240–5.

9. Rauscher FH, Shaw GL, Levine LJ, Wright EL, Dennis WR, Newcomb RL. Music training causes long-term enhancement of preschool children's spatial-temporal reasoning. Neurol Res. 1997;19:2–8.
10. Graziano AB, Peterson M, Shaw GL. Enhanced learning of proportional math through music training and spatial-temporal training. Neurol Res. 1999;21:139–52.
11. Schlaug G, Jancke L, Huang Y, Staiger JF, Steinmetz H. Increased corpus callosum size in musicians. Neuropsychologia. 1995;33:1047–55.
12. Rauscher FH, Shaw GL. Key components of the Mozart effect. Percept Mot Skills. 1998;86:835–41.
13. Rauscher FH, Shaw GL, Ky KN. Listening to Mozart enhances spatial-temporal reasoning: towards a neurophysiological basis. Neurosci Lett. 1995;185:44–7.
14. Sarnthein J, vonStein A, Rappelsberger P, Petsche H, Rauscher FH, Shaw GL. Persistent patterns of brain activity: an EEG coherence study of the positive effect of music on spatial-temporal reasoning. Neurol Res. 1997;19:107–16.
15. Steele KM, Brown JD, Stoecker JA. Failure to confirm the Rauscher and Shaw description of recovery of the Mozart effect. Percept Mot Skills. 1999;88:843–8.
16. Atherton M, Zhuang J, Bart WM, He S, Hu X. A functional MRI study of high-level cognition. I. The game of chess. Brain Res Cogn Brain Res. 2003;16:26–31.
17. Rueckert L, Lange N, Partiot A, Appollonio I, Litvan I, Le Bihan D, et al. Visualizing cortical activation during mental calculation with functional MRI. Neuroimage. 1996;3:97–103.
18. Prabhakaran V, Rypma B, Gabrieli JD. Neural substrates of mathematical reasoning: a functional magnetic resonance imaging study of neocortical activation during performance of the necessary arithmetic operations test. Neuropsychology. 2001;15:115–27.
19. Attie JN. Hayes Martin Lecture. The physician (ARZT) and the arts. Am J Surg. 1996;172:618–24.
20. Hyman SA, Michaels DR, Berry JM, Schildcrout JS, Mercaldo ND, Weinger MB. Risk of burnout in perioperative clinicians: a survey study and literature review. Anesthesiology. 2011;114:194–204.
21. Koopman C, Pelletier KR, Murray JF, Sharda CE, Berger ML, Turpin RS, et al. Stanford presenteeism scale: health status and employee productivity. J Occup Environ Med. 2002;44:14–20.
22. Middaugh DJ. Presenteeism: sick and tired at work. Dermatol Nurs. 2007;19:172–3. 185.
23. Pilette PC. Presenteeism in nursing: a clear and present danger to productivity. J Nurs Adm. 2005;35:300–3.
24. Turpin RS, Ozminkowski RJ, Sharda CE, Collins JJ, Berger ML, Billotti GM, et al. Reliability and validity of the Stanford Presenteeism Scale. J Occup Environ Med. 2004;46:1123–33.
25. West CP, Huschka MM, Novotny PJ, Sloan JA, Kolars JC, Habermann TM, et al. Association of perceived medical errors with resident distress and empathy: a prospective longitudinal study. J Am Med Assoc. 2006;296:1071–8.
26. Shanafelt TD, Bradley KA, Wipf JE, Back AL. Burnout and self-reported patient care in an internal medicine residency program. Ann Intern Med. 2002;136:358–67.
27. Fahrenkopf AM, Sectish TC, Barger LK, Sharek PJ, Lewin D, Chiang VW, et al. Rates of medication errors among depressed and burnt out residents: prospective cohort study. BMJ. 2008;336:488–91.
28. Davies PJ. Alexander Porfir'yevich Borodin (1833–1887): composer, chemist, physician and social reformer. J Med Biogr. 1995;3:207–17.
29. Oldani M. Alexander Porfir'yevich Borodin. 2nd ed. MacMillan Publishers Limited: London; 2001.
30. Jacobi E: Albert Schweitzer. In: Grove Music Online. Edited by Root D. Oxford University Press. http://www.oxfordmusiconline.com.proxy.library.vanderbilt.edu/subscriber/article/grove/music/25204 Accessed 31 Jan 2011.
31. Slonimsky N KL, McIntire D: Albert Schweitzer, Baker's biographical dictionary of musicians, centennial edition. Slonimsky N KL (ed.). New York: Schirmer Books; 2001. pp. 3251.
32. MacDonald H: Berlioz, (Louis-) Hector. In Grove Music Online. Edited by Root D. Oxford University Press. http://www.oxfordmusiconline.com.proxy.library.vanderbilt.edu/subscriber/article/grove/music/51424pg20 Accessed 31 Jan 2011.

Chapter 6
Combined Degree Opportunities

Melvin C. Makhni

Key Points
- There are many dual degree paths to choose from.
- A second degree can be pursued alongside or subsequent to the MD.
- Dual expertise will help physicians better manage the complex environment of healthcare in the twenty-first century.

Introduction

Physicians can no longer insulate themselves from the complexities of healthcare. The challenges facing medicine, such as insurance and malpractice reform, must be addressed at least partially by medical professionals, rather than being managed solely by politicians, businessmen, and lawyers. For better or worse, being a doctor today is no longer about simply mastering the fundamentals of medicine.

To ensure that the interests of patients and physicians are represented, doctors must develop the expertise that will allow them to engage in discussions that dictate the trends in these fields. For medical trainees, combination degrees appear to be the portal of entry into this expertise. Increased enrollment into these programs

M.C. Makhni, MD, MBA Candidate (✉)
Harvard Medical School, Harvard Business School
e-mail: melvin_makhni@hms.harvard.edu

R.D. Urman and J.M. Ehrenfeld (eds.), *Physicians' Pathways to Non-Traditional Careers and Leadership Opportunities*, DOI 10.1007/978-1-4614-0551-1_6,
© Springer Science+Business Media, LLC 2012

Table 6.1 Summary of most commonly pursued combined degrees

Secondary degree	# Additional years	Standardized testing	Reasons to pursue	Common career opportunities
PhD	3–6	GRE	Research interest Scientific credibility	Academic medicine Industry research Management
MPH/MPP	1–2	Varies	Public health interest Policy interest	Policy analysis Health economics Preventative medicine
MBA	1–2	GMAT	Healthcare leadership Wealth generation	Hospital administration Consulting/Management Non-profit sector
JD	2–3	LSAT	Policy interest Legal career	Legal consulting Malpractice law Public policy

reflects at least the perceived utility of enriching medical education with a secondary advanced degree. Across specialties, physicians face decreasing compensation as well as increasing career dissatisfaction. However, a second area of expertise allows for the possibility of pursuing additional interests alongside, or even instead of, a career in medicine. Multidisciplinary education for doctors will position them to not only better serve their patients in the current cost-cutting environment, but also achieve enhanced career satisfaction.

For those who consider supplementing medical education with a second degree program, there are several practical issues to consider. Understanding these issues will help facilitate the decision about which secondary degree to pursue in addition to when, how, and why to apply to such programs.

Choosing a Second Degree

The first step in completing a dual degree is choosing which additional degree to pursue. This decision depends primarily on current as well as expected future career interests. A list of the most commonly pursued joint degrees and the opportunities they provide is shown in Table 6.1. While individual schools offering such programs may have information about their specific programs on their websites, it is otherwise difficult to learn more about these options, since very little is published regarding these combination opportunities (See list of "Additional Resources" at the end of the chapter).

PhD Degree

The PhD is one of the most common second degrees completed by physicians. This track, requiring an average of 3–6 additional years of education beyond standard medical training, was traditionally designed for those who aspire to integrate basic science research into their future clinical practices. This can be an exciting prospect to intellectually curious medical students, for this opens the possibility of developing laboratory advances which can be effectively translated to improve patient care. In addition to providing an education into the process of scientific research, this title could further establish academic and scientific credibility, increase one's future potential for receiving grant funding, improve possibilities for upward mobility in one's department, and allow for transition to industry within the healthcare setting if so desired. It is important to note, however, that this degree is not essential to physician scientists; many physicians performing basic science research in fact do not have PhD's. Further, it is difficult for even the best time managers to concurrently run a successful clinical practice and a booming research laboratory. This leaves many MD/PhD's focusing the majority (if not all) of their academic energy on being a physician or a scientist.

Students completing MD/PhD programs traditionally complete the first 2 years of medical school before completing the PhD portion, and then return to their final 2 clinical years of medical school rotations armed with their PhD degrees. Similar to single degree PhD programs, the number of years until completion depends heavily on project success, expectations from advisors, and luck. Entrants can expect to earn the joint degree in less time than they would if they pursued each degree separately; however, this is not always the case, and so a maximum of up to 6 years of full-time study must be allotted to the PhD portion. Unfortunately, students may perform their PhD in a certain field of interest, and then enter their third year of medical school and become attracted to a different specialty to which their PhD may have less direct application. Further, the career of a physician requires between 7 and 14 years from starting medical school to becoming an attending clinician, so it is important for those contemplating whether or not to pursue a PhD to understand that their journeys through medicine may ultimately be more rewarding, but may be significantly longer, as well.

Some students may be attracted to the prospect of being compensated for up to the complete cost of tuition and living expenses during their years in both the PhD and the medical programs. This could allow students to defray on average over $150,000 of debt (not to mention the additional interest that compounds over the 20 years of repayment!). However, there is an opportunity cost to spending the extra years performing research; MD/PhD students earn their doctorates several years later than their single degree counterparts, and hence relinquish those years of salary that they would have otherwise received. While it may come as a relief to not be burdened with excessive debt during medical school, the long-term financial benefits of tuition relief are offset by this cost of deferring a full attending salary, and should therefore not be a factor in determining whether or not to pursue this dual degree.

MPH/MPP Degree

The Masters in Public Health (MPH) and Masters in Public Policy (MPP) are other very common degrees sought by members of the medical community. Earning an MPH or MPP requires 2 years, but many medical schools with joint programs now offer an integrated degree track, which allows students to earn these second degrees with only one additional year of education. Students in these programs often finish their first 3 years of medical school before enrolling in their first degree of their masters program, and then split their fifth year of education between both schools. The MPH degree is for students interested in such fields as epidemiology, health economics, or preventative medicine. Through this program they are able to learn the skills necessary to become influential not only in the realm of research, but also in policy affairs as well. Those interested in public policy may also be interested in the MPP. Graduates of this degree possess skills in economic and policy analysis and are well suited for healthcare related roles in government and the public sector.

MBA Degree

Another secondary degree of recently increasing popularity is the Masters in Business Administration (MBA). Similar to the MPH, this degree can also be completed in 1–2 years in addition to the 4 years of medical school, depending on whether or not the degrees are integrated by a particular institution. The dual MD/MBA degree is pursued by students with a wide range of goals. Some believe that they can benefit more individuals at once by serving in hospital leadership positions or by establishing sustainable health delivery systems in the developing world. Others hope that this education will prepare them to translate their research innovations from bench to bedside, or to tackle the problem of uncontrolled healthcare costs on the national scene. Another subset of applicants may desire the MBA in order to maximize their earning potentials in private practice, or even in careers outside of clinical medicine such as consulting, finance, or industry.

Although a primary motivation for financial gain is present in only a small subset of joint degree applicants, it sometimes engenders suspicion of the motives of all MD/MBA candidates. Most students in this joint degree track continue in the field of medicine and enroll in residency programs, yet those pursuing an MD/MBA must be prepared to be asked about their motivations, and about often whether or not they intend to stay in medicine. This degree combination is unique in that medical students who attain it may be asked to defend their reasons for gaining the extra knowledge and perspectives from this degree, rather than boast of it to a readily accepting audiences – practically, this may include audiences of residency interviewers, colleagues, and patients.

JD Degree

Another dual degree option is the MD/JD track. While many recipients of both of these degrees have completed the JD later in their careers, the combined program is gaining popularity. This lengthens medical training by 2–3 years, again depending on the individual institutions. Individuals pursuing this track may intend to be legal scholars in the clinical realm, or they may wish to pursue fields such as malpractice law, patent law, forensic medicine, or public policy. This is arguably the only degree which will open career options that are not otherwise attainable without a second degree. Medical professionals can enter into research, business, public policy, and even perform tasks such as legal consulting simply with an MD, but if the intention is to become a practicing lawyer, the JD degree is a necessary prerequisite.

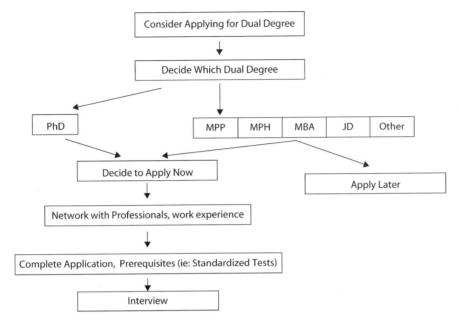

Fig. 6.1 Pathway to a joint degree

The Application Process

Application into dual degree programs can be done concurrently with application into medical school, during preclinical years, during residency, or after becoming a fully trained physician. Since there are so many opportunities to enrich one's medical career, one should only apply to a second degree program after considering the prospect of that degree in one's future. Without a clear idea about how the second degree can be utilized, one runs the risk of realizing too late that time and money could have been spent more fruitfully on a different pursuit – whether it is a different degree program, independent research, personal life experiences, or simply completion of medical school. A summary of a sample pathway to a joint degree is outlined in Fig. 6.1.

The first step in the application process is determining for which degree one should apply. The best way to truly understand the utility of this second degree is to spend time working in the field of interest and interacting with professionals in the field. For example, performing laboratory research and meeting researchers in the academic and industry settings will give one the best overview of the different paths available to MD-PhD degree holders. Before venturing into an MBA, it is crucial (and often mandated by programs) that one must work in a management setting. Serving as an intern in hospital administration or on a healthcare non-profit abroad can also be supplemented by individual meetings with MD-MBA's in the field.

The easiest way to do this is by contacting professionals within one's network. It is also possible to simply look up and contact individuals in the field for further information. These work experiences and professional interactions will not only help provide clarity about the dual degree, but they will also provide strength and diversity to one's application. Individuals met through these processes may also be approachable for letters of recommendations into the dual degree programs.

Completion of the degrees simultaneously is becoming an increasingly popular option for students, as more institutions have been offering such joint programs. This has allowed students to have opportunities to enter second degree programs with little background experience in these fields. In essence, these programs may make it easier for qualified medical students to acquire these second degrees. Or perhaps there is a selection bias, with applicants from the medical school being more uniformly qualified as compared to the overall candidate population. Regardless, one has an empirically higher chance of being accepted into the secondary degree from within the institution's medical school than from outside of it.

Programs often require all potential applicants (including joint degree MD candidates) to apply through the conventional admissions process. This entails completion of all standard prerequisite requirements, including standardized tests (i.e., GRE, GMAT, LSAT), application essays, and interviews by the same committee that determines the acceptances of all other candidates into each of the respective programs. However, this process varies by school; some programs allow their joint degree candidates to forgo the application process for the secondary degree and enroll directly from the medical school into the joint degree program. Details of each program should be considered on an individual basis by consulting the website or administrative office for each dual degree program in question.

For the application essays and interviews, it is important for all applicants to have a very clear understanding of how they wish to incorporate a second profession into medicine. Interview questions will often touch upon the busy nature of physicians simply trying to maintain their clinical practices, so one must be prepared to talk about future time management strategies. Less time invested in clinical practice can leave one open to criticism of delivering sub-optimal patient care, so this is another issue that dual degree candidates must be prepared to address in the application process and be mindful of throughout their careers.

Pre-medical students should apply into programs if they are certain that they wish to pursue both degrees. However, adding a second set of essays and interviews much could make the process more challenging. Most medical schools offering dual degree programs allow students in the non-clinical and even clinical years to apply into these programs, so there is rarely a need to rush into the application process. An exception to this generality is MD-PhD programs, because admission to both programs prior to entering medical school may allow for possible subsidization of educational expenses from the outset of the program.

If you are currently in residency training or a practicing physician, the entire process will be more cumbersome. Having been away from formal education for years, it will not be trivial to gather letters of recommendation, especially if you are a practicing physician who has been relatively isolated in private practice. It will also be time-consuming to stretch already full schedules to make time to write several essays and study for standardized tests, which have likely expired even if they were taken during previous years of education. In addition, it will be a more difficult process to incorporate into essays and interviews why one would want to add a new facet to his or her career, especially if the physician had been focusing primarily solely on clinical practice. That being said, the "MD" stamp on an application is also a powerful line on any resume, as long as one has relevant experience in the field and a sincere desire to pursue the second degree.

When to Pursue a Second Degree

A second degree can be completed alongside medical school or pursued later in one's medical career. Rarely, applicants to medical school have already completed their first advanced degree; these individuals have usually changed career paths from their first specialty towards medicine. They may have realized medicine to be their "true calling," or realized that they could further their career ambitions with a better understanding of the medical profession.

Many academic institutions created joint degree tracks which allow students to pursue modified, accelerated programs to more efficiently earn both graduate degrees before residency. The decrease in tuition expenses by 1 year can be a considerable factor for the average medical school student who graduates with 20-year loan repayment plans. Completing both degrees together also provides the benefit of convenience by allowing one to continue the momentum of being a student rather than having to leave a clinical practice to return to the classroom and once again pay tuition. Most importantly, earning an additional degree alongside the MD provides an opportunity for students to gain valuable perspectives, which can be nurtured and even implemented throughout residency and early years of practice.

The current trend is towards this integration of secondary programs into medical education, but there is also another trend towards physicians pursuing additional qualifications at later stages in their professional careers. Many "return to school" during residency or during their tenures as attendings, most often for the shorter Masters programs. After passing through residency, it could be tempting to return to school for a second degree "later," after finally having had the chance to solidify family relationships and earn enough salary to be free from old educational debts. By this time, however, a physician may have amassed a substantial practice – breaking this financial and career momentum to enroll in a second degree program could be a daunting task.

Applying into a second degree after completing several years of medical training may practically be more difficult but could arguably allow one to receive more benefit from the education. Years of practice experience will allow one to tailor the information learned to specific clinical interests. Information learned from the degree can be applied directly to one's career interests after graduation from the degree program, rather than years later if one is yet to complete residency. Practice experience could also provide the insight that the original degree sought may not actually be the one best suited for one's career goals, and that a different degree program, or simply independent study, would be best. Additionally, those completing joint degrees often are required to acquire their secondary degree from the same institution as they receive their medical education. However, later completion of the secondary degree would allow for more flexibility in this regard; a physician could apply to programs of the caliber and geographical region desired, or even enroll in flexible evening or online classes in order to avoid a complete departure from work.

Deciding Whether or Not to Apply for a Second Degree

Will a second degree be a transformational experience? It might, actually. It may impart a new skill set and more importantly, a new set of perspectives and reasoning that can be leveraged to achieve career goals and concurrently enhance career satisfaction. But at the end of the day, a secondary advanced degree is simply another sheet of paper that can be framed and hung on a wall. The MD alone is very powerful – if requires great sacrifice and hard work, and therefore denotes a certain degree of respect. It alone may open a breadth of career options to supplement or supplant a life in medicine. Most of what is learned from a second degree could very well be learned on one's own, without investing the time or money into a formal degree program. Further, most of what is learned will not ever be directly useful in one's future career, especially if an individual decides to remain primarily as a physician.

A second degree may be expensive, or with resourcefulness and good fortune it could be completely subsidized. It also requires between 1 and 6 years of time, depending on the degree path chosen; that means that students may find themselves reporting to others in the clinics who were once junior to them. Also, support from mentors may or may not be present. The rise of dual degrees in fields outside of the traditional MD/PhD has yielded some physicians who praise the utility of such education, as well as others who decry it for encroaching on the purely clinical focus needed to provide optimal direct clinical care.

Despite these costs of investing in further education, dual degree programs in the United States are evolving to better prepare physicians to tackle the pressing issues in today's healthcare environment. The attainment of multiple advanced skill sets is an attractive option for medical students, for it opens limitless possibilities within the field of medicine, and well beyond its confines. These programs allow for the exciting opportunity to experience a new intellectual culture, benefit from the wisdom of a second set of faculty and mentors, and develop unique cross-disciplinary perspectives on sophisticated, real-world problems. Such broad educational achievement allows doctors to serve as bridges and leaders across fields, and enables them to pursue related interests in fields intersecting medicine, such as research and global health, which they may have fostered before focusing on their medical training. The increased education and awareness could also allow for more effective secondary roles of physicians in hospital leadership, consulting, public policy, private practice, teaching, and so much more.

A secondary intangible benefit of a dual degree is the low-stress opportunity to step back from rigorous study of medicine and to learn something new and exciting. Many medical students have arrived from college straight to medical school, and then directly to residency – all without taking any time away from their studies. While a second degree is not exactly a vacation, it does present a detour opportunity before continuing a life of immersion in the field of medicine. Most degrees, while they may be time-intensive, will not be as dominating on one's schedule as studying for the USMLE Step I exam, third year of medical school, or residency. So, relative to a career in medicine, a second degree could be seen as a "break" to a medical student. This extra free time allows for the opportunity to halt the momentum of medical training and analyze personal and career priorities so that students can confirm their underlying desire to become a physician, and also finalize their choice of medical specialty. It could also be exciting to spend time interacting with highly qualified individuals with different personal and career goals, and different motivations and personalities. Even the material presented in courses, whether directly practical to a physician's future professional life or not, would likely be interesting as well.

The typical medical student faces little downside in applying into dual degree programs – especially the shorter masters options. For example, a second-year medical student approaching the dual degree application deadline may be conflicted whether or not to apply. Provided that the student has a baseline interest in the secondary field, connecting with students currently in and recently graduated from the combined program of interest can help one understand at least whether or not the time spent in the program could be interesting and educational. If so, one should simply apply! There is a trend towards an increasing number of medical students taking a fifth year off for extracurricular pursuits during medical school, whether in research or second degrees. Either way, residency programs often appreciate the increased investment in education. The time and money invested may seem daunting, but it is important for students to understand that they will likely spend the next several decades as a practicing physician. In the grand scheme, 1 year of time and tuition are relatively inconsequential, especially after having already invested 20+ years and likely hundreds of thousands of dollars in education. Instead of asking why to apply, it might be more helpful to determine if there are compelling reasons why not to apply.

A practicing physician interested in a second degree will likely have a more difficult decision to make. These individuals are less likely to pursue the more time-intensive PhD than their pre-medical and medical student counterparts. These candidates are likely to be at a later stage in their personal lives. Having children to provide for, for example, would make further investment of time and money much more difficult. Being at a later stage in their professional lives as well, they also have to consider the value of temporarily abandoning a clinical practice that they may have painstakingly built over the recent years. The change of momentum is difficult even with a masters program, since the investment in these programs becomes 2 years (rather than one additional year consumed by many dual degree programs).

A summary of the benefits and drawbacks of obtaining a dual degree is listed in Table 6.2.

Table 6.2 Benefits and drawbacks of dual degrees

Benefits of dual degree	Drawbacks of dual degree
Exciting	Financial cost of tuition
Intellectual development	Possibly irrelevant to medical career
Additional set of mentors	Opportunity cost of time
"Break" from medicine	Perception that one is not committed to patient care
Additional career opportunities available	Possibly decreased compensation for alternative career opportunities
Possibility for career change	Possible sacrifice of career depth for breadth

Conclusions

With so much change around the field of medicine, it is nearly impossible to predict the future landscape of healthcare. The only certainty is that it will become exceedingly complex. The roles of physicians will continue to evolve, and those physicians who can adapt to the new demands will watch their value to society rise.

For those excited to respond to these changes by defining their own professional role rather than occupying one that is pre-defined, it may be worth the investment of time, effort, and money to acquire a secondary degree alongside the MD. For those students who have never found their dream job, this is an excellent route to creating one that is designed specifically for them. It is for those who have found role models at the intersections of fields, and also for those who have searched but never found a mentor with the exact career that fits their individual goals; perhaps the career trails for these students have not yet been blazed.

Application of a dual education towards a dual career will be both difficult and time-consuming. This track is for individuals who have never been intellectually satisfied by simply doing the bare minimum required. For those who have found themselves asking questions that reach beyond the confines of medicine, a combined degree program may enable them to discover new, innovative solutions. It attracts those who are excited by uncertainty, as well as those who can handle the nebulous challenges that the future holds. In essence, for those students in college who led a varsity sports team, played in a band, founded a company, took classes outside their major "just for fun," and still managed to maintain vibrant social lives – dual degree programs may provide the tools necessary to help shape the field of medicine in the twenty-first century.

Additional Resources

MD-PhD Dual Degree Training. http://www.aamc.org/students/considering/research/mdphd/start.htm.
Directory of MD/MPH Educational Opportunities. http://www.amc.org/students/mdmph.
National Association of MD/MBA Students. http://www.md-mba.org/.

Lazarus A. MD/MBA: physicians on the new frontier of medical management. Tampa, FL: American College of Physician Executives; 1998.

Bohmer R. Designing Care: Aligning the Nature and Management of Health Care. Boston, MA: Harvard Business Press; 2009.

Parekh S, Singh B. An MBA: the utility and effect on physicians' careers. J Bone Joint Surg Am. 2007;89:442–7.

Desai A, Trillo R, Macario A. Should I get a Master of Business Administration? The anesthesiologist with education training: training options and professional opportunities. Curr Opin Anaesthesiol. 2009;22:191–8.

Scheinfeld N. Dermatologists with dual MD, JD degrees: a few comments on my life and those of other dermatologists with MD, JD degrees. Clin Dermatol. 2009;27:311–6.

Albert T. Dueling Degrees: Why some doctors are getting a JD. American Medical News. http://www.ama-assn.org/amednews/2002/01/28/prsa0128.htm, 2002.

The American College of Legal Medicine. http://www.aclm.org/

Rosner B, Nayak J, Minnery B. The complete guide to the MD/PhD degree. Alexandria, VA: J&S Publishing; 2004.

M.D.-Ph.D.: Reference. www.thefullwiki.org/M.D.-Ph.D.

Schafer A. The vanishing physician-scientist? Ithaca, NY: Cornell University Press; 2009.

Eisenberg M. The physician scientist's career guide. New York, NY: Springer Science+Business Media; 2010.

MD/MPH–DO/MPH Guide. www.amsa.org/AMSA/Homepage/About/Committees/CEH/MDMPHGUIDE.aspx.

Chapter 7
Finding Fulfillment Outside of Medicine

Edward L. Amaral

> **Key Points**
> - No matter where you are in your medical career, it is never too late to pick up a hobby.
> - There is a wide array of hobbies one can pursue: a hobby will challenge you, help you relax and yet create a sense of accomplishment.
> - More information is available on the internet, through local and national organizations, specialty publications, friends and colleagues.

As you progress in your medical career, be it as a student, trainee, junior or senior practicing physician, you will find that time is at a premium, especially leisure time. You will need to get involved with something completely different, something that will get your mind off anatomy and chemistry, off pneumonia or cancer workups and off staff meetings, sick patients and bills. But having the mind of a physician, it will be necessary to keep it active. I can't think of a better way to do this than by becoming involved with a hobby. A hobby will challenge you, help you relax and yet create a sense of accomplishment. It may take development of different modalities to reach your goal such as doing something creative, something educational completely unrelated to medicine, or some athletic endeavor that varies with the season. The most important thing is to get started! This can be achieved by asking friends and colleagues how they got started. Many school systems have "Nite-Life Courses" available to the citizenry of their region. The Internet can also be a valuable source of information. In short, "if there's a will, there's a way." Make up your mind, and forge ahead!

E.L. Amaral, MD, FACS (✉)
Department of Surgery, University of Massachusetts School of Medicine,
70-2 S.Quinsigamond Avenue, Shrewsbury, MA 01545, USA
e-mail: poppy99@massmed.org

R.D. Urman and J.M. Ehrenfeld (eds.), *Physicians' Pathways to Non-Traditional Careers and Leadership Opportunities*, DOI 10.1007/978-1-4614-0551-1_7,
© Springer Science+Business Media, LLC 2012

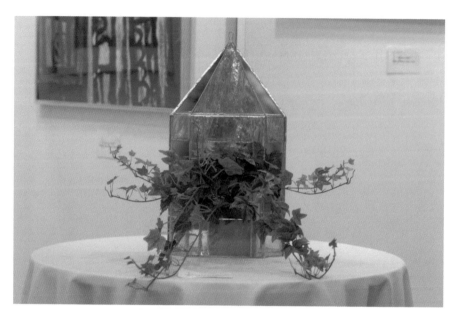

Fig. 7.1 Hanging Planter

I relate the following history to show that life's events can and often do alter one's interests and needs as life goes on. Being the son of a Dad who had active TB, sports were forbidden when I was a child back in the late thirties on – unless done covertly. As a result, I became involved with "Hobbies" early on. These included playing the piano, all aspects of photography, including processing and printing, and building things out of wood. I even built my own table saw. I joined the US Air Force after my surgical residency and added ceramics and golf to my interests while there. Upon entering private practice, I switched from piano to the electronic organ and added skiing and tennis to my "repertoire." At this point in my life, my time was almost totally consumed by my practice, my family (two boys and a girl), and meetings. When time and finances permitted some years later, my wife and I traveled.

One year, we took a trip to Paris where I visited the Cathedral of Notre Dame. It was there, in the rear of this magnificent church, that I saw the famous Rosetta Window with its sparkling, beautiful stained glass! I didn't know it then, but I was hooked! Sometime later I took a "Nite-Life" course in stained glass at a local high school taught by a wonderful, devoted teacher. My prime hobby was thus launched (Figs. 7.1–7.7).

If it was not for my family, my friends, and my hobbies, there were times when I would have gone mad, especially after losing my spouse of 35 years. With retirement, one can have too much time on one's hands. The kids are gone, one cannot play golf during a New England winter, but you would still have a different hobby to fall back on. Having reached retirement age and despite maintaining honorary hospital staff appointments, the significance of having hobbies in my life has become more apparent. I cannot emphasize this enough to the readers of this most informative book.

Fig. 7.2 "Cross of Hope"

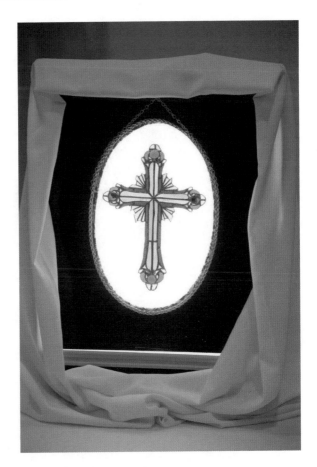

The following are statements by other physicians about the role that hobbies have played in their lives. I'm sure you will find them varied and interesting.

Physician #1

As an outdoorsman, I have always found wildlife fascinating. The beauty of the moment you see in an animal in its natural state is what I try to recreate when performing taxidermy. I have done this hobby since I was ten years old. I feel my hobby has helped me in my professional life in many ways. It involves motor skills which I also use at work as a surgeon. I also feel it has helped me see things in a three dimensional way which helped me with laparoscopy. This hobby helps me keep my mental sanity. I come home and see my work and I appreciate the time I obtained the specimens as well as the time spent creating my mounts. I feel any hobby is important during residency and afterwards to keep interests outside medicine (Paul Arcand, MD, Surgeon; Figs. 7.8–7.12).

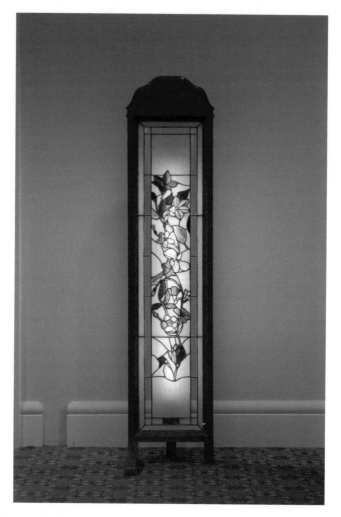

Fig. 7.3 Free-standing floral arrangement

Physician #2

It was a bird in a parking lot that did it.

I needed relief from the Chicago winter and the pressure of medical school so we had driven down to the Florida Everglades during vacation break. While pulling over to have a picnic lunch, we caught a glimpse of a bird that didn't look real. It was red, blue, green, and yellow, and it resembled a kindergarten child's rendition of a fantasy bird. I went to the gift shop and bought my first field guide to identify the "male painted bunting".

Birding is a natural extension of the thought processes we use in medicine. Despite the impression of birders being stuffy snobs, they are kind, smart people who enjoy an intellectual game similar to differential diagnosis, with the exception that if you reach the wrong conclusion, it doesn't matter at all and usually everyone joins in the laughter. The pattern

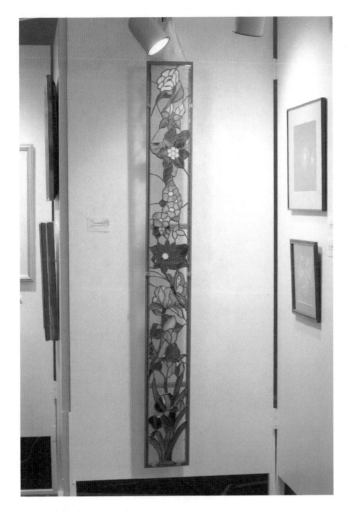

Fig. 7.4 Window sidelite insert

recognition is both visual and auditory. Birding brings you outdoors, away from the demands of our lives and can lead to interesting destinations in both warm and cold climates. I have friends who come along just to meet the birders themselves, a group spanning diverse ages and occupations. It is a hobby that can reward and challenge you for the rest of your life (Cynthia B. Brown, MD, Neurology).

Physician #3

A life devoted to caring for patients with advanced cancer and their families has been a relentless challenge. Most of my family has died from cancer including my mother when I was twelve years old. Even I have had cancer! There are three things that have kept me

Fig. 7.5 Enlargement of sidelite for detail

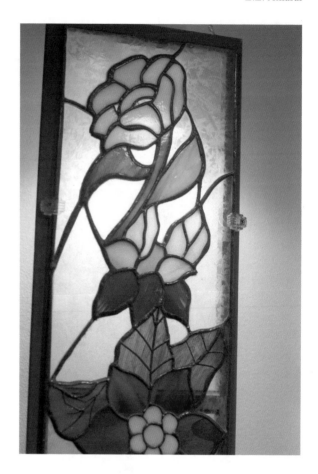

going through the years – the love of family, friends and colleagues – the sense that I was truly there for my patients and good at caring for them – my art!

All of my life I have been able to visualize things and to construct things with my hands. I don't know why? It just comes naturally. It is a gift for which I am most grateful. It is a source of great pleasure to see emerging on the canvas oil paintings that enable a meaningful moment in the life of a flower or a person, a time and place to live on even after death.

My focus is an integration of realism with impressionism. No medium other than oil can convey the graphic emotion that I seek to find. A picture which when mounted on a wall and in floodlight must convey in the observer the sense of "Wow," of "Wonder". Life is brief but the visual symbol for the life can last forever! (Jack T Evjy, MD, Oncologist; Figs. 7.13–7.15)

Physician #4

I have been interested in art since about age thirteen. I did largely figurative and portrait images. When I was an intern I would go out into the countryside with my young family and paint watercolor landscapes which I exhibited in the Medical Center art shows at Rochester.

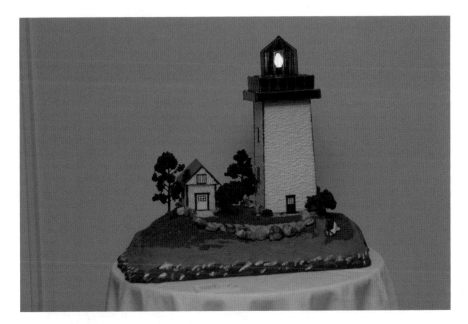

Fig. 7.6 Lighthouse

I remember making more money selling my art at these exhibits than my monthly salary as an intern which was only $50.00. The wonderful thing about doing art was the great contrast to what I did as a physician. I had two passions in life: medicine and art. I choose to do the most creative things in medicine: medical research, and building a new department in a new medical school. When I was in my early sixties, I decided to take art courses at the Worcester Art Museum. This led to many exhibitions, gallery associations and inclusions of my art in institutional and private collections. Art is an entirely creative undertaking and it complemented my efforts at creativity in Medicine. Now I am in my 80's and have just retired from Medicine. I have not retired from art, however, and I hope to continue to follow this passion for as long as my eyes and my brain make it possible. I strongly believe that medical professionals need to develop an interest outside of medicine that can keep that creative spark alive before and after retirement (Barry Hanshaw, MD, Pediatrician; Figs. 7.16–7.19).

Physician #5

Practicing the "Art of Medicine" is an ever increasing challenge as the continuum of time moves forward. We are expected to know and do more in less time with better outcomes. Burn out, depression and callousness can develop as we attempt to satisfy everyone but ourselves. As physicians, at any stage of our career, we need to remain cognizant not to lose the "be" in being human as I believe this a key characteristic that allows us to have compassion to treat others, courage to make difficult decisions, sacrifice our own desires when necessary and retain the ability to love our profession. The need to refresh my spirit and energy was a learning process of balancing professional responsibilities and personal needs

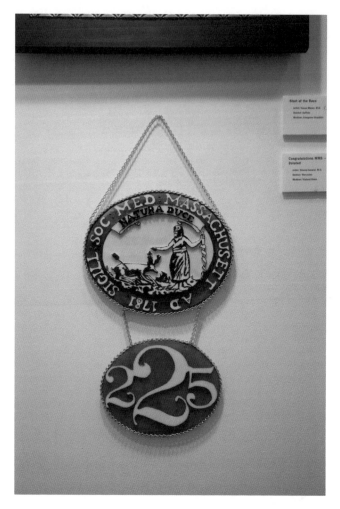

Fig. 7.7 Commemorative piece from the 225th Anniversary of the Massachusetts Medical Society

and remembering that in the grand scheme of this world, when nature is in balance calmness and beauty is created. To find harmony between all my interests, I began creating jewelry from tiny glass seed beads using various bead weaving techniques. Weaving one bead at a time into a piece of jewelry is convenient as I can work on a piece at any time and start and stop a project anywhere along its creation as well as bead at meetings and conferences. The ease of portability of my chosen art medium is perfect and having the ability to work on a project without time constraints gave rise to my jewelry's name "Therapeutic Jewels, by Dr. Claudia". It is therapy for me to be creative; to feel the tiny beads in my fingertips and see piles of loose beads be connected into a piece of beauty and wearable art. While beading, my mind is relieved of stress which is conducive for writing poetry and other works. By incorporating naturally polished beach stones collected while kayaking along the Maine coast, I can merge bead weaving and my more active related interests. I consider a healthy fusion of our intellectual and emotional well beings to be an essential component that allows us to be better and happier physicians. Tapping into our creative side, through whatever

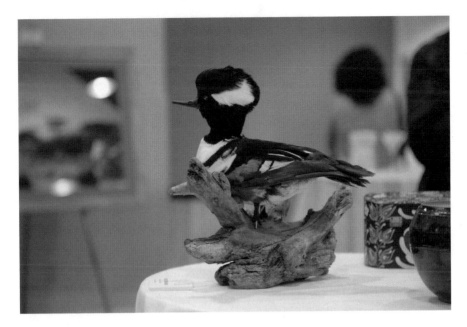

Fig. 7.8 Hooded Merganser

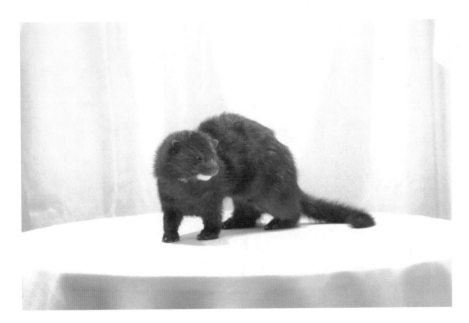

Fig. 7.9 Mink

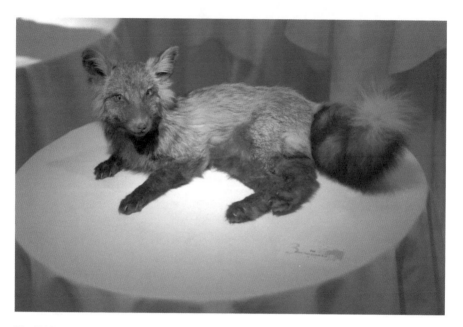

Fig. 7.10 Fox

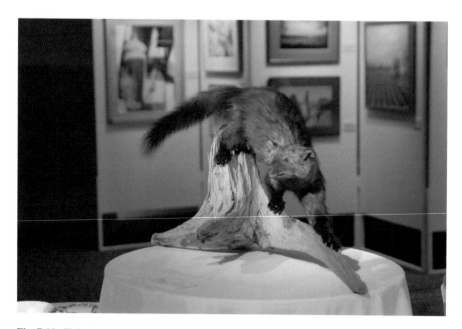

Fig. 7.11 Fisher (cat)

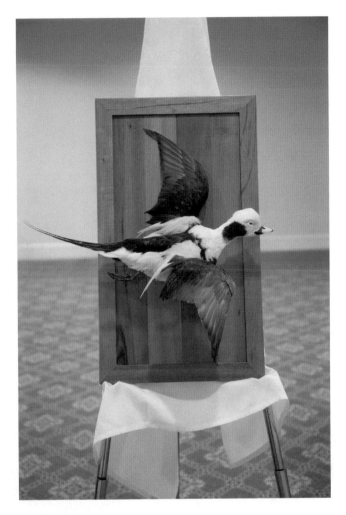

Fig. 7.12 Long tail duck

medium, I feel is essential to finding inner balance. "To heal one needs to feel, To feel one needs to listen, To listen one needs time, Time allows one to share, To share is to care…and caring heals". Taking time to feel and listen to our needs makes our journey through life not only healthier, but much more rewarding (Claudia Koppleman, M.D., Internal Medicine; Figs. 7.20–7.22).

Physician #6

I am a cardiologist in full-time practice, now for 28 years. However, before I entered medical school I had a difficult time deciding between a career in medicine or astrophysics. Although my decision was eventually to become a physician (a decision I have never regretted), I have never lost my enthusiasm for astrophysics. Therefore, when I finished medical

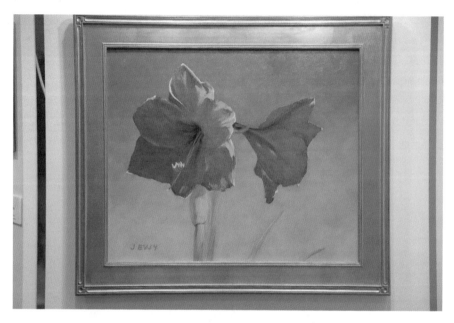

Fig. 7.13 Day Lily

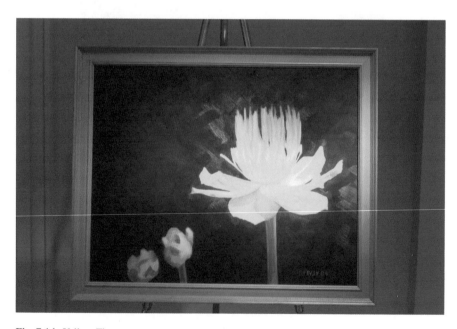

Fig. 7.14 Yellow Flower

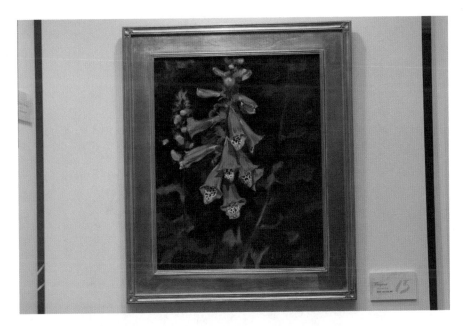

Fig. 7.15 Foxglove

school, I went right back to doing what I have always loved as an alternate activity. During my internship I purchased mirror blanks, and ground the optics for a large 16 inch primary mirror telescope. Then, I made all the mechanical parts, which I finished by the end of my residency.

Over the years, I have continued to build larger and better telescopes, and have been quite active in the astronomical community. In fact, I currently have the largest home-made telescope and observatory in the country. With these telescopes I have not only been able to have a great hobby that relaxes me from the stresses of medical practice and satisfies my craving for astronomical observations, but I have also been able to pursue my other life-long interest: participating in astronomical research. Having an intense intellectual hobby such as astronomy has given me an ideal diversion from the pressures of medical practice. Thus my original difficult choice of career has turned into a blessing, as I have been able to do both activities. I, of course, deeply enjoy the practice of medicine and cardiology. But as any clinician knows, no matter how much you enjoy medical practice, it is very much a demanding and exacting profession. It is good to have an alternate activity that helps clear the mind and places problems in perspective. This activity can be many things: athletics, intense areas of study, other hobbies. For me, it is the pleasure of coming home from a hard day of work, opening my dome to the cool evening air, and gazing out deep into the universe (Mario Motta, MD, Cardiology; Figs. 7.23–7.27).

Physician #7

For patriotic reasons, my interest in gardening began in adolescence during World War II. Though my results were modest, I took great pride in them, and I derived a great deal of satisfaction from my effort. I had to give up gardening when I went away to college. It was

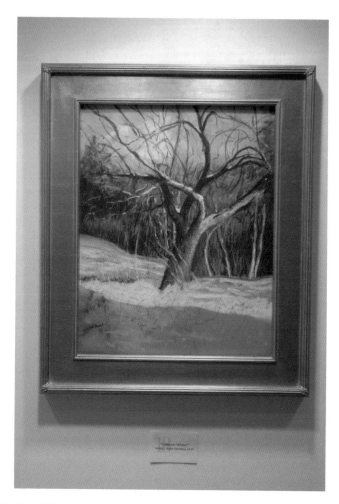

Fig. 7.16 Eastham Winter

not until I became a homeowner forty-two years ago, that I had the opportunity to rekindle my interest in gardening. The interest continues to grow to this day (no pun intended).

Gardening to me is communion with nature – a metaphysical experience associated with a sense of serene pleasure. I like getting dirty; it is an escape from the cleanliness that is almost an obsession with physicians. I even enjoy the "surgical scrub" that ends the gardening session for the day.

In a certain sense, gardening is a sport; one does not always win. There are successes to celebrate and failures to mourn. But the mourning resembles pathos more than it resembles grief.

Gardening is a convenient hobby. I can garden in almost any kind of weather. I do not have to schedule it because of a need for a partner and to hope for good weather as may be the case with tennis or golf. I can choose to do it alone. I can fit it into my schedule to suit me as to allow for the accommodation of other priorities.

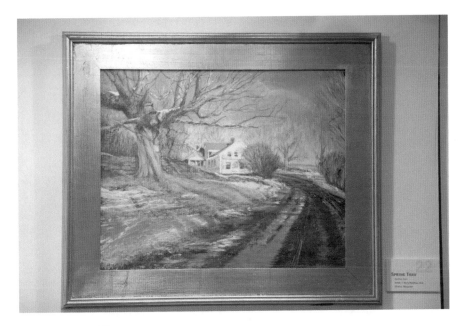

Fig. 7.17 Spring Thaw

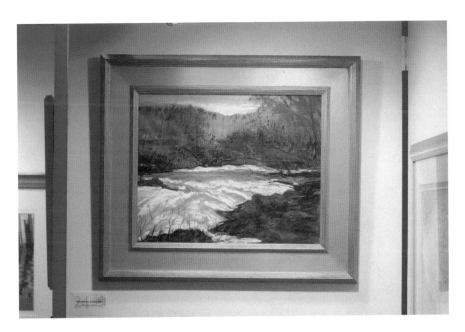

Fig. 7.18 Winterberries at Tower Hill

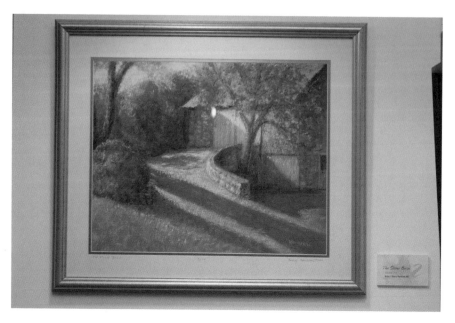

Fig. 7.19 The Stone Barn

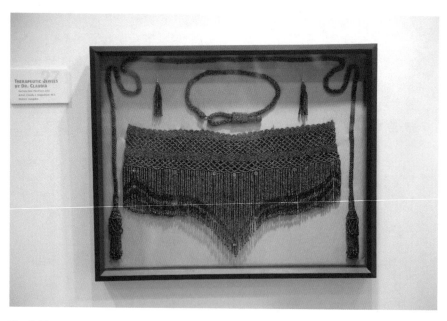

Fig. 7.20 Therapeutic Jewels

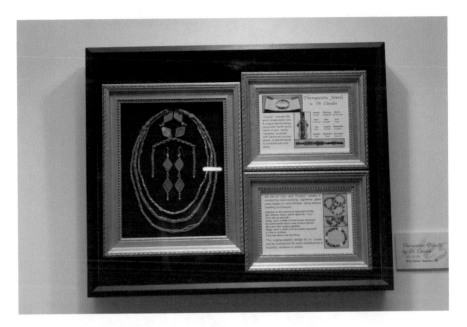

Fig. 7.21 Therapeutic jewels

Gardening is not just grunt work. It can have elements of an intellectual pursuit. There is much to learn about plant morphology, physiology and pathology and soil science. There is a need to know the qualities of the different microclimates that exist in your own garden in order to make the proper selection of suitable location and desired plant materials.

Designing a garden can be an artistic endeavor. Successfully combining suitable materials (plants, trees, shrubs, ground covers etc.) in proper sizes, shapes, colors and textures with walkways, sculptures, gates, arbors, benches, and water features such as ponds and fountains can result in a very pleasing composition (George Santos, MD, Ophthalmologist).

Physician #8

My hobbies are woodworking and particularly, woodworking on a lathe. I became interested in those beginning in grammar school and high school shop classes. Because of the requirements for substantial equipment and tools, those hobbies are difficult to pursue while in medical school or training. But once I was past training and had somewhat more time and space, I could actively pursue them again and even take more shop classes. Having a hobby that used my hands added a dimension to my everyday life that was different from my profession which was, basically, cerebral. Also, woodworking helped furnish my house. Later, I became more interested in lathe work which was less practical but allowed freer expression. These hobbies were relaxing just because they were so different from my work. Some colleagues have told me they would be at a loss to fill their time and feared boredom in retirement. However, when I retired, I was happy to be able to devote more time to my hobbies (Peter Schneider, MD, Nuclear Medicine; Figs. 7.28–7.30).

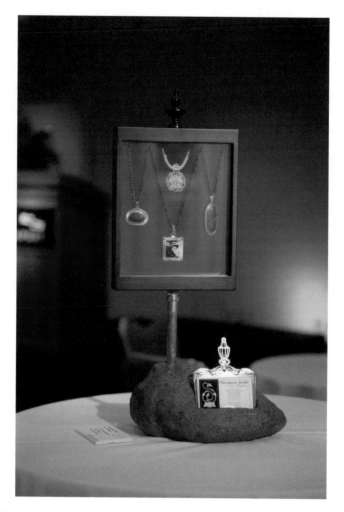

Fig. 7.22 Therapeutic jewels

Physician #9

I certainly agree with many who advise that hobbies and other interests outside medicine
was important. This is probably more important for surgeons who often work more hours
than residents these days. Given the often all-consuming nature of our chosen profession,
some diversion is healthy.

Woodworking allows me to be creative with my hands (the surgeon in me is showing) and
have an aesthetically pleasing and functional end result such as a piece of furniture. My
workshop is a peaceful sanctuary with little outside interruption (my wife and kids don't
like saw dust) (Mark Stoker, MD, Surgeon; Figs. 7.31–7.32).

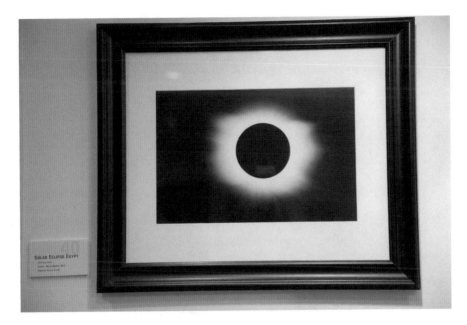

Fig. 7.23 Solar eclipses – Egypt

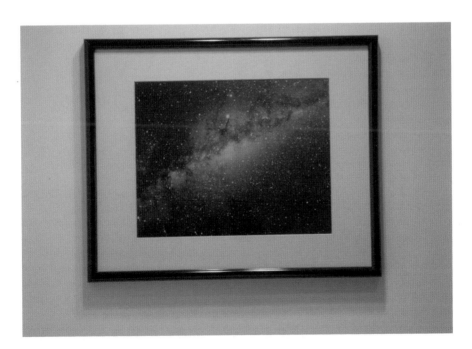

Fig. 7.24 Milky Way from South Africa

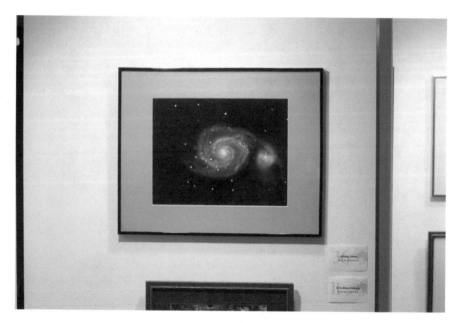

Fig. 7.25 Colliding galaxies

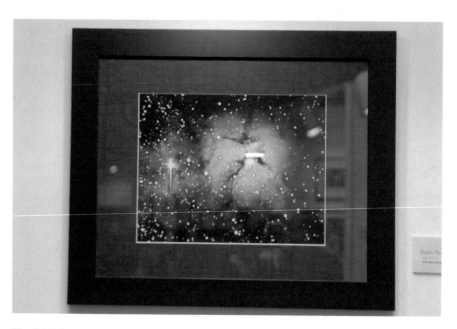

Fig. 7.26 Stellar Nebula

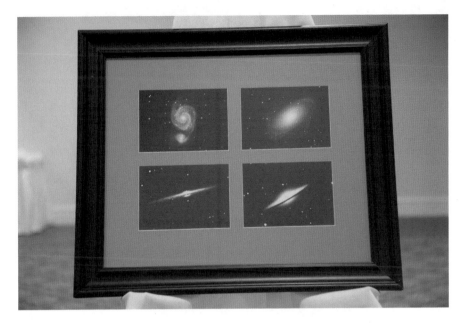

Fig. 7.27 Four galaxies

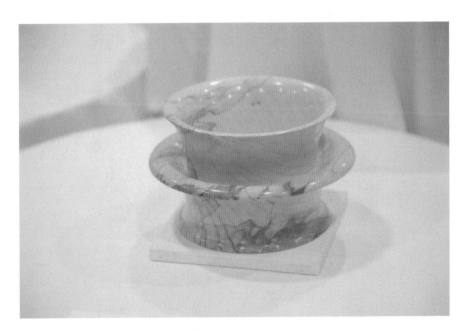

Fig. 7.28 Turned wood bowl (Spatled Elm)

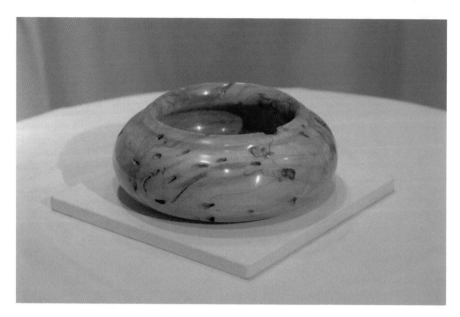

Fig. 7.29 Turned Wood Bowl

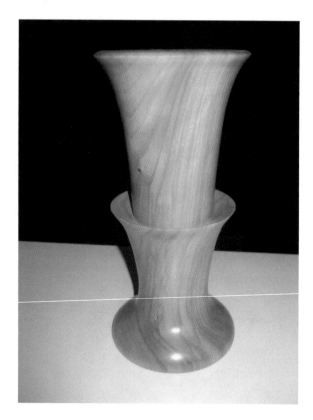

Fig. 7.30 Vase

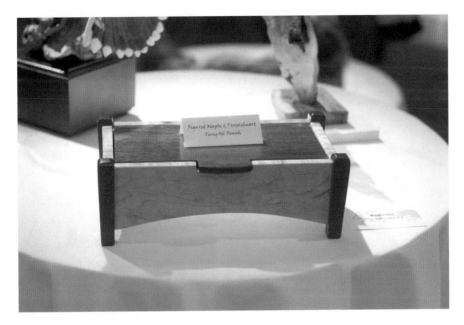

Fig. 7.31 Figured Maple and Purple heart box

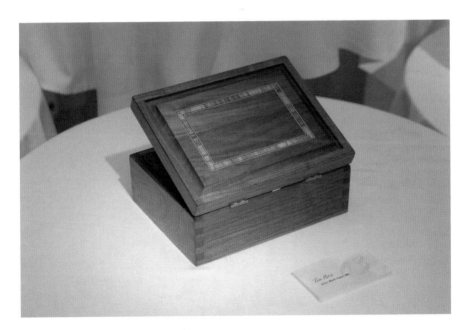

Fig. 7.32 Tea box

Physician #10

I am a 62 year old neonatologist who graduated from the University of Michigan with a BSE in Science Engineering and an MS in Bioengineering. My studies in bioengineering fostered my interest in Medicine.

As frequently happens in medicine, my daily life had been monopolized either by family or work. However, as our children became more independent and spent more time on their own activities, it became apparent that I should find an interest, a hobby that could offer me a respite from my professional life. Initially the usual outside activities of golf and swimming offered me alternative pursuits. Around ten years ago during a family vacation to the west coast, I used a newly purchased camera to capture some of the beautiful regions we had visited. While I had never viewed myself as being particularly creative, I eventually found myself quickly learning all aspects of photography from taking the photo to "developing" it on the computer to displaying the art at exhibits. Technological advances in photography have made the field more accessible to the amateur. I was able to unite my engineering skills from forty years ago with the new technology of digital cameras and printing paraphernalia that include high definition computer screens and ever-improving printer technology. The old engineer and physician became an artist with an entirely new world to pursue.

I now spend my free time by exploring new options for taking pictures – primarily outdoor scenes which include wildlife, architecture and landscapes. I have become involved in not just the process of taking the photos, but have developed skills in photo editing and display. At a course at the local Art Museum, I learned to mount, matt and frame my own photos. I am now able to participate in all aspects of creating and displaying my art so that I can share with others my perspective of unique beauty: birds in flight, flowering plants, unique architecture and structures. This has led me to discover places I would have otherwise not visited and created an entirely new passion to follow (Stuart Weisberger, MD, Neonatologist; Figs. 7.33–7.36).

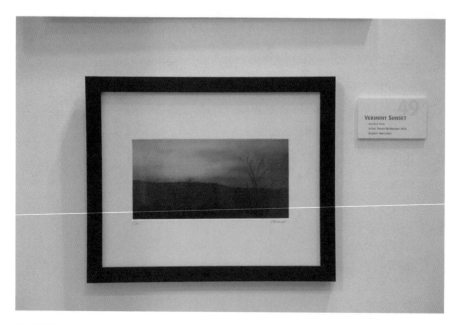

Fig. 7.33 Vermont sunset

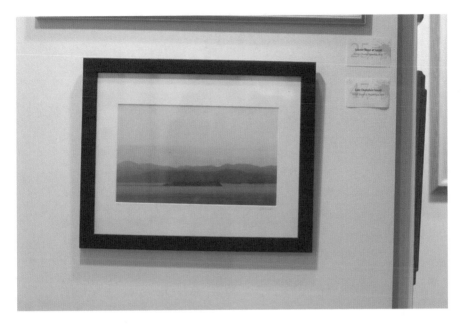

Fig. 7.34 Lake Champlain sunset

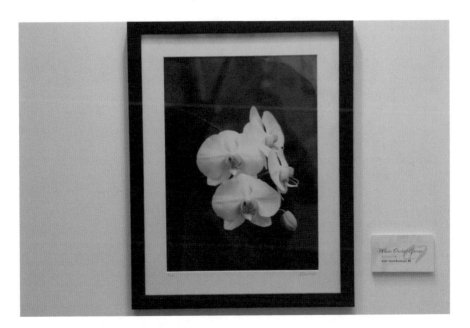

Fig. 7.35 White Orchid group

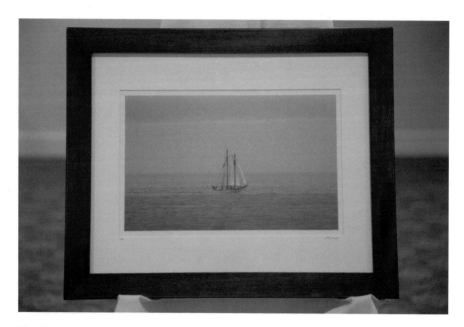

Fig. 7.36 Sailboat from Bar Harbor, Maine

Conclusion

Now you have heard ten personal stories from physicians who practice in different fields of medicine, giving you varied yet similar reasons why they became involved with their particular hobbies. All needed "something" besides medicine and family to maintain their equanimity, to fulfill their lives, and to feel "complete"! I hope these brief tales will pique your interest and curiosity and lead you to seek and find your particular hobby.

To get some ideas or more information about your current hobby, just do an internet search by typing "Hobbies" – you can learn a lot on your own, and likely will be surprised (and a bit overwhelmed) by the amount of information that comes up. Also talk to your friends and colleagues about your interests – others may share your passion for a particular hobby. Consider joining a hobby/activity group through your local community or a recreational or professional organization, and subscribing to relevant publications. Finally, you can inquire at a local college or university regarding educational opportunities that are related to your hobby(s).

Part II
Business, Consulting, and Industry

Chapter 8
Managerial Development

Stan N. Finkelstein and Richard M.J. Bohmer

Key Points

- Evolving trends in healthcare delivery are creating need and opportunities for individuals who are competent clinically, and also have an excellent understanding of the organizations within which they work.
- Individuals can pursue management education during medical school, residency, after clinical training, or even after having established clinical or scientific careers.
- Aspirants toward certain medical leadership positions will find a full management degree program to be beneficial, while others may find a set of specialized classes to meet their objectives.

Introduction

Healthcare delivery has become increasingly organizationally complex over the last 2 decades. More patients, often suffering from multiple coexisting diseases, are requiring more sophisticated therapies. Faced with greater demands, healthcare delivery organizations are responding by using multidisciplinary teams. At the same time organizations are grappling with staff shortages, both in absolute numbers and in particular subspecialties. They are looking to other providers to share the work of

S.N. Finkelstein, MD
MIT Engineering Systems Division and Harvard-MIT, Division of Health Sciences
and Technology, Harvard Medical School, Cambridge, MA, USA
e-mail: finkelstein@hcp.med.harvard.edu

R.M.J. Bohmer, MBChB, MPH (✉)
Harvard Business School, Soldiers Field Road, Boston, MA 02163, USA
e-mail: rbohmer@hbs.edu

R.D. Urman and J.M. Ehrenfeld (eds.), *Physicians' Pathways to Non-Traditional Careers and Leadership Opportunities*, DOI 10.1007/978-1-4614-0551-1_8,
© Springer Science+Business Media, LLC 2012

care delivery, further increasing team diversity. In this context, some physicians are looking to management training to help them navigate and optimize more complex organizations.

A Master of Business Administration (MBA) degree program offers excellent enrichment opportunities for individuals in various stages of a physician's career development. Acquiring the degree has become increasingly popular among medical students and also among physicians with established careers. Many others have taken the opportunity to enroll in management related courses in order to enrich their capabilities, but do not choose to pursue the additional graduate degree.

Numerous physicians in our academic community already hold MBA degrees. As most joint MD/MBA degree programs are relatively new, most of these individuals waited to enroll in the program until well after they completed clinical training. They represent a wide range of clinical specialties that include internal medicine, pediatrics, surgical specialties, and anesthesiology. Many continue to be active as clinical practitioners, while also serving in other roles as senior managers, and in those roles, contribute their managerial capabilities to advance the mandate of the organizations in which they work.

Enrolling in joint MD/MBA programs has recently become popular locally. For example, like most others, Harvard's combined program requires 5 academic years to complete and currently enrolls 12–14 students per year (a little less than 10% of the medical class) who were selected from a larger applicant pool. Students must apply separately to Harvard Medical and Harvard Business Schools and in practice most are already admitted to the medical school before they apply to business school. Once admitted, they enter the joint degree program. Interest in the program has grown from year to year. We strongly encourage our students to enter and complete residency training upon graduation with both MD and MBA degrees, before pursuing the wide range of professional opportunities that will become available to them.

Holders of MD and MBA degrees are finding outstanding career opportunities outside, as well as within academia. They serve as leaders of healthcare service organizations, as government policy officials, as corporate executives, entrepreneurs, and business consultants. Alumni of both Harvard Business School and Harvard Medical School who are holders of both degrees are currently represented in all of these career roles.

We have the privilege of directing the MD/MBA combined degree program that is joint effort between Harvard Medical School and Harvard Business School. Our program evolved from a student initiative that took place during the 1990s that encouraged the development of an academic course in management to be offered as an elective to first and second year medical students. The students aspired to gain understanding of how the constraints of the organizations in which they would go on to practice would affect the medical care they deliver. The MD/MBA joint program at Harvard was officially launched in 2005.

In this chapter, we will offer insights gained from teaching healthcare management in business school and in medical school and from advising medical students and physicians about their career development. We will attempt to provide some answers to frequently asked questions listed in Table 8.1.

Table 8.1 Frequently asked questions about healthcare management

Why pursue advanced education in management?
What content of the education may be particularly relevant to physicians' careers?
When during one's career development to pursue the additional degree?
What career opportunities graduates can expect to pursue?

Why?

Combined MD/MBA programs have been established to develop the next generation of leaders who are jointly skilled in the disciplines of medicine and management and who will apply their capabilities to complex issues of healthcare delivery. Students who opt for these joint programs decided to pursue this pathway early in their career development. Roles in which joint degree graduates can serve include traditional leadership roles as senior managers or physician executives. It can also include new career positions, including those of Chief Medical Officer and Chief Information Officer, which have been established in some healthcare delivery systems.

Equally important motivation for medically trained persons to acquire management training is to understand and to be able to cope with the rapidly evolving challenges of healthcare delivery. It is increasingly difficult, as an individual doctor, to be able to deliver high quality care without a deep understanding of the system in which he or she practices. Indeed, many physicians already need to incorporate various managerial tasks into their daily routines. As the fundamental unit of care delivery becomes the microsystem [1] rather than the individual practitioner, tomorrow's physicians will need to be able to shape the systems of care in which they work, and to adapt to the new models of medical care delivery that are occasioned by quality improvement initiatives and payment reforms. Even if a doctor does not aspire to become a senior manager, he or she will benefit by developing leadership skills and adapting them to the contexts of their everyday professional activities.

An important question to address is whether an individual's need for enrichment would be best satisfied by enrolling in a full MBA degree program. Or, would it suffice to become versed in specific managerial topics whose content is suited to an individual's roles and ultimate career goals and take courses, such as those offered by business and medical schools, professional societies and some independent education providers. For example, those who aspire to become a healthcare CEO or pharmaceutical company executive could well opt for the full degree. On the other hand, persons whose main roles are practitioners of medicine, but who lead practice units could do well to select classes in specific enrichment topics, such as team leadership, safety and quality improvement methods, or financial control. Some physicians who hold MBA degrees are also active contributors to health services research. However, the MBA degree is not generally considered to be a pathway to a career in research.

What Content?

Like medicine, the academic field of management is comprised of a portfolio of underlying academic disciplines. These disciplines, in turn contribute to sets of professional skills that students of these professional degree programs aim to acquire. Which of these skills may be desired or needed by physicians seeking enrichment in management depend on the stage of one's career, their current roles and future professional aspirations.

Broadly speaking, the topics on which MBA students focus can be thought of as falling into two categories: outward looking and inward looking. The former relate to an organization in its market context and include strategy and competitive markets, capital markets and sources of funding, and marketing and customer relations. The latter include operations, organizational culture, financial reporting and control, leadership and human resources management, and change management. Both of these sets of topics build on foundational knowledge drawn from a number of the social sciences, for example economics, individual cognitive and group psychology, and social anthropology.

Through study of topics such as these MBA degree programs, graduates are encouraged to develop key skill sets, of which the five mentioned below are some of the most important. Those physicians who complete MBA programs will receive grounding in all of these. Others who seek enrichment, but not necessarily an academic degree might consider pursuing course work in a selected set of these, such as human resource management or finance and accounting. Some MD/MBA programs offer specialized content that emphasizes case studies in health-related settings. We suggest that individuals whose careers will be devoted to healthcare can also learn much from educational content that draws on experiences outside of healthcare.

Developing Organizational Strategy

Positioning a delivery organization in its market is a pivotal task for a leader and requires an understanding of market dynamics and competition. Clearly articulating a delivery organization's role, the value it creates and the needs of the population to which it intends to bring this value is a critical task for senior leaders, even in single payer systems in which hospitals serve defined populations.

Designing Operations

The delivery organization's operations are the mechanism by which the value mentioned above is actually created for patients. Designing operating systems that reliably and safely deliver patient care is another core managerial task. This is much more than implementing standardized care protocols. It includes creating appropriate organizational structures, matching staffing models and staff development to the requirements of the care, deploying and managing teams, managing workflow, coordinating care, and developing reporting systems that track performance and safety.

Funding Operations and Exercising Financial Control

Funding a delivery organization's current operations or planning investments in new technologies and services is the core of a third set of skills that include raising and allocating capital and employing the tools of financial control. In some countries, such as the United States, this work is made more complicated by the existence of multiple payers or concurrent payment models.

Negotiation and Conflict Resolution

Conflicting goals and opinions are a fact of life in any large practice or in a hospital juggling the missions of clinical care, research and teaching. A fourth set of essential skills relate to leading negotiations and resolving the conflicts that are all but inevitable in modern healthcare delivery organizations. An associated set of skills is required for managing human resources and dealing with disruptive professionals.

Innovation and Performance Improvement

An important change in healthcare management over the last two decades has been an increase in attention to innovation and performance improvement. Managers have looked outside of healthcare for models to guide these efforts; systematic approaches to performance improvement such as Total Quality Management, the Toyota Production System, Six Sigma and Crew Resource Management, and models of innovation such as those used by the company IDEO. Selecting and deploying a systematic approach to learning and improvement is a fifth key skill set.

The concept of the "general manager" unifies the skill sets listed above. But what topics and skills might practitioners interested in understanding management but not wanting a full MBA consider useful? In part, this will depend on the practitioner's current role and her or his aspirations. Practitioners running their own practices, especially where these are multi-physician practices, will have a slightly different set of needs than those employed in a large delivery organization such as a general hospital as noted in Table 8.2. The former need predominantly to understand the mechanics of running an independent enterprise (irrespective of whether it is for-profit or not-for-profit), while much of the management work of the latter will focus on improving the performance of a unit or division within a larger, often multi-focused, enterprise.

Table 8.2 Management topics for physician executive development

Private, independent practice	Employed

• Finances and financial control
• Human resource management
  – Hiring and firing
  – Giving and receiving feedback
  – Succession planning and staff development
• Contract negotiation and conflict resolution
• Marketing
	• Team configuration and leadership
	• Approaches to quality measurement and system improvement
	• Change management

When?

Currently there is a wide range of options, described in Fig. 8.1 for when medical students and physicians can pursue enrichment in management. Opportunities include taking management-related academic subjects during medical school and pursuing combined MD/MBA degree programs from which graduates receive the two degrees concurrently. Also, full time or part time programs of study for the second degree can be taken at any time during one's career. In addition, some residency training programs now incorporate opportunities to enroll in management classes or opt for managerial rotations as requirements or during elective time.

Medical School

The earliest is during medical school. In the US, the Accreditation Council for Graduate Medical Education (ACGME) and the American Board of Medical Specialties (ABMS) include communication skills and systems-based practice in their core competencies. In the UK, the National Health Service has similar expectations in its list of competencies. The aim is to prepare students to work effectively in a complex training-hospital environment. Students are given the opportunity to understand the fundamentals of organizational and team behavior. For example, building, running, or being an effective participant in a team entails more than simply assembling a group of clinicians. Medical school is an ideal place to learn how complex systems work, and the ways in which they may fail and thereby cause patient harm.

Residency

During residency, junior physicians are already expected to take on managerial responsibilities. They lead small teams of interns and students and must interact successfully with complex care systems. The skills they need at this juncture include

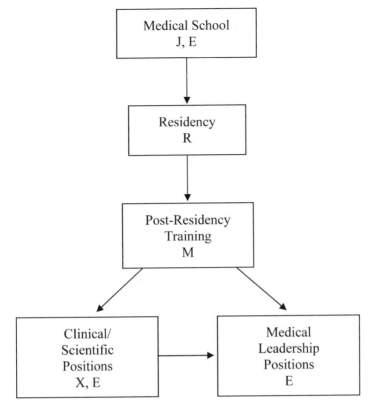

KEY:

J = Joint MD/MBA Degree Program

M = Full MBA Program

X = Executive MBA Program

E = Enrichment Courses in Management

R = Elective Rotations, Management Focused

Fig. 8.1 Pathways for management education for physicians pursuing medical leadership positions

the fundamentals of leadership, negotiation, and conflict resolution. Because they are at the forefront of some of the most difficult care of patients with complex conditions, they also need to understand how to prevent harm through human-factors design and by applying the principles of high-reliability organizations.

A number of residency training programs now expose the trainees to initiatives in clinical quality assurance and process improvement. Although the focus is mainly on the junior physician improving his or her own practice, residency is also an opportunity to gain experience in formal approaches to process improvement, such as the tools of continuous quality improvement.

In Practice

Numerous opportunities remain for enrichment in management when physicians are newly involved in private practice, or already established in their careers. Over time, managerial tasks such as operations design, organizational and financial control, and human resources management become increasingly relevant. Still other managerial works such as strategy setting, marketing, and raising capital are most relevant when physicians take more senior positions in a hospital, group practice, or other organization.

Physicians are often considered to be attractive candidates to enroll in full time and part time MBA degree programs. Many of the most selective full, 2-year MBA programs are said to value work experience before entering business school, and medical practice experience should certainly satisfy this expectation. Many physicians have populated the so-called "executive MBA" programs that provide for completion of degree requirements over a period of years. These latter programs offer a wide range of arrangements that include taking classes during evenings, on weekends, or full time on a short-term basis.

One challenging decision experienced practitioners often face is whether or not to interrupt a clinical career to enter a full time or executive MBA program. The career benefits of an additional credential must be weighed against the opportunity cost of leaving practice for an extended time. The opportunity cost – both in terms of lost income for the individual and lost manpower for his or her partner – tends to increase with increasing seniority. There may come a point in a doctor's career development when a full MBA is no longer worthwhile and shorter more focused executive development programs are preferable.

What Careers?

We believe strongly that, in the future, all doctors will be expected to have acquired a rudimentary understanding of how to work within, and improve the performance of healthcare delivery organizations. Indeed, a number of physicians have already opted to pursue enrichment in management, and continued in clinical practice roles. Those wishing to make the leadership of an organization, the main focus of their careers will likely need an MBA degree, while those who plan to stay firmly rooted in clinical careers may look to other management education opportunities that fall short of a full MBA degree program.

Though one prominent institution, the University of Pennsylvania has been offering medical students to join a combined MBA degree program for 40 years, the growth and popularity of combining medicine with management is a relatively new phenomenon [2, 3]. We have not been able to identify any systematically collected information on the career trajectories of those who have chosen these pathways.

The trend in medical leadership favors the expectation of formal management education among leaders of large health-related organizations. As of 2005, some 6% of U.S. medical school deans held MBA degrees [4]. Graduates of combined MD and MBA programs serve currently as chief executives of two of Boston's large teaching hospitals. These are model roles for the next generation of medical leaders, who will face the evolving challenges in the delivery of high performance, high value healthcare. We strongly encourage aspirants of these kinds of careers to complete medical residencies before undertaking significant managerial roles within an organization.

Medical entrepreneurship is another avenue that is attracting medical students and physicians to make use of both medical and management education. Some who have worked actively in the research laboratory seek to commercialize scientific advances related to their own work and are finding the skill sets to be complementary. Opportunities here can also include physicians with interests in so-called, "social entrepreneurship," building new organizations charged with implementing new models of care, with application to industrialized countries or the developing world.

Yet another group of physicians are those who look toward enrichment in management in order to pursue careers as leaders within medical product industries, management consulting or health-related finance. Serving in these roles early in one's career development may prove to be highly worthwhile experiences for those who go on to undertake senior leadership positions in organizations having direct involvement in the delivery of healthcare.

Conclusion

Many physicians and medical students have already benefited from enrichment in management by enrolling in classes or pursuing full MBA degree programs. Such learning is highly consistent with the trends in healthcare leadership that are creating opportunities for individuals who are clinically competent and also have an excellent understanding of the organizations within which they work. A vast array of educational programs from which to choose is available. Individuals are strongly encouraged to give serious consideration to selecting the ones that will be the best fit with the stage of their careers, their career aspirations and their plan for ongoing career development.

References

1. Nelson EC et al. Microsystems in health care: Part 1. Learning from high-performing front-line clinical units. JT Comm J Qual Improv. 2002;28(9):472–93.
2. Barzansky B, Etzel Sl. Educational programs in US medical schools, 2004–2005. JAMA. 2005;294(9):1068–74.
3. Sherrill WW. Dual-degree MD-MBA students: a look at the future of medical leadership. Acad Med. 2000;75(10 Suppl):S37–9.
4. Larson DB, Chandler M, Forman HP. MD/MBA programs in the United States: evidence of a change in health care leadership. Acad Med. 2003;78(3):335–41.

Chapter 9
The Pharmaceutical and Medical Device Industry

Jack T. Watters

Key Points

- Pharmaceutical industry presents many career paths for physicians and many opportunities to evolve and grow within a company.
- Career paths for physicians include basic science and basic or clinical research, policy development, government affairs, medical relations, or a combination thereof.
- Experience in basic or clinical scientific research, pharmacology, physiology, and patient care can be very helpful for a successful career in the pharmaceutical and medical device industry.

Introduction

Physicians are dedicated to the idea of helping people live longer, healthier lives. And no sector outside of clinical practice offers a better opportunity to fulfill this goal than the pharmaceutical industry.

I started in the pharmaceutical industry after my training as a physician because I wanted to be involved in clinical research. I was deeply interested in it and saw the work being done in pharmaceutical research and development as a natural outlet for my interests and abilities.

My curiosity was piqued during pharmacology lectures in medical school on the development of new medicines. I was fascinated by the idea of medical progress – of investigating new treatments and developing cures for diseases. But there were

J.T. Watters, MD (✉)
Pfizer Medical Department, Pfizer Inc., 219 East 42nd Street, New York, NY 10017, USA
e-mail: jack.t.watters@pfizer.com

R.D. Urman and J.M. Ehrenfeld (eds.), *Physicians' Pathways to Non-Traditional Careers and Leadership Opportunities*, DOI 10.1007/978-1-4614-0551-1_9,
© Springer Science+Business Media, LLC 2012

Table 9.1 Career options for physicians in the pharmaceutical industry

Basic science: Clinical researchers, drug safety experts, clinical pharmacologists, research-team leaders, clinical-trial managers

Clinical trials: Research designers and developers, statisticians, project managers

Development, marketing, distribution: Liaison to government/regulatory agencies, marketing and sales strategists, project managers, policy analysts and coordinators, advocacy team leaders

Public affairs and communications: Spokespersons, liaison to patient and physician groups, legal advisors, licensing and intellectual property managers, director of public health programs

few opportunities to pursue clinical research at the time in Edinburgh, Scotland, so I moved into the pharmaceutical industry in Europe.

My first job was as a clinical monitor on a large cardiovascular intervention study involving 6,500 patients in six countries. I monitored the study in Israel, Germany, Italy, and parts of the United Kingdom, with regular site visits to each of these countries.

The project was exciting, challenging, and rewarding. It gave me my first experience in the pharmaceutical industry, and I was hooked. Now I am just one member of a huge community of physicians who have made a similar discovery about how fulfilling a career in pharmaceuticals can be.

The impact of the development of new medications and therapies on healthcare is enormous. It is a vital pillar in the global health system. Over the last 50–75 years, the pharmaceutical industry has been one of the most dynamic and fast-growing of all industries in the private sector. Today, the industry employs nearly 700,000 people and supports another two-and-a-half million more jobs.

The pharmaceutical industry relies heavily on physicians in a wide variety of positions – ranging from science and research to policy development and governmental relations. A list of the categories of physician involvement in the pharmaceutical industry is shown in Table 9.1. For some physicians, the move from clinical care to pharmaceuticals provides a rewarding mid-career change. For others, it represents a natural way to spend the last few years before retirement. And for others, it represents an appealing path, straight from medical training. In short: Whatever your stage of professional development, the pharmaceutical industry provides many fulfilling career options.

The hundreds of thousands of people who come to work each day in pharmaceutical-related jobs are contributing in a tangible way to the quest for new ways to treat, cure and prevent the most feared diseases of our time. Pharmaceutical companies around the world are working on more than 800 potential medicines to treat cancer. And another 2,000 experimental medicines are in line to treat conditions ranging from Alzheimer's to hypertension.

Thanks to the contributions of this industry, people live a decade longer today than they did in 1950. Deaths from heart attacks have been cut in half in just 10 years. HIV/AIDS is no longer a death sentence, but is now a manageable condition. Those diagnosed with cancer have a much better chance today of extending their lives – even beating cancer completely – with the help of an ever-expanding list of new treatments.

The obvious end result of our work in pharmaceuticals is that we help improve people's lives, but the benefit extends far beyond individuals. In the end, we contribute to society as a whole. A healthier society is a more productive and fulfilled society and certainly a prosperous one. Everyone who works for a pharmaceutical company is in some way contributing to this high-level quest – and that can provide a great degree of career satisfaction.

As I look back on my years in the pharmaceutical industry, I am reminded of several key factors that have kept me energized, fulfilled and motivated by the work. The first is the feeling of widened influence. I firmly believe I have been able to impact more lives by helping advance medicine development than I could have in clinical practice. Second is the idea that a modern healthcare system must have several key elements in place to succeed, and robust pharmaceutical research and discovery is one of them. I have come to think of this industry as vital to our continually evolving understanding of human health. And finally, I have found that the pursuit of integrity can make all the difference in building a fulfilled pharmaceutical career. Those who succeed in the long-term in this industry are those who place a great emphasis on integrity, at all levels— from the research bench to the corporate board room.

Physicians and the Pharmaceuticals: A Natural Fit

One of the most stimulating aspects of jobs for physicians in the pharmaceutical industry is the scale and complexity of the drug-development process itself. Studies have shown that it takes more than a billion dollars and approximately 10 years (see Fig. 9.1) to bring new medicines to market – largely due to the intricacies of research, development and testing, and the multiple levels of the regulatory approval process. In today's environment, discovering and producing a new medicine is in some ways more challenging than sending people to outer space. Not every project succeeds – in fact, the majority of development projects fail before they get to the market stage. But the enormity of the end goal, the vast levels of partnership and collaboration required, and the many exciting twists and turns on the path toward drug approval make for an exciting professional journey.

As a research and science based industry, pharmaceuticals provides a natural fit for physicians. Science is ever-present as a back-drop for the work – no matter what level of an organization one works within– and the work can be intellectually stimulating. Your colleagues in this business are likely to be highly skilled people: The demand for their talent is great.

Because the work is so multi-faceted, pharmaceuticals presents many career paths for physicians, and many opportunities to evolve and grow within a company. One may become involved in science and research, policy development, government affairs, medical relations, or any mix of these— and other – disciplines during one's pharmaceutical career.

Depending on their background, many physicians in industry may choose to work in hands-on scientific roles, including bench science and clinical research.

The Research and Development Process

Developing a new medicine takes an average of 10–15 years.

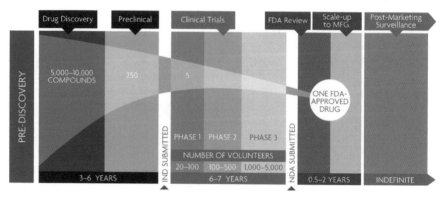

Fig. 9.1 The research and development process [from Pharmaceutical research and manufacturers of America, drug discovery and development: understanding the R&D process: www.innovation.org]

Some work as drug safety experts, monitoring drug absorption, distribution and metabolism in clinical trials, responding to adverse events, and tracking overall research trends and results. Physicians in these roles often have backgrounds in epidemiology. Others work in clinical pharmacology, where they help develop compounds for testing in the earliest stages of the research process. Known as Phase I, the goal of this level of research is to establish that a compound is safe for human testing. Physicians in these roles may have completed a clinical pharmacology fellowship.

Pharmaceutical industry physicians may also work in active roles in the later stages of drug development, known as Phases II and III. In these phases, clinical trials are larger and involve testing of patients with disease. As research strategists, these physicians may design studies, write protocols, interpret data and create clinical plans for drug development, managing a project from start to finish. They also may serve as operational managers, overseeing the business side of clinical trials. Physicians working in these phases often have clinical backgrounds and expertise in the disease being studied.

After a drug is approved, much work remains, including development of plans for marketing and distribution, and continuing liaison with government/regulatory agencies around the world and various patient and physician groups. Physicians may work in a variety of marketing-oriented positions, from helping develop and implement marketing strategies to serving in a liaison capacity between the scientific and sales/marketing sides of a pharmaceutical company's operations.

Physicians may also work in what is often referred to as "regulatory affairs," serving as members of policy-making and legislative-advocacy teams or as liaisons to government and regulatory agencies.

In recent years, there have been increasing opportunities for physicians in public affairs and communications. Physicians in these positions serve as spokespersons for a pharmaceutical company, articulating its vision and mission and working actively to build partnerships with patient and physician organizations and the public. Some physicians with an interest in law find satisfying careers working in the licensing and intellectual property divisions of a company.

The bottom line is that the variety of career paths is great: For any medical student or resident interested in the pharmaceutical environment, one does not need to look far to find an option. Practicing physicians who don't want to continue working in a clinical environment seek inspiration beyond their current professional roles, in order to expand unused skills or find a new career challenge.

Compensation and benefits can be lucrative in the pharmaceutical industry, and the opportunity for career progression and advancement is substantial. Many very successful pharmaceutical executives began their careers as medical doctors.

Additionally, today's pharmaceutical industry provides many opportunities for those interested in traveling and working internationally, or working with colleagues from other countries. We live in a truly global pharmaceutical product sales and marketing environment, and the result is that most large pharmaceutical companies have a presence in every corner of the globe. As an employee, you may have the opportunity to spend a portion of your career stationed in London, Tokyo, or Rome; and it is likely that you will find yourself in meetings and teleconferences that frequently include international participants.

How Patients Benefit from Your Work

The greatest impact of your work in a pharmaceutical company, of course, will be in the extension of life-saving medicines and therapies to literally millions of people. Development teams work for years on these therapies, and those that are ultimately approved can alter the course of disease dramatically among the world's populations.

Here are just a few examples of how the work of a pharmaceutical-company physician can directly impact patients:

- *Director of a clinical trials unit.* One of the most natural transitions for physicians to make is moving from clinical practice to clinical trials management. Clinical trials are one of the fundamental building blocks of drug development, and they allow physicians the opportunity to utilize much of their medical training – from pharmacology to epidemiology. Clinical trials put physicians in a position of both conducting research and directly impacting lives – as clinical trials often offer new hope for the sometimes seriously ill patients who volunteer for them.
- *Manager of a research team working on a new compound.* The path of a new medicine in development is seldom linear; it is more like a zig-zag, which eventually may lead to a successful new product. In the earliest stages of drug development,

physicians can play a crucial role as managers of various components of the research and discovery process. Research team leaders coordinate important details and provide the strategic vision and adjustments to ensure that work continues to move forward – despite setbacks. As a leaders in this stage of drug development, physicians utilize their scientific, clinical, and management skills and make many of the early decisions that eventually help turn therapeutic possibilities into realities for patients.

- *Director of a community health program.* Most of today's pharmaceutical companies recognize their obligation to help strengthen the healthcare system, which they rely on for their commercial success. As a result, many offer public health programs and charitable initiatives designed to "give back" to the community, often in partnership with not-for-profit organizations. As the director of special program to fight obesity in urban populations, for example, you might lead an effort that combines the resources of your company with those of a physician specialty society, a state health department and a public school system. Such public health programs touch millions of lives each year and can have enormous impact on the health of communities.

- *Policy liaison to a product-development team.* Once new compounds have successfully completed Phase I, Phase II, and Phase III testing, they enter another complex phase of development in which a host of business-oriented decisions must be made. The final coordination of manufacturing, marketing, sales, distribution, intellectual property and licensing has many implications for patient access to new drugs. As a physician policy director within a pharmaceutical company, you may be called upon to provide input and advice on a wide range of policy issues related to the new drug's distribution and use. Your work as liaison and expert on policy from government agencies such as the Federal Drug Administration (FDA) or physician groups such as the American Medical Association (AMA) help ensure that the new drug is effectively supported and dispensed by the medical community and safely used by patients.

Education and Background

A broad base of skills is needed for success as a pharmaceutical industry physician. Starting with medical school, a strong background in anatomy, physiology, and pharmacology is helpful. As a member of interdisciplinary teams in the pharmaceutical environment, your ability to understand the relationship between drugs, the human body, and basic medical care will be invaluable.

Specialized medical knowledge can be extremely helpful. The completion of specialty fellowships can position you for pharmaceutical jobs that require expertise in particular disease states. Common areas of specialty expertise include oncology, cardiology, neurology, and psychiatry – but specialists in a wide range of disease states are in demand. Practicing physicians who are board-certified in a specialty are attractive candidates for industry recruiters.

Experience in clinical research is extremely helpful for a career in pharmaceuticals. It is beneficial to gain this experience in medical school or residency, but clinical research experience at any stage of one's career will help position you for a transition to industry – especially for positions on the scientific side of pharmaceutical operations.

Experience with patient care can also be a huge benefit for those interested in a pharmaceutical career. Patient care is a component that many scientific researchers lack; it is helpful to have professional experience and an understanding of the kinds of patients who may end up taking the drugs you will be helping to develop.

Interested medical students and residents should begin making connection with the pharmaceutical industry early, while in school, in order to begin building a network and to gain a better understanding of career paths. Visit websites and read professional materials available at your school's career counseling center. Pharmaceutical companies often have scholarship programs available for students and residents – applying for these programs is an excellent way to make an early connection. Seek out and make connection with pharmaceutical representatives you may encounter during symposiums, presentations, and during visits to your school or health institution.

The challenge of transitioning to pharmaceuticals can be greater for practicing physicians – especially if they have been clinically active for a long period of time. Many have not had to search for a job or evaluate their career options. Practicing physicians should begin with networking – seeking out colleagues connected in some way with the pharmaceutical industry, and engaging proactively with pharmaceutical representatives. Working with a recruiter is also an excellent idea for physicians who want to transition from clinical practice into industry.

Related Careers in the Medical-Device Industry

While this discussion has centered on the pharmaceutical industry, a related industry – the development and manufacture of medical devices –also holds promise for medical students, residents, and other practicing physicians.

The development of medical devices – ranging from simple surgical tools to complex radiological imaging equipment – is, like pharmaceutical research, a key element in the advance of modern medicine. Those who work in the development of medical devices are contributing in a tangible way to the management of patients and their health.

The medical device industry has a huge impact in the United States. Statistics show that the industry was responsible in 2008 for nearly 423,000 jobs, $24.6 billion in annual payroll, and almost $136 billion worth of products sold.

The medical-device sector has grown substantially in recent years, offering new job opportunities for medical professionals. Between 2005 and 2008, the number of workers employed by industry increased 12.5% and the total worth of products sold also increased 11.6%. Salaries in the medical technology industry are well above the national average.

Like the pharmaceutical industry, jobs in the medical-device industry can be quite diverse, ranging from research and development, product design, engineering, production, and quality control to corporate management, sales, and regulatory and legal affairs.

Many of the same educational factors that are important for a career in pharmaceuticals can help you succeed in medical devices. These include a strong background in the sciences, and particularly in engineering.

Specialized medical knowledge can be extremely helpful, and the completion of specialty fellowships can position you for medical-device jobs that require expertise in particular disease states. Experience in clinical research is also a strong plus.

Conclusion

The pharmaceutical and medical-device industries offer the opportunity to be a part of a something much bigger than each of us as individuals: the quest for medical treatments and cures that can end human suffering and save lives. Along the way, you will work with talented colleagues in a fast-paced, dynamic, stimulating environment. That makes this career path a great choice for medical students, residents, and practicing physicians.

Additional Resources

To learn more about a career as a physician in the pharmaceutical industry, visit:

Pharmaceutical Research and Manufacturers of America (PhRMA). www.phrma.org
United States National Institutes of Health (clinical trials website). www.clinicaltrials.gov

Career Building Sites

PharmaceuticalCrossing.com. www.pharmaceuticalcrossing.com/
HireRX. www.hirerx.com/
CareerBuilder.com. www.careerbuilder.com/
Medzilla. www.medzilla.com/
BioSpace.com. www.biospace.com/

Medical Device Industry Careers

To learn more about a career as a physician in the medical-device industry, please visit:

Advanced Medical Technology Association (AdvaMed). http://www.advamed.org

Chapter 10
Healthcare Consulting

Jason Sanders

Key Points

- Healthcare consulting offers an unparalleled development opportunity.
- To make an informed decision you should experience a day in the life of a consultant firsthand.
- You can transition to consulting at different time points in your career.

In addition to medicine evolving as we replace old paradigms with new ones, your individual careers may also change over time, in unpredictable ways (Dean Jeffrey Flier, Harvard Medical School 2008 graduation).

We don't simply ask how we can *afford* healthcare. We show how to make it *affordable* – less costly and of better quality (Clay Christensen et al., The Innovator's Prescription).

Introduction

Most physicians who do consulting are not "born consultants." They may have paraded black doctor bags and stethoscopes in childhood, but rarely do family photos reveal an idolization of PowerPoint decks or laptop computers. In fact most consultants, whether physicians or not, are wayfarers, passing through the hallways of professional services firms en route to long-term careers elsewhere. For physicians these destinations may be venture capital, hospital management, pharmaceuticals, or even a return to clinical practice. What draws people to the management

J. Sanders, MD, MBA (✉)
Consultant McKinsey & Company, 75 Park Plaza, 3rd Floor, Boston, MA, 02116, USA
e-mail: jasonsanders@post.harvard.edu

R.D. Urman and J.M. Ehrenfeld (eds.), *Physicians' Pathways to Non-Traditional Careers and Leadership Opportunities*, DOI 10.1007/978-1-4614-0551-1_10, © Springer Science+Business Media, LLC 2012

consulting profession is an unparalleled development opportunity: achieving impact with clients, tackling complex problems, gaining experience rapidly across industries and functions, and becoming leaders. A minority of physicians will explore non-healthcare sectors, but those who dive into healthcare will create and implement solutions to some of the most challenging issues of our generation.

Consulting Success Story

Bob Kocher, MD, is a Principal at McKinsey and Company where he leads the McKinsey Center for Health Reform, and a Non-Resident Senior Fellow at the Brookings Institution Engleberg Center for Health Reform. He previously served in the Obama Administration as Special Assistant to the President for Healthcare and Economic Policy and a member of the National Economic Council. In the Obama Administration, Dr. Kocher was one of the leading architects of the healthcare reform legislation focusing on cost, quality, and delivery system reform. Prior to joining the Obama Administration, he served as a Partner at McKinsey & Company where he led McKinsey Global Institute's healthcare economic research, authoring the landmark "Accounting for the High Cost of US Healthcare" and a 2009 update, and where he served private and public sector healthcare clients. "I've spent many years studying the economics and economic incentives of the US system and how it compares to others around the world. I also worked in about 20 different countries on healthcare policy and strategy, giving me familiarity with how other systems approach similar challenges. These experiences enabled me to gain a great deal of perspective around how to address cost, quality, and access to inform the US debate."

Dr. Kocher received undergraduate degrees from the University of Washington and a medical degree from George Washington University. He completed a research fellowship with the Howard Hughes Medical Institute and the National Institutes of Health. He went on to complete his internal medicine residency training at the Beth Israel Deaconess Medical Center and the Harvard Medical School. He is Board Certified and licensed in Virginia.

Is Consulting for You?

Medical school clerkships show you what doctors really do, from well-child visits to joint replacements. You see the highlights, the low points, and the bread-and-butter work in between. Each type of experience influences your ultimate residency choice, according to a personal weighting scale.

Similarly, business internships show you what consultants really do. Yet physicians have little time to sample consulting jobs compared to business majors or MBA students. Premedical students tend to dedicate their free time to scientific research or healthcare-related volunteer work, and often go straight from college to

Table 10.1 Starter list of resources for finding volunteer consulting opportunities in healthcare

- Hospital/health system senior managers (e.g., chief medical officer), department chairs, medical directors
- Community health centers
- Local companies: e.g., pharma, biotech, medical devices, healthcare IT
- Hospital/health system technology transfer office
- Non-profit organizations: e.g., patient advocacy, public health, research foundations
- Residency program director and office of graduate medical education
- Medical school advisers, office of enrichment programs, and alumni office
- Local business schools, especially those with combined MD/MBA programs
- Local public health schools, especially those with combined MD/MPH programs
- Local medical association or specialty society chapters
- Physician colleagues and mentors

medical school, which is jammed with basic science courses and patient care. How then can a physician make an informed decision about consulting?

First, try to spend 4–10 weeks interning at a consulting firm; easier times to do this are the summer before your last year of medical school or residency. An alternative is to attend a 1–2 day recruiting workshop hosted by a consulting firm, often targeted at MDs and PhDs.

Second, look out for "volunteer" consulting opportunities as a medical student or resident, as you already have the capabilities and knowledge, when combined with independent initiative, to make an impact in healthcare organizations. For example, a local nonprofit organization for pediatric cancer awareness and research might need help planning its 3-year growth strategy; the medical director of the emergency department might need help reducing door-to-discharge times by redesigning the patient triage process; and a biotech company might need help doing diligence on a potential new compound to add to its neurology pipeline. In fact, you may discover that such "informal" consulting suits you perfectly since it is easier to combine with a clinical career. A list of volunteer consulting opportunities to consider is shown in Table 10.1.

Third, make the most of indirect information: reach out to the growing network of doctors who have business and consulting experience, keep up with newspapers and journals, and read books such as this one.

Day in the Life of a Consultant

Let us start with the highlights: recommending a change in strategy to the CEO of a large hospital; dramatically improving public health measures in an under-resourced country; increasing the number of new drug treatments that make it to late-stage development at a pharmaceutical company; helping a health insurer create value for its members. The theme is impact, which in consulting speak means making a significant and immediate difference in the lives of individuals, institutions, and societies.

The unique opportunity to implement change at the system level draws physicians to consulting. Such impact can happen as early as your first month on the job, and your contributions to the team are not merely encouraged but expected.

As in any job, there are the low points too: waking up at 4 a.m. on a Monday morning to catch a 6 a.m. flight; getting delayed for hours in a small airport; taking your Blackberry to the beach to dial-in to a weekend conference call; redoing PowerPoint layouts late at night; copying and binding a mountain of presentation decks for an early morning meeting; discovering an incorrect assumption in the model 2 months into a project. Of course a demanding lifestyle, nonstop paperwork, and high-stakes thinking are no strangers to physicians. It simply is important not to lose sight of this reality check to the glossy appeal of consulting jobs, especially by comparison to mounting frustrations with the practice of medicine.

While the "fascinoma" cases are inspiring to medical trainees, seasoned physicians show how bread-and-butter patients and illnesses are the foundation of a clinical career. Just as a premedical student might follow William Carlos Williams' house calls in northern New Jersey, or John Carter's bedside initiations in the first seasons of *ER*, a potential consultant needs to understand a day in the life.

A new consultant is a full member of a project team that works with a client on a specific problem. This team comprises partner leaders as well as a project manager and other early-tenure consultants. You own a defined piece of the work over the course of the project, ranging from 2 weeks to several months. The major healthcare sectors are pharma, biotech, medical devices, health insurers, clinical providers, and health systems. Within a sector, consulting projects take one or more functional cuts: e.g., strategy, finance, operations, organization, marketing, and information technology. Putting this together, hypothetical projects could be to serve a global pharmaceutical company on a 3-month growth strategy study, with your workstream on the role of generic drugs, or to serve a health system on a 6-month organizational transformation program, with your workstream on standardizing clinical pathways.

The day typically begins with a team "check-in." You share a plan to push forward the solution to the problem; and your colleagues offer feedback, update their pieces of the work, run through the calendar, and discuss overall progress. The remainder of the day is execution, such as phone calls with experts, client meetings, external research, and quantitative analysis. Effective teamwork is critical, as you bounce ideas off your colleagues and join them in meetings and conference calls. PowerPoint continues to dominate business communication, and you synthesize observations, insights, and recommendations on "pages" to convey the solution as a "story." These decks are the background for progress review meetings every week or two, and ad hoc conversations with partner leaders and clients. The day finishes in the evening with a quick team debrief, when you agree on high-priority items to complete that night, and outline the next morning's schedule. An example of the day in the life of a consultant is shown in Table 10.2.

Consulting firms invest heavily in professional and leadership development. Your team will help you build skills in problem analysis, solution brainstorming and due diligence, oral and written communication, time management, team leadership,

Table 10.2   Illustrative day in the life of a consultant: Start and stop times may vary…

7:00 a.m.	Wake-up
7:30 a.m.	Check Blackberry for overnight e-mails
8:00 a.m.	Meet fellow associates and project manager to get breakfast en route to client site
8:15 a.m.	Set-up in "team room" and review plan for the day with project manager
8:30 a.m.	Analyze new business unit financial data
10:15 a.m.	Update Powerpoint charts and pages
11:00 a.m.	Present your "pages" during conference call with consulting team leadership
12:00 p.m.	Make final changes to the deck before client meeting
12:30 p.m.	Grab lunch
1:00 p.m.	Work through materials together with the client team and figure out next steps
2:30 p.m.	De-brief with consulting team about the client meeting
3:00 p.m.	Submit targeted requests for additional data
3:15 p.m.	Speak with partner from your last project to help him or her prepare for an upcoming meeting
3:45 p.m.	Conduct interview with an industry expert
4:30 p.m.	Synthesize and share takeaways from the expert interview
5:30 p.m.	Join conference call on emerging industry trends
6:00 p.m.	Discuss with consulting team any refinements to the working set of client recommendations
6:45 p.m.	Agree with consulting team on any work to be started/completed before tomorrow morning
7:00 p.m.	Break for dinner, gym, family, etc.
10:00 p.m.	Catch up on e-mails, push on any work for tomorrow morning
11:00 p.m.	Go to sleep

and client partnerships. Interspersed with the steady progress of client work are off-site training sessions, web-based tutorials, healthcare sector conference calls, and local office community events.

When to Take a Detour

Consulting is a flexible career move, offering multiple points of entry. The bulk of any new hire cohort at a large firm join after an MBA program, but larger numbers are doing the same after PhDs, MDs, JDs, and MPHs. You also will meet colleagues fresh out of undergraduate studies and others with significant clinical or industry credentials. If you lack prior business experience and are a medical student, completing the MD degree will make you a much stronger candidate. Once you have achieved this milestone, though, you can apply for consulting jobs at almost any time thereafter: whether after internship, after residency, after fellowship, or during clinical practice.

When to take a detour from your fellow physicians doing full-time clinical practice can be an agonizing decision. But first, if you absolutely are sure that clinical practice is not for you, the timing decision should be an easy one. For everyone else, making detailed pros versus cons lists and speaking candidly with advisers are critical to making the best decision – one that you can live with. Below are a few frequently asked questions.

Do I Need to Complete Residency and Get Board Certification?

Finishing residency is a major and well-respected achievement, not to mention a de facto requirement for scope of clinical practice. It signifies a physician's commitment to the profession, to the highest training standards for safe and effective patient care. If this is an important personal goal, you should go full speed ahead.

From the consulting perspective, board certification is not a strict requirement either for entry or eventual success. It is nice to have, especially for certain projects, such as a pharmaceutical study on a new drug indication or a provider study on clinical quality. But there are people without board certification or even an MD degree who do this type of work every day, which is not a surprise when you step back and consider the sheer size of the U.S. healthcare industry.

A familiar quip is that physician mentors tend to recommend doing what they did: from "I left straight after medical school," to "you at least need to finish residency to be a real doctor," to " you should practice for a few years to enhance your credibility." The caveat is that many mentors trained during a different generation, when the "business" of medicine was not as formalized, and when consulting firms did not recruit physicians as heavily. Many doctors simply did not even think about consulting until after residency. You have the good fortune of more opportunities, but ironically this makes the decision even more difficult.

Should I Choose a Particular Specialty to Have a Dual Medicine and Business Career?

Anyone who enters the Match should thoroughly sift a host of factors when selecting a specialty. Ultimately the most critical ones are your clinical passions. At the end of the day, physicians from all specialties have gone into consulting, from primary care to urology. On the other hand, if you strongly are considering a dual business or administrative career, certain specialties may offer relative advantages. For example, the option to do shift work as a hospitalist or emergency medicine physician could allow you to do consulting simultaneously. Surgical training may spark insights into medical device development, and primary care experience will prepare you to counsel others on medical homes and accountable care organizations.

Will Additional Clinical Experience Help My Consulting Career?

You first need to think about your goals for a consulting career. Most physicians do work touching healthcare, but some have interests in different industries, such as banking, software, or consumer goods. If you want to stay in healthcare, the next step is to look at whom consulting firms are hiring: general management firms hire people from a variety of backgrounds, and even healthcare boutique firms hire a sizeable number of nonphysicians. Of course clinical experience is highly attractive to these firms, but it is not a prerequisite. Hence, the general recommendation is to pursue clinical practice for as long as you are passionate about it, but not necessarily as preparation for consulting. In fact, many of the basic consultant skills and terminology can only be honed on-the-job, regardless of your prior experience. Aside from the special considerations above about board certification, you should revisit your career options each year, balancing the personal satisfaction and incremental benefits of clinical practice against its opportunity costs.

Industry Overview

Management consulting arose during the early twentieth century. Its pioneers were dubbed efficiency experts as they helped clients apply management discipline to emerging private corporations. Today consulting has expanded into a global business with deep expertise across all types of industries (both private and public) and functions. Healthcare consulting is growing at a strong pace, driven by the rising percentage of United States GDP spent across the healthcare value chain.

The healthcare consulting landscape is best understood at the structural level before turning to specific firms. The principle business models are large strategic management firms versus smaller boutique firms. The former tend to serve all of the sectors mentioned above (from pharma to health insurers to health systems), and the latter focus on a specific sector (e.g., pharma). Also while the large firms have expertise across all of the functions mentioned above (e.g., strategy, operations, financial performance), the latter focus on select functions. In fact, firms dedicated solely to information technology account for a large share of the market, given the rising prominence of applications such as electronic medical records (EMR), computerized physician order entry (CPOE), and integrated billing systems. As the overall industry trends toward greater specialization, consultants likewise are focusing in a healthcare sector and function earlier in their careers: e.g., pharmaceutical R&D organization or hospital lean operations.

Your biggest decision is whether to transition to consulting, but once you have crossed that bridge choosing the right firm for you is worth some legwork. Major consulting firms with healthcare practices include Accenture, Bain & Company,

Booz & Company, The Boston Consulting Group, Deloitte, McKinsey & Company, Oliver Wyman, and PricewaterhouseCoopers. For smaller firms, you can contact the Association of Management Consulting Firms at www.amcf.org. Most consulting firms are partnerships, and whenever possible you should meet people across all tenure levels, whether at dedicated recruiting events or through informal networking. You need to find the people with whom you feel most excited to work, day in and day out. For each firm, other factors to consider include: reputation, office locations, travel expectations, client breadth and depth, functional expertise, distinctive ideas, development opportunities, career paths (e.g., full-time versus part-time), and special programs (e.g., global rotations or new client service initiatives). In addition to in-person conversations and company web sites, you can get further information via third-party resources such as Vault industry guides (www.vault.com) and Modern Healthcare (www.modernhealthcare.com), which might be available in hard copy at a university library.

How to Apply

Larger firms have streamlined application processes, whereas boutique shops may rely more on networking. The application cycle typically begins in the fall for start dates the following summer, but interviewing can proceed into the late spring or early summer. The essential components are a resume and interviews. The interviews may involve several "rounds," leading up to final interviews with partner leaders in the specific firm office location you wish to join. The case study is a common interview format used to test your analytical and communication skills. It is a bread-and-butter business problem designed to simulate the types of thinking you will need to do on the job: e.g., a medium-sized manufacturer in Indiana wants to understand why its profits are declining. Sample cases are available on consulting firm web sites or through third parties such as Vault. If you decide to apply, be sure to reach out to your mentors and other physicians who recently have joined consulting firms. Should you decide to pursue a career in consulting, a summary of the steps you might consider is listed in Table 10.3.

Table 10.3 What to do next

- Figure out whether consulting makes sense for you
- Decide when is the right time in your career path to try consulting
- Gather information on different consulting firms
- Practice several case studies before your interviews
- Stay in touch with your network of physicians who are making similar decisions

Additional Resources

25 Top consulting firms, by Wetfeet.com, January 2008.

Ace your case®: consulting interviews, by Wetfeet.com, 3rd edn, January 2008.

Consulting for PhDs, lawyers, and doctors, by Wetfeet.com, January 2008.

Largest Healthcare Management Consultants: 2010, ModernHealthcare.com.

Say it with charts: The executive's guide to visual communication, by Gene Zelazny, February 2001.

The innovator's prescription: a disruptive solution for healthcare, by Clay Christensen, Jerome H. Grossman, and Jason Hwang, December 2008.

Vault career guide to consulting, by Laura Walker Chung and Eric Chung, December 2007.

Vault guide to the case interview, by Mark Asher and Eric Chung, December 2007, December 2007.

Vault guide to the top 50 management and strategy consulting firms, by Naomi Newman, September 2010.

Chapter 11
Physicians in Management

Richard Marshall

Key Points

- Management roles can be divided into leading other clinicians and taking on management responsibilities outside of the direct line of clinical responsibility.
- Most physicians who become involved in management use a combination of progressively increasing levels of responsibility and training to achieve their goals.
- Prior leadership and management experience is paramount, and in some cases a physician may benefit from a formal education such as a master's degree in business, administration or public health.

Introduction

At some point during their career, most physicians seek ways to enrich their experience beyond full-time clinical practice. Many physicians have had leadership roles prior to beginning their medical training. You may have been the captain of a sports team, the head of a debate team, or the manager of your A Capella group's trips to regional competitions. You may have been the social chairperson of your dorm in college, or headed up a student group that tutored inner-city children. In medical school, you may have served on committees to re-examine the curriculum, and as a resident, you may have been involved in a house officer's organization.

R. Marshall, MD (✉)
Department of Pediatrics, Harvard Vanguard Medical Associates,
165 Dartmouth Street, Boston, MA 02116, USA
e-mail: richard-marshall@vmed.org

R.D. Urman and J.M. Ehrenfeld (eds.), *Physicians' Pathways to Non-Traditional Careers and Leadership Opportunities*, DOI 10.1007/978-1-4614-0551-1_11,
© Springer Science+Business Media, LLC 2012

If you find yourself described above, you may find a role in management a natural fit when you decide you want something more than a full-time clinical life. In this chapter, I will describe the range of management opportunities that physicians sometimes decide to pursue. I will also discuss ways to prepare for a role in management, and pathways for taking on such roles. I hope to leave you with confidence that physicians are often well suited for managerial roles, that those roles have challenges and opportunities for growth that differ from those available in clinical practice, and that the transition to, or addition of, managerial roles to clinical practice life can often be accomplished fairly easily.

Management Roles of Interest to Physicians

Management roles can be divided into two main groups. One concerns leading other physicians, and often other clinicians. I will discuss several examples: managing a small office; leading a clinical group in a larger organization (a team leader or local chief); leading a larger clinical group, such as physicians in a single specialty in a multi-site group practice, or a large hospital based clinical department; and leading the physicians for an entire entity, such as a large medical group or hospital. The second group of roles involves management outside the direct line of clinical responsibility. Examples of these include roles in health plans, or roles on the business side of clinical groups or hospitals, such as site administrator, chief operating officer, or chief executive officer (CEO).

In most small offices, one physician emerges to lead the group. My first managerial role came about in this way. I started a new practice with two other physicians of a different specialty, who became busy with clinical work more quickly than I did. After about 4 months of practice and a few crises such as the resignation of our bookkeeper, it became clear that one of us needed to lead the practice and make sure the office functioned properly. Since I was less busy, we decided I should take that role. It was that simple.

The range of responsibility in a small office is extensive. The managing physician usually oversees both managerial and clinical staff. When things are going well little oversight is required, but the resignation of the business manager to take a more lucrative job, the filing of a workmen's compensation case by a nursing assistant who strained her back assisting a patient, or the flooding of the office during a torrential rainstorm can turn what seemed like a quiet job into an onerous responsibility. Fortunately, all of the physicians in the group can be called upon to help. They know that the survival of their practice is up to themselves alone; no large organization is there to pull them back from disaster. Terms of office for managing partners usually last several years, but more often than not, other partners step forward to play the role over time, as all group members recognize both the burden and the importance of the role.

By comparison, local leadership roles in larger medical groups have a much narrower range of responsibility. The local leader is often responsible for managing schedules, productivity, and achievement of quality goals. Management of underperforming clinicians is another important task. While the scope of responsibility is

Table 11.1 Reasons to become involved in management

- Solve problems for your patients
- Solve problems for your group
- Create innovative solutions to problems that others adopt
- Increase the variety of responsibilities in your work life

narrower, there is less of a sense of urgency about these responsibilities from other group members. Such issues can be seen as a matter of interest to management, but not to other clinical staff, who see their role in purely clinical terms. Still, these roles are ideal for a physician to discover what it is like to lead other physicians and clinicians, due to the support from the infrastructure of a larger group.

More significant leadership roles in medical groups usually have a larger scope of responsibility. The head of a specialty in a large medical group often has responsibility for setting practice standards for the specialty. Standards could range from what characteristics are sought in new hires, to the implementation of evidence-based medicine or new procedures in the practice, to the implementation of utilization management initiatives for patients with a new health plan. In this role, one must often work through lower layers of management to succeed. Collaboration with administrative staff from the business side of the organization is usually critical for success.

Leaders of hospital-based clinical departments often have a similarly wide scope of responsibility, with a broad agenda that covers such topics as management of clinical staff with performance issues, implementation of hospital-wide initiatives, and department financial success. If the hospital is an academic institution, the breadth of the role is even larger, often including the management of research and teaching responsibilities. Once again the person in this role will need to rely on more junior leaders, usually divided by functions, such as research, teaching, quality and safety, etc., to succeed.

The role of chief medical officer (CMO) or Chief of Staff sits at the top of the ladder of clinical leadership roles. In this role, one has overall responsibility for the performance of the clinical staff. In addition, one represents the clinical staff in management circles, and to one's own boss, usually the CEO of the organization.

The CMO or Chief of Staff role is a daunting responsibility. In managing the clinical staff, the leader usually has department chairs or directors to assist with the task. But in terms of being the interface between the business side of the organization and the clinical staff, he or she is often alone, when, for example, explaining to the company's board the reasons for lower than expected productivity in a given year, or to the clinicians, the rationale for a business decision that involves switching thousands of managed Medicare patients from one health plan to another, requiring each physician to support the move with his or her own patients. On the other hand, if the local newspaper publishes quality scores showing the group or hospital leading all other organizations in the state, or the leader realizes that due to personal effort ten underperforming physicians were worked out of the group in a single year, he or she can feel a great sense of personal efficacy as a leader. A summary of reasons why many physicians become involved in management is listed in Table 11.1.

Leaving the Line of Clinical Responsibility: Roles on the Business Side

Some physicians find the management and leadership roles related to clinical lines of responsibility too limited. To be effective in the way they wish, they choose to become more involved in the business side of healthcare and clinical practice.

Physician roles in health plans offer one such opportunity. Initial positions in health plans often involve responsibility for utilization management, quality improvement, provider relations, or a combination of the above. These positions may be of great interest to physicians who want to have a broad impact on healthcare policy and decisions. They allow one to act across the entire population of health plan subscribers. While clinical expertise is still required, a broader sense of benefit for the population served comes into play, which must be balanced against the needs of an individual patient, those with a specific diagnosis, or a particular physician group.

Leadership roles in health plans depend significantly on the size of the plan. For some plans that insure large numbers of patients, the role can have aspects of overseeing the health of the general public. Interaction with government and public health officials, the press, and representatives of consumer groups can become a major role.

Involvement on the business side of physician groups and hospitals has similar features. Often a physician moves to these roles because they have a greater interest in change and improvement than they are afforded managing clinicians. Responsible for their unit's overall performance, they have at their disposal the full range of resources within the group for achievement of their goals. Examples of such positions are becoming a site administrator, becoming a chief operating officer, or a CEO. Once again, if the hospital or medical group is large, and the role is at a high level, the physician can feel he or she can impact the health of the general public through their role. Conflicts can arise between one's identity as a clinician, which remains even if one no longer practices, and one's role as a business leader. Similarly, conflicts can arise between the role of a physician business leader and clinical leaders within the same organization. Nevertheless, many of the strongest current leaders in healthcare in the United States have played the role of physician business leader/CEO.

Career Pathways: How Do I Get There from Here?

Most physicians who become involved in management use a combination of progressively increasing levels of responsibility and training to achieve their goals. Of the two, experience is the more critical.

It is relatively easy to gain the needed experience, and a list of options is presented in Table 11.2. There is a lack of leaders for clinical work. When opportunities arise, a person needs only to agree to take on the responsibility. Early examples of this might include agreeing to represent your group to a meeting called by a

Table 11.2 Easy ways to get management experience

- Join a group in your office to solve a cross-functional problem, such as improving the work flow for flu vaccines in the fall
- Join a committee in your professional group working on an issue, such as a reimbursement issue with health plans
- Speak up about a concern you have in your practice, and then take responsibility for coming up with a solution

health plan to explain new coverage rules, or taking responsibility for figuring out new roles for your staff when you hire your first RN to assist you in the practice. If you do well at such tasks, you will soon find that larger roles are available, perhaps taking responsibility for a search committee for a new physician for the group, and then mentoring the person selected. Such roles prepare you for considering broader tasks, such as a stint as managing partner or local leader of your group.

Training is also readily available. Leadership training or management training courses, lasting approximately a week, are ubiquitous. Talk to current physician leaders about how they learned their job; they may provide you with resources for further training and be willing to serve as a mentor as you explore expanding or changing your role. There are also a large number of executive MBA programs which can prepare you for larger levels of managerial responsibility.

However, training is not always needed. Many of today's physician leaders followed the simple path of progressively accepting greater and greater levels of responsibility, and finally found themselves as CMO or Chief of Staff of a large group. I followed this path in a large medical group, working my way up from team leader to a site chief, then a specialty chief, and finally chief medical officer. The entire process took about 10 years. Along the way I availed myself of opportunities within the group to attend trainings about quality improvement, human resources issues, and leadership training. More and more medical groups have such programs, the one at Mayo Clinic being best developed and most extensive.

Executive training, a masters degree in healthcare administration or public health, or an MBA is more useful, of course, to those who want to ascend the ladder of leadership on the business side of healthcare. Others working in that area often have such training, and you will need a certain level of expertise around financial management and economics to succeed in those areas.

Special Considerations

An Example of the Work of the Physician Manager: Problem Physicians

While many of the tasks described for physician managers could be performed by others, the management of problem physicians belongs particularly to them. Physicians, like anyone else, can develop performance problems at any point in their career. The most common cause of performance problems are personal issues, such as the development of physical or mental illness, stresses in relationships, or serious illnesses of family members. Substance abuse is another significant cause of performance problems. Maintaining a busy practice while experiencing such issues is often not possible; issues such as increased complaints from patients or delays in completion of medical records can sometimes signal the presence of a much more significant problem. Physician managers are responsible for identifying such situations, and for helping resolve them. Fortunately there are many resources for problem physicians in most states, oriented toward supporting the physician in dealing with his or her problems and returning to effective practice, often with a time of removal from practice.

While such responsibilities may seem difficult, it is critical that physician leaders carry them out carefully and compassionately. Similar to the successful management of a complex and difficult patient, all of one's knowledge, analytical capabilities, and communication abilities are required for achieving an optimal outcome. Successful conduct in this area can spare patients poor care and the physician in question a lost career.

The Question of Continuing to Practice

Physicians spend a significant portion of their young adult life preparing for their eventual career. Because of the many years invested in becoming a physician, and the years after starting practice required to further develop one's skills, relinquishing practice must be done only after careful consideration. The vast majority of physicians in clinical leadership positions continue to practice, though often on a very part-time basis. It is often said that continuing to practice elicits a positive perception in the eyes of those whom one manages. It seems just as likely that continuing to practice helps maintain one's own self-esteem. Practice provides an anchor which the physician manager can use as a guidepost when they face such unfamiliar tasks as representing clinicians to a board of trustees. Maintaining this piece of one's identity, earned at such great cost, is usually highly beneficial to the physician manager.

Conclusion

Roles in management and leadership offer a way for physicians to expand both their scope of responsibility and their impact beyond one on one care of patients. Good physician leaders with vision and a desire to lead are greatly needed if we are to deliver high quality healthcare at a reasonable cost to all our citizens. Healthcare particularly needs leaders from those traditionally underrepresented: women, people of color, and people from various sexual orientations and cultures, to help craft a healthcare system sensitive to everyone's needs. While these roles provide significant challenges, they also carry with them important opportunities that physicians cannot find in clinical practice alone. I encourage all readers to explore these opportunities, and to take on those which fit your personal desires and circumstances.

Additional Reading & Resources

Briscoe F. Temporal flexibility and careers: the role of large-scale organizations for physicians. Ind Labor Relat Rev. 2006;60:88–104.

Developing Physician Leadership. American College of Physician Executives. www.acpe.org/Education/index.aspx.

Leatt P. Physicians in health care management: 1 Physicians as managers: roles and future challenges. Can Med Assoc J. 1994;150:171–6.

Practice management 101 for physicians. Medical Group Management Association. Blog.mgma.com/blog/bid/23264/Practice-Management-101-for-Physicians.

Stoller J. Developing physician leaders, a call to action. J Gen Intern Med. 2009;24:876–8.

Chapter 12
Physicians and Entrepreneurship

Peter R. Russo

Key Points

- For a variety of reasons, an increasing number of physicians are pursuing entrepreneurial opportunities. There are unlimited opportunities for entrepreneurs who can bring innovative solutions to meet the growing demand for better outcomes and more affordable healthcare choices in the US and globally.
- A critical skill for a would-be physician/entrepreneur is the ability to identify and assess opportunities. In order to be worth pursuing an opportunity must have an identified customer, a compelling value proposition, and a viable business model.
- One large surprise for many physicians/entrepreneurs is the fact that the single biggest factor between success and failure in a new venture is the "people issues." First-time entrepreneurs are well served to work with a trusted mentor.

Introduction

One way in which many physicians immerse themselves into the world of business is by becoming entrepreneurs. In fact, every physician that manages his or her own practice might rightly call themselves entrepreneurs, but for the purpose of this chapter, I will refer to entrepreneurs who launch ventures that scale beyond

---

P.R. Russo, MBA (✉)
Boston University School of Management, Boston University, Bedford, MA 01730, USA
e-mail: prrusso@bu.edu

R.D. Urman and J.M. Ehrenfeld (eds.), *Physicians' Pathways to Non-Traditional Careers and Leadership Opportunities*, DOI 10.1007/978-1-4614-0551-1_12,
© Springer Science+Business Media, LLC 2012

Table 12.1 Most common reasons physicians pursue entrepreneurship

•   Seeking wealth or a better lifestyle
•   The challenge of creating and building a venture
•   Having a greater impact on the lives of others
•   Solving a problem that has become frustrating
•   Drawn to an opportunity

that of their own practice of medicine. In fact, the majority of the individuals whose biographical sketches are outlined later in this book are great examples of physicians/entrepreneurs.

What is *entrepreneurship*? While there are many definitions used to describe the word, my favorite is that first espoused by Howard Stevenson at the Harvard Business School. "Entrepreneurship is the pursuit of opportunity without regard to resources currently controlled." This is in contrast to the job of a manager, who is typically tasked with the efficient deployment of resources that he/she has been given control over.

Probably the first question that a physician might ponder is "*Why* become an entrepreneur?" There are a variety of reasons that we typically hear a physician/entrepreneur reference when we ask this question. I have described some of the most common ones below. Most entrepreneurs will say that they were motivated by a combination of these factors (see Table 12.1).

Seeking Wealth or a Better Lifestyle

This can also be described as the "grass is greener" phenomenon. Many physicians find frustration in the practice of medicine at some point, whether it is the desire for a better work/life balance, greater control over the decisions that they make every day, or a desire to earn greater rewards. Many of the MD/MBA candidates that we work with express such feelings. Among all of the opportunities in the business world, entrepreneurial pursuits seem particularly attractive, because of the perceived lack of bureaucracy. Yes, there are tremendous opportunities in the world of entrepreneurship and a trained physician may be well poised to capitalize on them. And also recognize that the world of entrepreneurship comes with many frustrations, long hours, and seemingly arbitrary decisions made by those necessary for our success. Do your homework and truly understand what you are likely to face.

The Challenge of Creating and Building a Venture

For an MD who has set high standards for his or her personal achievement, the task of creating and building a venture can be a truly exhilarating experience. Turning a vision into reality, improving outcomes for large numbers of patients, creating jobs and economic value are all exciting outcomes. This is clearly evidenced by the fact that so many successful entrepreneurs, who are able to "cash out," cannot wait to get involved in their next venture.

Having a Greater Impact on the Lives of Others

When discussing this topic with entrepreneurs who once practiced medicine, I often hear them speak about the number of lives that they are able to positively impact through their ventures, compared to what they were able to accomplish treating patients. Directing the activity of an assembled resource base certainly has the potential to bring a physician's skills "to scale" and impact large numbers of patients. Dr. Devi Shetty, founder of the Narayana Hrudayalaya hospitals in Bangalore, has gone from being a renowned heart surgeon to having impacted the lives of tens of thousands of patients by making healthcare affordable to them.

Solving a Problem That Has Become Frustrating

Those of us who are drawn to the world of Entrepreneurship are particularly attracted to the idea that large or chronic problems in society are solvable, with a new approach. That belief lies in the heart of most entrepreneurs, and this is no more evident than in the field of medicine. We hear many stories of physicians/entrepreneurs who saw something wrong with the way medicine was currently being practiced and had a better idea. Jonathan Gertler, whose biography appears later in this book, describes his first startup, a company that introduced an embolic entrapment device, in these terms.

Drawn to an Opportunity

This reason is really almost a "catch-all" category, in that it is often identified in conjunction with one of the others here. What I am referring to is a physician who had no conscious desire to enter the world of entrepreneurship, but who finds themselves involved in an opportunity too compelling to pass up. This may happen as the result of research that they are doing, or a consulting project that they are involved in or because the "spare time" endeavor that they are tinkering with requires too much of their time to pursue properly, but it is too exciting to walk away from.

This is not a "one time" decision for many physicians. Sometimes, a physician will become involved in an entrepreneurial venture and enjoy the interaction so much that they decide to give up the practice of medicine. Equally common is the physician who becomes increasingly confident of their skills as an entrepreneur and more aware of the value that they can bring, and for any one of the reasons above, begin to think of themselves as more of an entrepreneur than a physician.

Where Does an Entrepreneur Look for Opportunity?

Whether we are working with the life science sector or any other area in our economy, entrepreneurs look for opportunities where change is taking place. New "rules of the game" tend to even the playing field for a new player. This "change" might take place as the result of new laws or regulations, and will often take place as the result of new technology. When thinking about opportunities and technology, keep in mind that there are as many opportunities created by finding innovative ways to *use* new technology developed by others as there are by introducing new technology of your own.

To illustrate my point, just consider two fundamental areas of technology innovation that are having a huge impact on the life science sector right now, the mapping of the human genome and information technology. The fact that the intersection of these technologies is enabling rapid and affordable gene sequencing has created countless opportunities in the areas of drug development and personalized medicine.

The undeniable fact is that there is a limitless demand for better outcomes and more affordable healthcare choices in the US and globally. Entrepreneurs who are able to think of innovative ways to deploy technology to deliver these solutions will have an eager audience.

While the world of technology is changing quite rapidly, here are a few of my "favorite" areas where I expect to see a number of successful entrepreneurial startups:

- Digital (and portable) medical records.
- Expert medical systems that allow diagnosis to be performed largely through software.
- Increased availability and allocation of "telemedicine."
- Aggregated databases that link medical procedures and their cost to outcomes.
- Low cost rapid diagnostic devices.
- New drug delivery systems that are both affordable and customized to the treatment.
- The use of bioinformatics to reduce the time, risk and expense of developing new biopharma products.
- New developments in material science that will allow the development of medical devices that are more compatible with the human body.

What Makes an Opportunity Worth Pursuing?

Let us assume that you are interested in becoming an entrepreneur. What qualifies as an idea worth pursuing? I would have to honestly say that we see more would-be entrepreneurs than viable ideas. Generally, I like to challenge the entrepreneur to describe a problem that needs solving, name a customer who has the problem, describe a solution that solves the problem, and identify a way that they can charge enough for their solution to more than cover the cost of delivering it. We call the collective set of answers to these questions a *business model*. Every viable business has constructed a viable business model. The steps to constructing a business model are briefly outlined below.

Constructing a Business Model

- *Identify a problem and solution and a customer.* This combination allows us to describe a *value proposition*, how a venture creates value for its customers in terms of measurable outcomes. A value proposition must involve the creation of real value in the eyes of a customer whom we can identify. This customer may be the patient, or the payer, or another key decision maker.
- *Define how we will charge for our solution, and how much we will charge.* Obviously, what we can charge for our product or service will be limited to the value we create, but we may also be limited by factors such as competitive solutions, affordability, and willingness to pay. How we will charge should consider whether our customers will pay by use, pay by subscription or membership fee, or whether we will need to subsidize our equipment to acquire the customer and sell them a disposable.
- *Identify the key capabilities that we will need to deliver this solution to our customer.* This list will include manufacturing, product development and our sales channels. We need to consider which of these represent potential strategic advantage to us and which might be outsourced. As a new venture, we must acquire all of these resources, either through building them internally or through outsourcing them. Our plan might consider outsourcing initially and bringing processes into the company once we have sufficient volumes.
- *Perform an economic analysis of the model.* This is normally done by constructing a spreadsheet model of the business. Identify the costs associated with all of the capabilities outlined above, in terms of both unit cost and required investment. Compare that to the revenues we are likely to generate. Perform sensitivity analysis. Certain key variables will emerge that have the greatest impact on the financial success of the venture. These are "key success factors" and they are an outcome of the business model decisions we make.
- *Evaluate the business opportunity from the perspective of the investor.* Given the business model that we have constructed, can we make a compelling case to potential investors that this is a good use of their capital? Can we describe a scenario in which this business will achieve sufficient success that they can see a return of their capital investment plus a fair return? Only when we can answer this question in the affirmative do we have a viable business opportunity worth pursuing. For social ventures, a surprising amount of the above is still relevant. Even to the extent that we are seeking grants from foundations, we should think in terms of the return that we are offering them, compared to the many other places they can deploy their money.

How Do You Keep a Good Idea to Yourself (Protecting Your IP and Other Barriers to Entry)

For any venture that has identified a compelling value proposition and a viable business model, the one thing that is certain is that it is going to have competition. Not only is it unlikely that no one has thought of your idea, but once you demonstrate it in the marketplace, others are sure to want to follow. One key issue, therefore, in the strategic evaluation of a new concept is what barriers exist for "me too" competitors. The more formidable the barriers to entry that you can erect, the more likely that you will enjoy a sustainable competitive advantage and the profit and growth advantages that come along with that. Barriers to entry can take multiple forms. If I can control the distribution channels through which a product is distributed, or be the first one through a long regulatory approval process, I may enjoy a near monopoly for some time. But often, for technology-based products, these barriers come in the form of intellectual property protection. A primer on intellectual property is beyond both the scope of this chapter and my expertise. I will, however, touch on a few key issues that entrepreneurs should understand.

Much of the technology used in life sciences comes from university-based research and the majority of university-based research is government funded. Since the Bayh-Dole Act was passed, universities can own and control the IP developed with this research and they also must share the proceeds with the inventor (see Chap. 1).

Intellectual property is generally protected one of four ways, depending on the nature of the property and the rights to be protected:

- *Patents* are granted giving the right to exclude others from utilizing your invention for a period of 20 years (which can be extended under certain circumstances). In order to receive a patent, your invention must be both novel and nonobvious. They are generally expensive to obtain, maintain and defend. (Even a fairly basic patent will cost in the tens of thousands of dollars). In order to protect their right to file a patent, an entrepreneur will often file a "provisional patent," a far less expensive alternative, which will essentially "hold their place in line" for 1 year, while they can determine whether their invention is really worth anything. The patent for Lipitor is a good example of a very valuable one, about to expire.
- *Copyrights* protect original works, whether they are musical, literary, pictorial or software. They are often used in the software industry to protect code, documentation, and databases. They are inexpensive to file for, the grant is automatic, and the term of a copyright is at least the life of the author plus 70 years. Copyrights can be registered at any time, but must be registered before you can file a suit. Many of the most valuable copyrights are in the film and entertainment business. You will see a copyright designated as © or "Copyright © 2011 by Peter Russo. All rights reserved."
- *Trade Secrets* are a very effective way of protecting your intellectual property. Essentially, you only share with someone what they "need to know," and when you do, you bind them to confidentiality with some form of nondisclosure agreement.

There are many best practices for trade secret protection, and perhaps the most famous (and valuable?) trade secret is the Coca-Cola formula.

- Trademarks are the way that you protect the words, images, sounds, etc. that customers will use to identify your company and its products. While filing is not mandatory, they tend to be inexpensive to file, and their term is indefinite. The Coca Cola logo and the Nike "swoosh" are two examples of valuable trademarks, which are usually designated with a ®, ™ or "Reg. US Pat. & Tm."

It is imperative that any entrepreneur who is pursuing a venture for which intellectual property is an essential element get good legal counsel early. Mistakes made here may be impossible to reverse. Also, it is important not only that you are able to keep other from copying your intellectual property, but that you are able to defend yourself from others who claim that you are infringing upon theirs. A sound IP strategy will address both.

How Does an Entrepreneur Finance a Venture?

One of the most important tasks of the leader of a venture is to not run out of money. No matter how compelling your opportunity is, without the necessary capital to bring it to fruition, you have no chance of success. With that in mind, I have three rules that every entrepreneur should keep in mind when they consider strategies to finance their venture (see Table 12.2).

Think of investors like customers. I am always amazed at how many entrepreneurs do a thorough analysis of their customer and market, in terms of market segmentation, prioritizing target markets, understanding the decision-making process, etc. and then take an entirely different approach to raising money. The fact that someone has money, or even invests in startups, does not make them a fit for your venture. Before any entrepreneur approaches a capital source, he should do his homework, learning their typical stage of investment, industry sector, investment size, and preferred time horizon and match that to the venture. It is also important to learn where your investors' money is coming from and what expectations they need to meet for their investors. Not only will this save you substantial wasted time, but calling on inappropriate sources of capital can erode your credibility. Any investor will do due diligence on a company before investing. You should do your due diligence on them before inviting them to invest. Speak with some companies that they have funded before. Remember: not all money is the same shade of green!

Table 12.2 Rules for financing a venture

- Think of investors like customers: do your homework
- Put yourself in the shoes of your investor
- Develop a "milestone strategy" for your venture

Put yourself in the shoes of your investor. In order to develop a compelling argument for an investor, you need to put yourself in their shoes. Try to understand your investor's expectations and motivations. How would they define a "good outcome"? What types of investments do they try to avoid? What are their greatest concerns? Once you understand these things, developing a compelling argument for them to invest in your venture will be far easier.

Thinking like an investor, would you prefer to invest your money with a stranger or with someone who was introduced to you by a trusted source? The answer to this question should be obvious. Try to avoid asking anyone for money without a "warm introduction," someone who will vouch for you and your venture. You can obtain such an introduction through networking, with advisors, law firms, people who have raised money from them in the past, etc.

Develop a "milestone strategy" for your venture. As a venture progresses through the various phases of commercialization, it will achieve a series of milestones, which are essentially inflection points, at which the probability of success is higher, and the riskiness of the venture is lower (which generally means that the valuation will be higher). These milestones might be such things as a proof of concept, early test results, positive clinical trials, regulatory approval, etc. In fact, the earliest milestones for a life science company might be so risky as not to be fundable except through grants or others not investing for financial profit. A common strategy for an entrepreneur is to identify the critical milestones for the venture and raise sufficient money to achieve that milestone (with some room for error, of course), and then raise money at a higher valuation when that milestone is reached, in order to achieve the next one, and so on. It is probable that the venture will be attractive to different investors each time.

The beauty of this strategy is that, by managing the risk for the investors, the entrepreneur can raise the money required to commercialize the venture at a higher average valuation. The problem with the strategy is that the entrepreneurs "manage" this risk by taking it upon themselves. If a company does not achieve a milestone, or if market conditions change, an entrepreneur might be left without money and with few options. To mitigate this risk, entrepreneurs can do several things, including raising more money than they think they need (always a good idea!) and by identifying, prequalifying and beginning to communicate with the investors we expect to approach at the next milestone.

Advice for Would-Be Physicians/Entrepreneurs

The physicians whose biographies appear later in this book offer some great advice for physicians who are thinking of entering the business world, whether they plan to be entrepreneurs or not. While I am not a physician myself, I have had the privilege of working with and mentoring a number of physicians over the years, and it from that experience that I offer the following advice (see Table 12.3).

Table 12.3 Advice for would-be physician/entrepreneurs

- Understand why you are doing this
- Be honest with yourself
- It is all about the people
- Network, network and network
- Expect that this will not be your only venture

Understand why you are doing this. This may seem obvious, but when asked, a surprising number of entrepreneurs have a difficult time answering this question. There are many possible answers, from wanting to make a difference in the world, to desiring a better lifestyle or attaining a certain level of wealth. There are three reasons why the answer can be critical. First, when you think about an entrepreneurial opportunity, your assessment needs to consider not just whether this is a real or viable opportunity, but also whether it is a good opportunity *for you at this time.*

Second, the role that you may choose to play in your venture will be a direct result of the answer to this question. There was a very interesting article in the Harvard Business Review in 2008 in which Noam Wasserman discussed the question that every entrepreneur must answer: "Would you rather be rich or king?" [1]. Which is more important to you – the ultimate success of the venture or your role in it? To honestly answer this question, an entrepreneur needs to truly understand what his goals are.

Finally, your own measure of success and your own satisfaction with your venture should be based upon a clear understanding of what your goals are. Launching a new venture requires bringing together a diverse set of constituents, from customers, to investors, employees and partners. Each will bring their own set of goals, it is important that you do not lose sight of yours.

Be honest with yourself. No entrepreneur is a perfect fit for all of the skills required to make their venture a success. Therefore, it is imperative that an entrepreneur understand what he/she can bring to the venture and what he/she needs to attract from the outside. This does not mean to imply that you will not be able to grow, but you need to be realistic about how quickly you can grow and how quickly the venture *needs* you to grow. You may decide that certain required skills are just not ones that you are likely to bring and the sooner you recognize that, the sooner you can bring those resources to the venture. As I will soon discuss, finding a good mentor is an important step for any would-be entrepreneur. Understanding yourself, and your own strengths and weaknesses will help immeasurably in choosing and benefitting from this relationship.

It is all about the people. Perhaps the biggest surprise that physicians/entrepreneurs I have worked with identify when describing the transition from medicine to Entrepreneurship is how much time and effort they need to spend on "people issues." Whether it is identifying the right people, attracting them to your venture or persuading them to do what you need them to do, this is a very challenging task. It is also not one that physicians have been well trained for. Nonetheless, the quality of the people whom you can attract to your venture and the leadership that you provide to them is probably the single biggest differentiator between success and failure. Understand how you will develop these skills and how you will constantly improve them, whether it is through education, mentoring or experience.

Network, network, and network. Whether you plan to launch a venture tomorrow or several years from now, begin to meet people who are in the space that is interesting to you. Attend events, do informational interviews, ask for career advice, bounce ideas off of people, and especially, ask them to refer you to people in their own network. Whether you seek input from potential customers, strategic alliance partners, investors, advisors or employees, your best source will be the personal network that you build. I should also say that, as a group, entrepreneurs are extremely generous when it comes to helping future entrepreneurs and you will be amazed at their willingness to share valuable insight and advice for little or no compensation. One important caveat, however, is that you should treat the time that people share with you as a valuable commodity. Understand why you are asking for their time, what you expect to learn and show your appreciation for their willingness to share it with you.

Expect that this will not be your only venture. It is possible that the first venture that you launch will be so successful that you will "live happily ever after" and never do this again. The empirical evidence suggests that this is unlikely to be the case. If your venture does not succeed, you are likely to try again, wiser for the experience. Especially if you venture is successful, you are likely to want to relive that success. Think of your venture as the start of a journey, not a single destination. This perspective can change your own set of goals end expectations significantly. Perhaps you aspire to be the CEO of a large venture backed medical device startup. If you have no prior business experience, it is not going to be easy to convince your investors that you are the right person for the job. However, if you are willing to bring in an experienced CEO once you have achieved a certain milestone, and play a lesser role this time, while you learn from your experience, there is no reason why you cannot achieve that goal next time.

Reference

1. Wasserman N. The Founder's dilemma. Harvard Business School Publishing. Harvard Business Review; Boston, MA. 2008.

Additional Resources

Bussgang J. Mastering the VC game: a venture capital insider reveals how to get from start-up to IPO on your terms. Penguin Group; Boston, MA. 2010.
Wasserman N. The Founder's dilemma. Harvard Business School Publishing. Harvard Business Review; Boston, MA. 2008.

Useful Websites

http://ecorner.stanford.edu/
http://www.entrepreneurship.org/en/resource-center/legal-and-strategic-challenges-for-life-science-and-biotech-companies.aspx
http://www.kauffman.org/advancing_innovation/life_science_entrepreneurship.aspx

Part III
Medicine at the Macro Level: Public Health, Global Health, and Public Policy

Chapter 13
Public Health

Paul Biddinger

Key Points

- The mission of public health is to provide for the best possible health of the community through assessment of community health needs, development of health policy, and assurance of the availability of preventive and health services for all.
- Many physicians find that the community focus of public health training and career opportunities is an outstanding complement to the individual patient focus of medical practice.
- Formal training in public health can allow physicians to better interpret the ever-growing body of medical literature and help translate it to their patients and colleagues.

Introduction

When asked, many physicians seem to have surprising difficulty defining the field of public health. To some, public health is a watchdog, monitoring health and intervening when disease outbreaks, environmental threats, or unhealthy behaviors threaten the well-being of the community. To others, public health is an authority figure, regulating the delivery and quality of healthcare. To still others, public health is a safety net, ensuring the provision of health services to some of the most vulnerable members of society, including children, the poor, and those with HIV/AIDS, among others.

P. Biddinger, MD, FACEP (✉)
Department of Emergency Medicine, Massachusetts General Hospital,
Boston, MA 02114, USA
e-mail: pbiddinger@partners.org

R.D. Urman and J.M. Ehrenfeld (eds.), *Physicians' Pathways to Non-Traditional Careers and Leadership Opportunities*, DOI 10.1007/978-1-4614-0551-1_13, © Springer Science+Business Media, LLC 2012

Table 13.1 Core functions of public health

"*Assessment*" means that public health needs to define and collect accurate and comprehensive data on the health of the community in order to identify and target health problems
"*Policy development*" means that public health must design, implement, and test effective strategies to protect and advance the health of their community
"*Assurance*" means that public health has a duty to ensure that all members of the community, particularly including marginalized and vulnerable populations, have access to health services and medical care

Similarly, when asked to define the value of a graduate degree in public health, physicians with and without degrees in public health will also give a variety of answers. Some may cite the significance of biostatistics training for future researchers; some may cite the importance of physicians' understanding of epidemiology. Others may note the value of the degree in rising to leadership positions in healthcare and government.

In fact, public health encompasses all of the actions and responsibilities above, and training in public health certainly can provide important technical and analytical skills that complement physicians' medical training. But what ultimately best defines careers and graduate study in public health is what makes the field of public health different from the field of medicine. In contrast to the mission of medical practice to provide the best possible care for the individual patient, the simplest definition of the mission of public health is to provide for the best possible health of the community.

At the most basic level, the three basic duties that public health must attend to are: *Assessment*, *Policy development*, and *Assurance*. These have been named the "Core Functions of Public Health" by the Institute of Medicine [1] and are outlined in Table 13.1.

In order to perform the Core Functions, the US Centers for Disease Control and Prevention (CDC) has also named the "Ten Essential Public Health Services" [2], which are listed in Table 13.2. Looking at this list of the essential services of public health, it is easy to see that a substantial diversity of medical, scientific, political, economic, and legal skills are required to provide these services to the community.

Because graduate programs in public health offer training in the diverse quantitative, analytical, and other skills required in public health, and because of the breadth of challenges and opportunities that can be found in the practice of public health itself, graduate public health education and careers in public health are a popular choice for many physicians and other medical professionals.

Why Pursue a Degree or a Career in Public Health?

While many physicians choose to pursue a career in public health or pursue a public health degree with a specific goal in mind, an infectious disease specialist may want to learn how to intervene to decrease the incidence of tuberculosis for example,

Table 13.2 The 10 essential public health services

1.	*Monitor* health status to identify community health problems
2.	*Diagnose and investigate* health problems and health hazards in the community
3.	*Inform, educate, and empower* people about health issues
4.	*Mobilize* community partnerships to identify and solve health problems
5.	*Develop policies and plans* that support individual and community health efforts
6.	*Enforce* laws and regulations that protect health and ensure safety
7.	*Link* people to needed personal health services and assure the provision of healthcare when otherwise unavailable
8.	*Assure* a competent public health and personal healthcare workforce
9.	*Evaluate* effectiveness, accessibility, and quality of personal and population-based health services
10.	*Research* for new insights and innovative solutions to health problems

Adapted from Centers for Disease Control & Prevention. 10 Essential Public Health Services. http://www.cdc.gov/nphpsp/essentialServices.html

there is a great variety of reasons why physicians may choose to pursue education or a career in public health. Interestingly, until the early 20th century the fields of medicine and public health were integrated, and there was no separate training for each. However, after publication of the Welch-Rose Report of 1916 [3], which argued for the need for a unique cadre of professionally trained health workers focused on the protection and preservation of the health of the population as a whole and on the prevention of disease, public health began to evolve as a discipline distinct from medicine. Where medicine has developed increasingly sophisticated methods to diagnose and treat disease, public health has evolved to design and test techniques of measuring the health of the community and of intervening to stop disease before it starts. Perhaps because of these differences in emphasis between the two fields, the chief reasons why physicians pursue public healthcareers commonly relate to the two greatest themes that currently distinguish the field of public health from the field of medicine: a focus on prevention and a quantitative focus on populations.

It is intuitive to physicians that preventing disease is preferable to treating it after it emerges. In fact, all of the 10 great public health achievements of the 20th century, as chosen by the CDC (Table 13.3) [4], relate strongly to the prevention of illness or injury. In the recent past, physicians who have despaired of seeing severely injured victims of all-terrain vehicle (ATV) crashes who are too young to control their vehicles have campaigned as public health advocates for age-limits for ATV riders. Physicians who have wished to decrease the incidence of HIV infections have campaigned for condom distribution and needle exchange programs. Physicians who have noted the alarming rise in obesity in the US have campaigned for healthier school lunches. Through these experiences translating clinical lessons into broader population-based interventions, many physicians have been drawn to career opportunities in public health. Some have joined their local or county board of health, or even served as health directors and health commissioners. Others have joined relevant state or federal public health committees. In many ways, physicians are often

Table 13.3 Ten great public health achievements 1900–1999

- Vaccination
- Motor-vehicle safety
- Safer workplaces
- Control of infectious diseases
- Decline in deaths from coronary heart disease and stroke
- Safer and healthier foods
- Healthier mothers and babies
- Family planning
- Fluoridation of drinking water
- Recognition of tobacco use as a health hazard

Adapted from Centers for Disease Control & Prevention. Ten Great Public Health Achievements in the 20th Century. http://www.cdc.gov/about/history/tengpha.htm

drawn to public health by a desire to protect the health of their patients and to try to prevent illness and injury before it happens.

In addition to being motivated by the prevention of disease, physicians also may become involved in public health as they strive to learn more rigorous methods to study and improve health across populations. Although there are different graduate programs available in public health (see Education below), all public health programs include focused training in biostatistics and epidemiology. Such training is useful whether or not they ultimately practice public health, and allows physicians to better function as physician-scientists and both appreciate and attempt to influence the factors that affect their patients' health that are outside the control of the individual clinical encounter.

As a Physician, How Can I Benefit Personally?

As mentioned above, some of the chief benefits of formal training in public health relate to the biostatistical and epidemiologic training that is part of the public health degree program. With formal training in biostatistics, physicians are better able to describe basic statistical concepts such as probability, random variation and probability distributions, apply common statistical methods, and communicate findings based on statistical analyses. With formal training in epidemiology, physicians are better able to identify appropriate sources of population data, understand basic epidemiology terminology and calculate basic measures, and evaluate the results of epidemiologic studies that they may encounter. No matter what the physician's ultimate practice setting, this training allows them to better interpret the medical literature and better translate it to their patients and colleagues. Further, public health training helps physicians become more sophisticated in their understanding of the value and limitations of medical tests and screening interventions such as PSA testing, mammography, and others.

For those physicians who aspire to begin, or are beginning a career in academics, the study of public health at the graduate level also allows them to better design and execute their own research studies, perform appropriate statistical analysis, and draw proper conclusions in the literature. Such physicians may be more likely to design successful studies overall and be less reliant on other colleagues for statistical analysis or study design.

In addition to the educational and academic benefits of pursuing formal training in public health, many physicians find special fulfillment in the pursuit of public health research and/or public health practice. A cardiologist may find equal pleasure in discovering new dietary interventions to prevent heart disease and in practicing clinical cardiology. Emergency physicians may enjoy serving their community through assisting with the development of plans to improve the region's health emergency preparedness. Pediatricians may feel that they are more connected with their community by serving on the local board of health and ensuring that breakfast is served to the poorest students each morning. Such activities outside of the hospital and medical office can serve to enrich a medical career.

Some physicians choose to make public health their primary career after their medical and graduate public health training. Options for these individuals can include, among many other options, serving as an Epidemic Intelligence Service (EIS) officer for the CDC for two years, serving as the health director or commissioner for a city, county, or state, or serving with the United States Public Health Service. In addition, many physicians have used the skills and experiences they have gained through public health education and practice to pursue careers in healthcare administration and leadership, policy design and development, and even politics.

How Can I Benefit My Patients?

A physician may find many different ways in which a graduate degree in public health benefits his or her patients. By becoming a more sophisticated reader of the medical literature, the physician will be more likely to appropriately interpret new data and apply this knowledge to patient care. By better understanding biostatistics, the physician also may be more likely to appropriately order and accurately interpret medical tests when evaluating a patient for a given rare condition. For example, a proper understanding of Bayes' theorem helps a physician use pre-test and post-test probabilities to determine when to order a given test for an unlikely disease, and how to act on the results of positive and negative tests when the test is ordered.

In addition, with a better understanding of public health, physicians can act as advocates for the community, and improve health for all of their patients. With persuasive data, skilled economic analysis and education in health risk communication, it may be possible for a trained physician to locally improve vaccination rates, to improve seat belt use, or to decrease health disparities and affect the lives of not only his or her patients, but their relatives, their friends, and their community.

Education, Other Background Needed

While it is sometimes possible to pursue a career in public health with a medical degree alone, many physicians choose to pursue specific graduate training in public health to augment their medical career and/or improve their practice of public health in the community.

The most common public health graduate degree program chosen by physicians is the Masters in Public Health (MPH). The MPH degree is traditionally a 2-year degree, though many universities have programs that can allow physicians to obtain their MPH in about 1 year. The MPH program encompasses the five core areas of public health: biostatistics, epidemiology, health services administration, social and behavioral science and environmental science. All MPH students must demonstrate competence in 12 core public health domains upon completion of their degree [5]; however, the MPH curriculum typically also allows students to pursue a specific concentration in either one of the core areas or in another specialty area of public health such as maternal and child health, nutrition, global health, public policy or others, depending on the institution. The MPH degree can be earned either in a Program in Public Health taught within a graduate school of a university (such as a School of Medicine) or at an accredited School of Public Health. Schools of Public Health commonly offer more concentrations, specializations, and/or degree programs than Programs in Public Health; however, both Programs in Public Health and Schools of Public Health are accredited by the Council on Education for Public Health (CEPH), which is an independent agency recognized by the US Department of Education. A list of accredited programs can be found on the CEPH website: www.ceph.org.

Some MPH degrees may be obtained in less than 2 years through intensive summer programs, night programs, or other flexible initiatives. In addition, some universities offer combined MPH degree programs with other degrees such as the MD, JD, MBA, and others. Several CEPH-accredited programs are offered on-line, but no matter what the format, all MPH programs must be at least 42 semester credit units in length. In addition, all MPH programs must have a culminating experience, sometimes known as a thesis or capstone experience. The specific requirements of the capstone experience can vary from program to program.

Sometimes, physicians choose to pursue Masters-level degrees related to public health other than the MPH degree. Examples of such degrees include the Master of Science in Public Health (MSPH), which is typically obtained by students whose coursework focuses more heavily on research, the Master of Healthcare Administration (MHA), and the Master of Science (MS) degree, which may reflect public health-related coursework from a nonaccredited School, among several others. While many students receive great benefit from coursework in non-MPH degree programs and/or nonaccredited programs, the US Public Health Service, branches of the US Military and some state and local governmental agencies require graduation from an accredited school or program for MPH-level jobs.

Beyond the Masters level, some physicians pursue a doctoral degree in public health. Most commonly, students who pursue a Doctorate in Public Health (DrPH) are anticipating a career in academics, research, and/or leadership in public health.

The DrPH is the highest degree in public health and requires a very substantial commitment of time and effort. The requirements for a DrPH typically consist of four semesters of coursework beyond the Masters level, and an additional research project culminating in a dissertation. It is also possible to obtain a Doctor of Philosophy (PhD) or Doctor of Science (ScD) in public health, though the degree opportunities and requirements vary by institution.

Vignette

An internist had been practicing for almost 10 years when he began to feel a need to seek out additional opportunities outside of his clinical practice. He began to volunteer to serve on committees at the state medical society (violence prevention and student health) that met three or four times per year. After 2 years of meetings, he came to realize that the biggest problems his committees usually faced were not problems that could be solved by individual physicians, but rather were problems that needed public health interventions to significantly improve. He therefore decided to run for election to his local board of health, and won a seat. From his position on the local board of health, he helped to secure a part-time violence counselor and a ban on sugary sodas in the local schools. He continues to serve on the local board of health, and is considering going back to obtain his MPH in order to enhance his skills and his ability to improve his community's health.

References

1. Remington RD et al. The future of public health. Washington: Institute of Medicine, National Academy of Sciences; 1988.
2. Core Public Health Functions Steering Committee (1994). Public Health in America. Washington, DC: Office of Disease Prevention and Health Promotion, USDHHS.
3. Welch WH, Rose W. Annual report of the Rockefeller Foundation Appendix V. Warsaw: Institute of Hygiene; 1916. p. 415–27.
4. United States Centers for Disease Control and Prevention. Ten great public health achievements – United States, 1900–1999. Morbid Mortal Weekly Rep. 1999;48(12):241–3.
5. Calhoun JG, Ramiah K, Weist EM, Shortell SM. Development of a core competency model for the Master of Public Health Degree. Am J Public Health. 2008;98(9):1598–607.

Additional Resources

American Public Health Association (APHA). www.apha.org.
Association of State and Territorial Health Officials (ASTHO). www.astho.org.
Association of Schools of Public Health (ASPH). www.asph.org, www.whatispublichealth.org.
Centers for Disease Control and Prevention (CDC). www.cdc.gov.
Council on Education for Public Health (CEPH). www.ceph.org.
National Association of City and County Health Officials (NACCHO). www.naccho.org.
United States Public Health Service. www.usphs.gov.

Chapter 14
Public Policy and Public Administration

Rahul Sakhuja and Palak Shah

Key Points

- Health practitioners can play an *essential role in shaping public policy* with their knowledge of how healthcare is delivered.
- Engaging in public policy allows physicians to *address systemic barriers to health improvement* and to impact populations of patients rather than one patient at a time.
- *Further training* in public policy *may prove useful* in pursuing this field. For a career in policy-related research, a PhD might be helpful, but for people interested in being practitioners, a Masters degree should suffice.

Introduction

Almost every decision that we make in healthcare is shaped by public policy. In our practices, there are patients in whom systemic factors preclude them from achieving an optimal health status, despite optimal medical therapy. Many physicians feel that independent of the number of patients treated, little impact is made on the prevalence of a particular disease. These experiences reflect the complex set of systemic factors that affect health. Engaging in public policy is one way in which to address the issues underlying these scenarios.

R. Sakhuja, MD, MPP, MSc (✉)
Department of Cardiology, Massachusetts General Hospital, 101 Trowbridge Street,
Boston, MA, USA
e-mail: rsakhuja@partners.org

P. Shah, MPP
Harvard Kennedy School of Government, Cambridge, MA, USA

R.D. Urman and J.M. Ehrenfeld (eds.), *Physicians' Pathways to Non-Traditional Careers and Leadership Opportunities*, DOI 10.1007/978-1-4614-0551-1_14, © Springer Science+Business Media, LLC 2012

To impact the health of patients, of course physicians must work with patients directly; however, physicians must also involve themselves in policy decisions at all levels. At a national level, public policies, such as Medicare, determine health insurance coverage and the means for patients to follow-up with physicians and prescribed testing. At a hospital level, policy-minded physicians conceive of quality and safety projects to continually improve patient care and outcomes. At a provider level, practice guidelines driving clinical decisions are only one of many examples of policy initiatives influencing care.

This chapter will focus on the path of pursuing public policy/public administration, what it means, what it might entail, and what one might do with such interests and/or training.

What Is Public Policy?

In trying to define public policy, most texts will quote multiple different definitions [1]. For example, one widely quoted definition derives from Thomas Dye's *Understanding Public Policy*. Dye defines public policy as "what governments do, why they do it, and what difference it makes" [2]. However, even his definition has evolved over time, from his first edition: "Anything government chooses to do or not to do" [3]. *The Encyclopedia of Public Administration and Public Policy* defines its component parts. "Public" reflects the voice of a group of people and "policy" consists of the rules and processes the public chooses to address their concerns. Therefore, "public policy refers to the process whereby the members of a geographic area or political unit make choices that address their areas and issues of concern." Consequently, the study of public policy consists of research and training around "the tools and processes associated with public decision making and priority setting" [4].

Ultimately, public policy has to do with setting public priorities and defining interventions and solutions, often governmental, to address these priorities. As mentioned above, the definitions are broad, reflecting the many career choices available to the people interested in public policy. In particular, public policy training can equip physicians to choose from a wider range of careers in the private, non-profit, or governmental sectors (Table 14.1).

Why Pursue Public Policy?

As a physician, if you perceive systemic barriers to improving the health status of your patients and seek the ability – beyond direct patient care – to solve health problems, you should consider public policy. Healthcare is always a crucial public policy issue. Clearly, with the recent passage of the Patient Protection and Affordable Care Act, healthcare policy will continue to be a focal point for many years to come.

Table 14.1 Examples of public policy endeavors for physicians by sector

	Domestic	International
Government		
Executive	Elected/appointed to run healthcare agents (Center for Medicare-Medicaid Services)	Advise/draft healthcare policies with the Ministry of Health
Legislative/ Parliamentary	Serve as top legislative advisor for congressional committees on health to draft healthcare policy	Represent World Health Organization to structure and enforce laws to promote health (e.g., immunizations)
Non-profit		
Think Tank	Research and/or design systems to curb drivers of increasing cost of healthcare and reform system of health insurance.	Research and/or design systems to reduce barriers to dissemination of generic pharmaceuticals in developing nations
Service provider	Create initiatives to assess and improve quality of care delivered in healthcare organization	Develop systems of care to curb disease at population level (e.g., HIV/AIDS, reduce maternal/ fetal death)
Advocacy agency	Assume leadership positions and set agenda for national specialty organizations (e.g., American College of Cardiology)	Create or manage an advocacy organization around specific health issues (e.g., UNICEF)
Private	Work within consulting agency on public sector issues (e.g., health reform implementation)	Work with pharmaceutical companies to garner political support, dissemination of information

It will be even more essential to have physicians, intimately familiar with patient needs and healthcare delivery, informing – if not leading – the process.

To address these growing needs and the growing impact of public policies on physician practice, public policy training is now being incorporated into medical school and residency curricula. There are a growing number of physicians in policy-setting positions at hospital, state, and national levels. While there were only two graduates per year from the joint program in medicine and public policy at Harvard prior to 2003, between 2003 and 2010, 33 medical students graduated from the program. Public policy training can distinguish you among your peers, since it remains a rare physician who pursues training or a career in public policy. That said, if you thrive most on individual patient interactions, then pursuing public policy might not be the appropriate course.

With respect to caring for patients, patient outcomes can be improved by physicians in public policy. For example, without public policies, certain vulnerable populations – the poor and the elderly – would not have Medicaid or Medicare, and therefore, would not have access to health insurance and a myriad of healthcare services. In fact, the new Administrator of the national Center for Medicare and

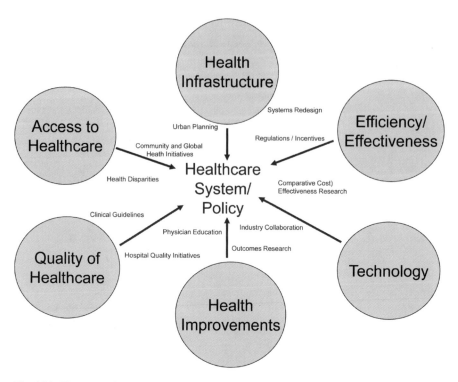

Fig. 14.1 Key areas of medicine impacted by public policy

Medicaid Services is a physician, setting health policy priorities for these large populations. Independent of the availability of novel technologies, without physicians advocating for certain diagnostic and treatment modalities or performing cost-effectiveness analyses, patients might not have access to these technologies.

Moreover, physician leadership in various capacities is also critical to the optimal care for patients. In particular, some physicians attend public policy schools to train in leadership or nonprofit management. Without physician leadership in nonprofit or governmental agencies, barriers to patient care may not be adequately identified and addressed. From patient care experience, a physician can likely suggest ways to structure systems or organizations to optimize patient care. That said, these skills are taught at both public policy and business schools. Depending on whether you are interested in managing a hospital, specialty organization (e.g., American College of Cardiology), advocacy agency, or international organization, one might look at both business and public policy programs in order to determine the best fit. Figure 14.1 demonstrates some of the areas in which physicians with public policy training can excel.

What Is a Master of Public Policy or Public Administration or a Master of Arts in Public Policy?

These are professional degrees for people interested in working on topics pertaining to public service. There are Master of Public Policy (MPP), Master of Public Administration (MPA) programs, as well as Masters of Arts in Public Policy (MA). For the most part, there is no clear difference between programs – an MPP at one institution is likely similar to an MPA or an MA at another institution. The entry requirements and flexibility with regard to required coursework may differ.

People who pursue these degrees seek skills to evaluate information to develop and assess alternative approaches to current and emerging issues. In addition, people hone skill to be leaders – to implement policies, projects, and programs that resolve important societal problems. Most commonly, medical students tend to return to complete their internship and residency, though not necessary depending on one's interests and goals. Often, after having become a board eligible physician, many people will seek policy positions in a variety of major domestic or international institutions thereafter. At some institutions, 1-year mid-career programs are available for physicians (and others) who have previously been in practice.

Applicants interested in doing research in or working on domestic healthcare policy issues often concentrate in healthcare policy. Others interested in starting organizations or joining advocacy or service provider organizations focused on health might also focus on nonprofit management. Still others who are interested in international health and the drivers of worse health outcomes might focus on political and economic development. Students commonly pursue coursework across these disciplines, in addition to "skill-specific" courses on negotiation, communication, leadership, and electoral politics.

Information on the particular coursework and opportunities at each school can be found on the websites of the specific institutions.

Do I Need a Masters Degree?

After 4 years of medical school and student loans, many students are understandably hesitant to sign up for additional schooling. However, while medical school teaches physicians how to think scientifically, public policy-based degree programs provide a systematic framework for approaches to large public dilemmas. Rather than focusing on science and physiology, public policy students think about economics, politics, resource constraints, as well as issues of fairness and equity. Very accomplished MD/MPP graduates, currently in senior leadership positions, have remarked that they continue to rely on the lessons they learned during their MPP.

One major reason to pursue a public policy degree is the breadth of coursework. Overall, these Masters degree programs crystallize the most essential skills for being an effective policy maker. Ultimately, there are some generalizable skills attainable from a public policy degree program – gathering and analyzing quantitative and qualitative information to solve new policy problems (policy analysis, regression analysis), using scarce resources to achieve policy objectives (management), and developing the ability to take responsibility for the top-level decisions about which issues should address (leadership). Medical students who majored in economics, and have a strong foundation in statistical analysis, often find that they still lack access to vital courses in management, communications, leadership, or economic development or health policy.

Another reason to pursue a degree is access to a network of classmates, who will likely hold significant policy positions in the future; that network is invaluable. Moreover, non-healthcare professionals often approach healthcare issues, both domestic and international, through a different lens than do healthcare professionals. Many MD/MPP graduates agree that exposure to non-healthcare professionals and their perspectives – on healthcare policy or political and economic development – have been an important aspect of their training.

Admittedly, you may be able to pursue similar career opportunities without a public policy degree. Many physicians transition into a policy job without school, and learn the necessary skills "on the job." However, both people with and without formal training have stated that a public policy degree offers systematic frameworks and skills to work in the political context, and agree that those with training find it easier to access and succeed in political, policy, and public-sector managerial positions. Moreover, it provides the time and connections to change one's career trajectory toward public policy and administration.

Ultimately, if one does decide to pursue an MPP/MPA, one of the major considerations is when to do so. Ideally, one would pursue the degree at the time that one is planning on working in public policy. First, the more specific one's goals are, the more apt one is to choose the appropriate institution and coursework to further one's career. Second, since the political landscape changes frequently in public policy, it is often helpful to pursue one's training at a time at which one will start using the knowledge. Finally, for most people, the skill set erodes rapidly with time without active use of the tools acquired.

Should I Get an MPP/MPA or an MPH?

Often, you can pursue public policy training at a school of public health or a school of public policy. Depending on the school, these degrees may be somewhat interchangeable in terms of the coursework offered. That is, one student could attend a school of public health, get an MPH, and obtain the similar skills as another student at a school of public policy. For example, both the Harvard Kennedy School of Government and the Harvard School of Public Health have coursework and areas of concentrations in healthcare policy. The differences are unique to the particular institution and the coursework offered therein. If you are interested in comparative effectiveness research in a given specialty, you may be more likely to find coursework at a school of public health, whereas if you are interested in a senior leadership position affecting how the healthcare reform is enacted, you may find more coursework at a school of public policy. This may not be the case at every institution.

However, there are some clear differences. In a school of public policy, most of your classmates come from non-healthcare backgrounds. Students are interested in many different fields of public policy (e.g., education, political and economic development). While some people find this distracting, others believe that solutions to problems in the healthcare sector might derive from processes that have worked in other arenas. Even in healthcare policy classes, most people are non-physicians. In speaking to many people who have pursued joint MD/MPP degrees, a consistent asset to public policy programs was the ability to see how non-physician colleagues thought about healthcare. This was particularly useful as it reflected the reality of most physicians working in public policy (i.e., most of their interactions were with non-physicians). In addition, the majority of students in schools of public policy are interested in developing and implementing programs to address an issue based on available analysis. On the other hand, most classmates in schools of public health are in the healthcare arena, many of whom are physicians. While some people find this insular, others find it helpful to discuss issues and network with like-minded people, many of whom they might continue to work with in the field. In addition, the majority of students in schools of public health are interested in creating strategies to generate and evaluate data and programs, which serves as the basis for implementation.

With regard to where to apply, there are many variables, many of which are particular to the individual applicant (e.g., where do you want to live?). Importantly, before applying, think about your goals – what are you going to use your training to do? Based on your goals, look through the offerings of particular institutions. In particular, based on one's background and learning style, one should evaluate how extensive the core curricular requirements are – particularly, what courses are required, what students think about the required courseload, and how many electives will be allowed. Then, talk to students who have pursued or graduated from joint degrees. You can find students at your medical school's alumni office or the alumni office of the public policy/public health schools. Last but definitely not least, look into the funding sources for each institution. For example, some institutions provide full scholarship upon admission, whereas others have multiple scholarships available for application.

Should I Get a PhD in Public Policy?

From speaking with physicians in prominent policy making roles, the consensus appears to be that for a career in research, a PhD can be very useful, though not an absolute requirement. If the primary focus of your career is going to be health economics research or medical anthropology for example, then considering a PhD in the social sciences in conjunction with an MD might be worthwhile to consider. On the other hand, for a career in public policy making, one doctorate – i.e., an MD – appears to be sufficient training, especially if pursue a Master of Public Policy/Administration.

References

1. Howlett M, Ramesh M. Studying public policy: policy cycles and policy subsystems. Toronto: Oxford University Press; 1995.
2. Dye T. Understanding public policy. 7th ed. New York: Prentice Hall; 1992.
3. Dye TR. Understanding public policy, vol. 1. Englewood Cliff: Prentice-Hall; 1972.
4. Schultz D. Encyclopedia of public administration and public policy. New York: Facts on File; 2004.

Useful Links

A list of public policy/administration schools by state is: http://en.wikipedia.org/wiki/List_of_public_administration_schools.

In 2008, US News and World Report ranked the Health Policy and Management concentrations at schools of public policy. http://grad-schools.usnews.rankingsandreviews.com/best-graduate-schools/top-public-affairs-schools/health-management.

Another rather generic website that also reviews what the different Masters degrees mean in general and a searchable database for schools is: www.gopublicservice.com.

The Association of Professional Schools of International Affairs also provides an overview of all of its accredited member schools. www.apsia.org.

The nonprofit foundation, the Kaiser Family Foundation, provides information, fact sheets, and tables and charts on major health policy issues facing the United States. www.kff.org.

Recommended Reading (in the Field of Medicine and Public Policy)

Blendon RJ, Benson JM. Understanding how Americans view health care reform. N Eng J Med. 2009;361:e13.

Blendon RJ, Benson JM. Health care in the 2010 congressional election. N Engl J Med. 2010;363:e30.

Bodenheimer T, Grumbach K. Understanding health policy: a clinical approach. 5th ed. New York: Lange Medical/McGraw Hill; 2008.

Claxton G. How private health care coverage works: a primer. A Henry J. Kaiser Family Foundation Report; April 2008. http://www.kff.org/insurance/upload/7766.pdf.

Cutler D. Your money or your life. New York: Oxford University Press; 2004.

Cutler DM. Equality, efficiency, and market fundamentals: the dynamics of international medical care reform. J Econ Lit. 2002;40(3):881–906.

Cutler DM, Rosen AB, Vijan S. The value of medical spending in the United States, 1960–2000. N Engl J Med. 2006;355(9):920–7.

Feldstein PJ. Health policy issues: an economic perspective. 4th ed. Chicago: Health Administration Press; 2007.

Oberlander J. Long time coming: why health reform finally passed. Health Aff. 2010;29(6):1112–6.

Staff of the Washington Post. Landmark: The inside story of America's New Health Care Law and what it means for all of us. Tennessee: PublicAffairs.

Starr P. The social transformation of American medicine. New York: Basic Books; 1982.

Williams SJ, Torrens PR. Introduction to health services. Part one: overview of the health services system. 7th ed. New York: Thomas Delmar Publishing; 2008.

Chapter 15
Global Health

Lena Ebba Dohlman

Key Points

- Choose a volunteer experience that is a good match for you; this includes selection of the volunteer organization, location, and an experience that will benefit your patients and be appropriate for your existing skills and knowledge.
- Benefits of a global health experience are many, including the satisfaction of helping people, an expanded world view, professional growth, and broadened medical knowledge.
- You can choose global health as a career at any stage of your professional life, and there are many organizations that can support your work.

Thinking About Working Overseas? (Fig. 15.1)

This was one of the most memorable experiences of my life. I have waited many years to go to Africa as a physician and to serve in some way. Health Volunteers Overseas has helped me to fulfill a dream and at the same time I know that the dream is not complete. I want to return and do more to experience the places, the people, the unforgettable moments that will always stay with me [1].

Have you thought about working in a medically underserved country in Africa, or wished you could have helped out during the recent medical crisis experienced by Haiti? Do you long to experience medicine with a focus on caring for patients, not

L.E. Dohlman, MD, MPH (✉)
Department of Anesthesiology, Critical Care & Pain Medicine,
Massachusetts General Hospital/Cambridge Health Alliance, Brookline, MA 02446, USA
e-mail: ldohlman@partners.org

R.D. Urman and J.M. Ehrenfeld (eds.), *Physicians' Pathways to Non-Traditional Careers and Leadership Opportunities*, DOI 10.1007/978-1-4614-0551-1_15,
© Springer Science+Business Media, LLC 2012

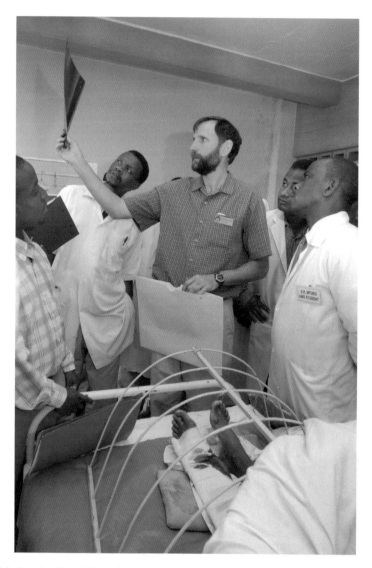

Fig. 15.1 Sustainable healthcare improvement through training, orthopedics overseas in Tanzania (photo by Karl Grobl. Courtesy of Health Volunteers Overseas)

the computer entries and insurance forms? Does international travel and meeting people from other cultures intrigue and energize you? If so, you should consider incorporating global healthcare into your career.

Perhaps, you have yet to take your first volunteer trip overseas and are not sure where to begin. Or you may already have enjoyed several international medical trips and want ideas about how to find other opportunities. This chapter was written to encourage and guide you in your search for a career that involves global humanitarian healthcare.

The chapter begins with an overview of interest in global health in the United States, and what medical needs of low resource countries might be addressed by this interest. The benefits and logistics of finding meaningful volunteer work will be discussed because physicians often begin work in developing countries with a volunteer stint. You will be encouraged to assess your personal motivations and needs as well as the needs of the country you will be working in. The importance of making realistic and well-thought out plans is emphasized. Some physicians may volunteer overseas once or twice before deciding to focus on other interests. Others will go on to make global health a major or even primary part of their career. The chapter will include a discussion on ways to make a full-time career in global medicine for those who know early that this is what they wish to do, or make the decision after several volunteer experiences. Whichever path is chosen, a successful experience working in a developing country should be enriching and mutually beneficial for the medical practitioner as well as the overseas site. The goal of this chapter is to help you be a successful humanitarian healthcare worker.

Global Health Today

"What's really hot now is global health." This comment, made in reference to job opportunities for MPH graduates, is a reflection of the rapidly growing interest in international health among US health professionals [2]. The opportunities to work or volunteer overseas and the resources for finding those opportunities, especially on the Internet, have grown dramatically in the past 2 decades [3]. This is wonderful for those medical students, residents, and practicing physicians who hope to become more involved in global health work.

The altruistic desire to go beyond our US borders to improve the lives of patients in resource-poor countries has existed for decades – but only among a select few. According to one survey, only 0.32% of physicians in the United States had been active in international health prior to 1984 [4]. In contrast, by 2008 half of U.S. medical schools had specific programs, offices or centers for global health, and nearly all have incorporated some form of global health teaching into their curricula. Many universities, schools of public health, and both private and academic hospitals have done the same. At least 30% of US medical student graduates have already had a global health experience by the time they enter their residency [5, 6]. The interest among residents is also very high, and for some the availability of global health opportunities is a significant factor in selecting their training programs [7].

What has led to this recent surge of interest in international health experiences? Recognition that our world is increasingly interdependent is certainly part of the reason. Millions of people are crossing international borders every day for tourism, work, or refuge.

The threat of emerging and drug-resistant infectious diseases, toxic materials, or contaminated food is perceived by many to be only a plane ride away. Noncommunicable diseases such as cardiovascular disease, high blood pressure, diabetes, and cancer are also becoming increasingly prevalent globally, even in low-income countries.

Many researchers and policy makers believe that solutions to health problems occurring in resource-poor countries will be useful to all countries [8]. It has also become clear that healthcare is deeply interlinked with global economic health and the political stability of all nations [9]. Improving the healthcare of all nations has the potential for minimizing international terrorism and political strife within and among nations [10]. Media focus on these far-reaching effects of global health problems has contributed to awareness of the world's health inequities.

The Millennial Generation of 18–29-year olds seems especially to have taken the global view to heart. Redubbed the "Global Generation" by some, they reportedly have a broader worldview and a greater interest in international events. As a group they have been said to be especially multicultural, accepting of differences and committed to being socially responsible [11]. For the members of the Millennial Generation, more than any previous generation, healthcare is global. Now in medical school and residency, their world view is likely one of the driving forces for the growing interest and support for involvement in global health.

Whatever the reasons behind the new passion for international health work are, all generations of physicians can benefit from the new wealth of information resources and opportunities to volunteer or work abroad.

Why Volunteer Overseas?

"The imbalance we are seeing in Africa today is that less and less manpower and equipment are available to treat more and more people. We are not talking Development here: we are talking Survival" [12]. This plea for help came from Dr Paul Fenton, a physician working in a teaching hospital in Malawi.

The most obvious reason to volunteer your time and expertise in a developing country is that there is an enormous need. The World Health Organization (WHO) in its 2006 annual report commented that "At the heart of each and every health system, the workforce is central to advancing health" and that the global workforce is currently in crisis. The workforce shortage was estimated at almost 4.3 million doctors, midwives, nurses and support workers. The poorest countries, especially in sub-Saharan Africa, are the hardest hit. The WHO called for international cooperation and stressed the importance of developing "capable, motivated and supported health workers" [13].

Anyone who has spent time working in a hospital or clinic in a developing country has witnessed firsthand how healthcare workers struggle to keep up with the impossibly long lines of patients waiting to be cared for. The author remembers being shocked as well as impressed that five or six physicians in an orthopedic clinic in Vietnam could routinely see one thousand patients a day. Healthcare providers in developing countries are mostly overworked and underpaid. Even physician salaries are often inadequate to support a family. Healthcare workers who are forced to work outside their regular jobs to make ends meet have less energy to devote to their patients and no time for continuing education. It is no surprise that doctors and nurses in the developing world are often tempted to leave demoralizing jobs if they are given the opportunity to immigrate to a better-paid position in a developed country. This increases the work burden even further for those who stay, and wastes training resources which are already woefully limited.

Add a health crisis such as an epidemic, a natural disaster, or a conflict to an already chronically stressed healthcare system and the system becomes totally overwhelmed. Patients who need urgent care for injuries, childbirth and surgical emergencies, infections, malaria, and other deadly conditions will simply die from lack of care.

With the right attitude and preparation, any healthcare worker in developed countries can find a way to make a significant contribution to the health and well-being of fellow human beings in the neediest of countries. Whether you are in primary care or a super specialist, there is a way to make a difference. That difference may happen immediately in the life of one patient you take care of, or it may take decades of dedicated work to improve the care in one clinic, hospital, or nation's healthcare system. The satisfaction of knowing you have reached out to help will be an important benefit to global health work but is only a small part of what you will gain.

The Benefits of Volunteering Overseas

"I had to get used to working solo, often recovering one patient in the corner of the operating theater whilst simultaneously anesthetizing the next. At times I was also the surgical assistant, midwife, pediatrician, hematologist, porter, and electrician. I learnt to cope with patients dying for lack of equipment, blood and drugs that we take for granted. But, it remains one of the most fulfilling and worthwhile times of my medical career." This was the assessment of Ian Fleming, an anesthetist from the United Kingdom, on his experience working in a hospital in Burundi, with the organization Medicines Sans Frontiers [14].

Medical volunteers from developed countries have over the years been generous with their time and funds in offering their assistance to patients and colleagues in low-income countries with weak healthcare systems. Volunteers have helped relieve the burden of routine clinical care and emergency care during environmental and manmade disasters. They have worked to strengthen the manpower shortages by teaching and mentoring young healthcare workers, running workshops and courses and designing curricula. These volunteers often face considerable challenges in cultural differences, ethical dilemmas, unfamiliar equipment and diseases, and even threats to their own personal safety. Despite the difficulties, volunteers often return home saying that they have received more than they gave.

Some of the benefits of medical work in a developing country that makes so many volunteer again and again when time and finances permit are listed in Table 15.1.

Many of these benefits will be taken home after the volunteer experience and will continue to resonate in the personal and professional life of the volunteer.

Table 15.1 Benefits of medical work in developing countries

- The satisfaction of helping people in need and making a difference
- Broaden medical knowledge through exposure to diseases and advanced stages of disease that are not often encountered at home
- Improved clinical and diagnostic skills that rely on physical examination, rather than expensive laboratory testing or imaging
- Expanded world view through exposure to another culture, and political and economic system
- Professional growth by awareness of public health issues and understanding the importance of communication
- Improved technical and procedural skills through exposure to high volumes of cases
- The satisfaction of giving back by sharing knowledge and skills
- The pleasure of practicing medicine with less "paperwork"
- Raised awareness of the waste of resources in income-rich countries and ways to conserve
- Enjoy meaningful adventure travel
- Enjoy the challenge of working in an austere environment and having to adapt and make do
- To interact (and often befriend) colleagues from another culture as well as fellow volunteers who share your altruistic views

Physicians often mention that they feel recharged in their enthusiasm for clinical medicine. They are more confident with clinical and teaching skills. Some physicians express being more interested in treating multicultural patients and practicing in underserved areas after overseas work [5, 7, 15]. Healthcare workers who maintain contact with colleagues they have worked with overseas feel enriched by a larger and more diverse circle of friends.

A young orthopedic resident expressed how an experience working in a mission hospital in South Africa affected him positively. "How do I write about an experience that has changed me forever? Going to Mthatha in July 2007 and working at Bedford Hospital was one of the most formative times in my Orthopedic training on multiple levels. Overall, this experience has reminded me why I ever became a doctor in the first place. It has fortified my desire to go into orthopedic trauma and has given me back my passion and focus, which the healthcare system here in the States can often take away" [1].

Dr Kelly McQueen wrote about her experience teaching at the Kilimanjaro Christian Medical Center (KCMC) in Tanzania. "The students' enthusiasm for learning was unparallel to any residency experience I had had to date. ...to be part of and contribute to such a program and tradition was extremely rewarding, and the personal returns were enormous...the sights, sounds, and feelings of East Africa and KCMC are stored in my heart like a nourishing inner spring" [16].

Getting Started

If you are looking to work overseas for the first time, it is strongly recommended that you look for an established program with which to travel. There are many advantages of joining a reputable aid organization or program even if you are an experienced volunteer. Competent organizations will have worked out relationships

Table 15.2 Considerations for choosing an overseas organization/site

- How much time can you afford to spend overseas? The shortest trips will be 1 or 2 weeks and often require you to pay all costs. With three or more months of commitment some organizations will cover travel and cost of living expenses
- Do you want primarily a "hands on" service trip or do you want to focus on education? The line between the two is getting increasingly blurred as more service organizations are realizing that education is key to sustainability of health improvement. Education oriented programs will often do clinical and skills teaching as well as lecture and classroom teaching
- Is safety an important consideration? Some organizations take pride in going to active crises zones with the understanding that injuries and even deaths of volunteers are a distinct possibility. Others pull out of countries when the US State Department issues warnings to US citizens and will only work in countries with a stable government
- Would you feel comfortable working in a country with political and religious beliefs which you don't share? Would you find it difficult to resist criticizing those beliefs? If so it might be best to choose another country or program
- Do you prefer to work with a faith based or secular organization?
- How flexible is your time for volunteering? Would you be able to leave for a disaster zone within a few days of being asked or will you need to plan your schedule many months ahead of traveling?
- Do you want to bring your family with you and will it be safe for you and your children. What will your spouse or partner do while you are working?
- Do you have special health needs and concerns that will restrict where you can go and for how long?
- Unable to travel? Have you considered supporting efforts overseas from home by collecting donated equipment, raising funds, or giving logistic support?

between key players and performed a needs assessment at the overseas site. Reputable groups will work to minimize the problem of too many independent groups and healthcare providers working uncoordinated in the same area. Most good organizations will also vet the volunteer and guide preparations, making it more likely that the trip will be a productive and successful one for everyone. Physicians have started their own programs, but success has depended on many years if not decades of commitment to a particular clinic or hospital. It is important that a volunteer not be a burden to already overworked physicians and nurses overseas by making unnecessary demands on their time for assistance with orientation, housing, equipment, and manpower when this can be taken care of by an established organization which understands the system.

As a volunteer, you will be a diplomat of your university or hospital, profession, and country as well as a caregiver and teacher. When deciding what type of organization to volunteer with, it is therefore helpful to take an honest look at your values, motivation, skills, and interests. Shared values, good communication, and reasonable expectations between the volunteer, aid organization, and overseas site will make success more likely. Fortunately, there are now so many programs and organizations available that anyone who is determined to get involved in global health should be able to do so and be successful.

Important points to consider when choosing an organization and site are listed in Table 15.2.

In searching for answers to these questions, you will find it helpful to speak to former volunteers, attend meetings where global work is discussed, research aid organizations on the internet, and network with others in your institution and medical association who are interested in global health.

Finding an Organization

Finding the right program or organization is difficult today only because there are so many from which to choose. A good place to start is within your own institution, whether that is a medical school, residency program, or hospital. Search for ongoing international rotations or trips and speak to former trip members to ask how they were successful in getting involved. Attend your medical association's annual meeting. They often have lectures, meetings, or other informational sessions about global work which afford the opportunity to network and ask questions. Research the internet. Good places to start are your institution's and your medical association's web sites. Look for organizations that are well known and respected or that have been in existence for several years and are run by academic institutions or as non-profit organizations. Seals of approval by charity watch dogs are another plus. Read the mission statement of organizations carefully. This will help you choose a program that is aligned with your values, skills and goals. If this is your first experience going overseas, find a program that will guide your preparations before leaving. It is especially important to bring an open mind and adaptable attitude. You can't fully know what the overseas experience will be like until you go but with realistic expectations you will almost certainly return feeling enriched and enlightened.

Global Health as a Career

Attractive, paid positions in global health can be difficult to find and are competitive but are certainly available to a determined physician with the right experience. Preparations for a career in global health can start as early as with the choice of a medical school. Although most medical schools now include global health in their curriculum, they vary in the type and amount of international health experiences offered. Larger universities with long-standing international connections and centers for global health often can provide more support for students interested in working overseas. The few medical schools that make global health a major focus are another option [17].

Global health training and formal international clinical rotations have until recently been less available in residency programs than in medical schools, but this is changing rapidly. Global Health residencies are offered in some programs and usually include time to get a Master in Public Health (MPH) [18]. Many medical associations have an international health interest group with information on their web site which sometimes includes residency programs that have global health programs [19]. Residency applicants should ask about details of the availability and support a program offers for international health rotations before making their ranking choices. Early networking with faculty who are known for their global health work can be very helpful for mentoring and recommendations for future positions.

Obtaining an MPH or other degree from a school of public health is strongly recommended but not required. Some will do this during or after medical school or residency, but it is also common for physicians to obtain an MPH in mid-career.

Fellowships and internships are offered with the World health Organization (WHO), Centers for Disease Control (CDC), the American Society of Tropical Medicine and Hygiene, and many academic and nonacademic organizations [20–22]. Searching the internet for international fellowships can be an excellent way for a young physician to get their foot in the door if global health work is their goal.

For more mature physicians, repeat volunteering with aid organizations such as Doctors Without Borders or the International Red Cross can occasionally lead to permanent positions [23, 24]. Some find it more practical to support their global health passion with a regular job at home and an arrangement to take extended time of unpaid leave every year to volunteer. For those who are determined to make a full-time career in global health, researching opportunities and networking are the keys to finding a position.

Conclusions

Many persons have the wrong idea of what constitutes true happiness. It is not attained through self-gratification but through fidelity to a worthy purpose. Helen Keller [25]

Volunteering overseas can be one of the most gratifying activities in a physician's career. Often the rewards are different than what is expected. Saving a life or improving a patient's quality of life overseas is of course very satisfying. Teaching a technique or treatment to a local caregiver who goes on to teach others within their country may initially feel like a small contribution but can lead to an enormous and lasting difference. When you return frequently to the same volunteer site and see positive changes over time which you may have brought about, it is immensely rewarding. Your advice and support to overburdened colleagues in a developing country can have a lasting impact by giving them a sense of optimism and confidence that the world has not forgotten them. Making positive connections with colleagues overseas that can become lifelong friendships is another benefit that is often mentioned by those who volunteer successfully. It can take time to understand what an overseas community wants and needs, but when you feel you have made the connections, understand what they need, and can empower them by providing the tools and means to help themselves, you feel you have changed the world to a better place.

As a global health volunteer you will be a caregiver, a teacher, and a diplomat of your profession and country. You will gain knowledge about medicine, cultures, and yourself. Working overseas is not for everyone, but if you have the interest and are willing to take a challenge, it may be the most rewarding work you will ever do.

Tips for Premeds and Medical Students

1. Learn a foreign language, or two, or three.
2. Get exposure to people of other cultures by traveling or by working with immigrants within the United States.
3. Find out what global health programs are available when applying to medical schools or residency.
4. Search for mentors who do global health work
5. Join the "Global Health Committee" of the American Medical Student Association and look up information on the Global Health Scholars Program. Check out their web site at http://www.amsa.org/AMSA/Homepage/About/Committees/Global. aspx.

Tips for Residents

1. Look for global health programs and mentors within your training program hospital and medical school.
2. Search your national society for global health committees and programs to become involved with.
3. Search the web for global health scholarships you can apply for including the Fogarty Fellowship.
4. Consider getting an MPH and look for public health programs focused on global health. Research the Association of Schools of Public Health at www.asph.org.
5. Take care of your own health when working overseas by following the advice of a travel clinic or the "health advice for travelers" section of the Centers for Disease Control (CDC) web site at http://www.cdc.gov.

Tips for Physicians Finished with Training

1. Find a medical volunteer program to spend time overseas.
2. Look for global health committees or programs in your national society, your hospital or medical school.
3. Give yourself a year to plan and prepare for your first medical trip.

4. Research the country you are visiting before you go. Find country health data on the World Health Organization web site at http://www.who.int/en/ and the CDC web site http://www.cdc.gov. Get a flavor of local events by searching the web for English language newspapers in the country you are visiting.
5. For long term involvement in global health, consider getting an MPH in global health or getting training in tropical medicine. Search the Association of Schools of Public health at www.asph.org and the American Society of Tropical Medicine and hygiene at http://www.astmh.org.

References

1. What we do-notes from the field-personal impact. www.hvousa.org. Accessed 30 October 2010.
2. A kaleidoscope of careers in public health. Boston Sunday Globe; 21 March 2010: Advertising Supplement.
3. Crump JA, Sugarman J. Ethical considerations for short-term experiences by trainees in global health. JAMA. 2008;300:1456–8.
4. Baker T, Weisman C, Piwoz E. US physicians in international health: report of a current survey. JAMA. 1984;251(4):502–4.
5. Drain PK, Primack A, Hunt DD, et al. Global health in medical education: a call for more training and opportunities. Acad Med. 2007;82:226–30.
6. Association of American Medical Colleges. 2009 Medical School Graduation Questionnaire: all schools report. Washington: Association of American Medical Colleges; 2009. http://www. aamc.org/data/gq/. Accessed 13 October 2010.
7. Drain PK, Holmes KK, Skeff KM, et al. Global health training and international clinical rotations during residency: current status, needs, and opportunities. Acad Med. 2009;84:320–5.
8. Narayan KMV, Ali MK, Koplan JP. Global noncommunicable diseases – where worlds meet. N Engl J Med. 2010;363:1196–8.
9. Kerry VB, Auld S, Farmer P. An international service corps for health – an unconventional prescription for diplomacy. N Engl J Med. 2010;363:1199–00.
10. WHO World Health Report 2007. http://www.who.int/whr/2007/overview/en/index.html. Accessed 30 September 2010.
11. The "First Globals": The emergence of a "global generation" and what it means. http://www. britannica.com/blogs/2009/07/the-emergence-of-a-global-generation-what-does-it-mean. Accessed 25 September 2010.
12. Fenton P. A plea for help from Malawi. World Anaesth. 1998;2(1):25.
13. The World Health Report 2006 – Working together for health. http://www.who.int/whr/2006/ en/. Accessed 28 August 2010.
14. Henderson K. Lessons from working overseas. Anaesthesia. 2007;62:113–7.
15. Gupta AR, Wells CK, Horwitz RI, et al. The international health program: the 15-year experience with Yale University's internal medicine residency program. Am J Trop Med Hyg. 1999;61:1019–23.
16. McQueen KA. A change in perspective: experience with the OTP in Tanzania. ASA Newsl. 1996;60:9–11.
17. Medical School for International Health-Ben-Gurion University of the Negev. http://www. cumc.columbia.edu/dept/bgcu-md. Accessed 14 September 2010.
18. Brigham and Womens Hospital Global Health Residency under the Division of Global Health Equity and Internal Medicine Residency. www.brighamandwomens.org/socialmedicine/ gheresidency.aspx. Accessed 10 October 2010.

19. The American Academy of Family Physicians. http://www-aafp.org/online/en/home/aboutus/specialty/international/opps/html. Accessed 10 October 2010.
20. World Health Organization. http://www.who.int/en/. Accessed 10 October 2010.
21. Centers for Disease Control. http://www.cdc.gov. Accessed 10 October 2010.
22. The American Society of Tropical Medicine and Hygiene. http://www.astmh.org. Accessed 10 October 2010.
23. Doctors Without Borders. http://www.doctorswithoutborders.org. Accessed 10 October 2010.
24. The International Committee of the Red Cross and its human resources. http://www.icrc.org/Web/eng/siteengO.nsf/htmlall/jobs. Accessed 10 October 2010.
25. Helen Keller. www.memorable-quotes.com. Accessed 14 September 2010.

Part IV
Academia

Chapter 16
Careers in Academic Research

Sheng F. Cai and Rebecca L. Aft

Key Points

- Research experiences can be beneficial for trainees and practicing physicians at all stages of their professional development.
- Individuals seeking a research experience can obtain funding support from medical societies, federal and private grants, and from residency training programs.
- The Medical Scientist Training Program is a combined degree M.D./Ph.D. program designed to fund and train physician-scientists. These physician-scientists are highly sought-after in academia, because they can fulfill roles in many professional areas, including basic science research, clinical research, teaching, and clinical medicine.

Introduction

The practice of clinical medicine, regardless of the particular field or specialty, relies on a continuously updated body of data that is acquired from the laboratory as well as from clinical trials. Diagnostic and therapeutic options are constantly being shaped and informed by the published literature. As such, the practice of medicine

S.F. Cai, BS
Medical Scientist Training Program, Washington University in St. Louis School
of Medicine, 41-41 41st Street, Apt 2P, Sunnyside, NY 11104, USA

R.L. Aft, MD, PhD (✉)
Department of Surgery, Washington University, 660 South Euclid Avenue,
Campus box 8109, St. Louis, MO 63110, USA
e-mail: aftr@wustl.edu

R.D. Urman and J.M. Ehrenfeld (eds.), *Physicians' Pathways to Non-Traditional*
Careers and Leadership Opportunities, DOI 10.1007/978-1-4614-0551-1_16,
© Springer Science+Business Media, LLC 2012

at the bedside and research in the academic setting are inextricably linked, one having a profound impact on how the other is conducted.

Medical students are often taught that a substantial proportion of the material covered in the medical school curriculum will become obsolete within 5–10 years after their graduation. Keeping abreast of the medical literature and approaching clinical and basic science data with a critical eye is an essential skill that should be expected of any physician. Thus, one key attribute of a good clinician is not only the ability to establish a solid foundation of medical knowledge, but also the ability to incorporate new information and apply it effectively to patient care. A working understanding of research in the academic setting can provide both trainees and practicing physicians, even if they do not intend to pursue a career in academia, the means to develop these essential skills.

Furthermore, physician-scientists, those with M.D., M.D./M.A., or M.D./Ph.D. degrees who receive extensive training in both clinical medicine and academic research, are uniquely positioned with their special training to facilitate the translation of findings made in the laboratory into novel therapeutics and diagnostics at the bedside and to bring unique clinical insights to the laboratory. The skills of these physician-scientists are versatile and heavily valued, and these individuals can fulfill a number of different roles along the spectrum of professional responsibilities from academic researcher to pure clinician.

Why Pursue Academic Research?

Academic research is a two-way street – skills learned in the laboratory can enhance clinical understanding and knowledge gained in the clinic can bring new insights to the laboratory. Overall, gaining hands-on exposure to the scientific method in the laboratory or in clinical research provides an invaluable opportunity to learn the limits of our scientific knowledge, the frontiers to be explored, and the tools available for specific research areas. In addition, involvement in research provides the opportunity to hone critical thinking skills, develop an understanding of statistics and other analytical modalities that are ubiquitous in the medical literature, and learn valuable technical skills that otherwise cannot be taught in the traditional medical curriculum. The motivation to pursue research in academia can depend on the particular stage of professional development as well as the specific niche that a trainee or practicing physician seeks to occupy. Academic research can range from basic biological science to translational research to correlative science studies associated with clinical trials to populations-based studies. Many students/clinicians have a specific area of interest and pursue research projects that are related.

For trainees, research has virtually become an integral component of the graduate and postgraduate curriculum. There are multiple avenues for research in the basic sciences as well as for clinical research at all levels of training. Several of the more common pathways will be discussed here.

Summer Research Programs/Elective Research Rotations

Most medical schools and residency programs have research opportunities and dedicated elective research rotations available to trainees as a component of the curriculum. Elective research rotations that can be applied toward academic credit during medical school are not eligible for compensation, but summer research programs are often funded either privately or by federal grants awarded by the National Institutes of Health (NIH). These funded programs provide students with a stipend to cover living expenses. Other research organizations such as the Howard Hughes Medical Institute (HHMI) allocate a proportion of their funds to support the research projects of both undergraduate and graduate students. In addition, professional medical societies, such as the American Medical Association, the American Academy of Pediatrics, and the American Society of Hematology, often provide competitive grants for residents and fellows to conduct research in their respective fields (See *Resources* below for funding sources).

These opportunities allow trainees to interact more closely with faculty in a particular field of interest that a trainee may be considering. One-on-one interaction with colleagues and mentors in a research setting is an ideal way for trainees to become introduced to a specific field. Not only do mentors have more time for teaching and in-depth discussion of pertinent issues in the research setting, but also investigators readily welcome fresh perspectives and new ideas from young trainees when approaching complex scientific and clinical problems requiring creative solutions. Students and residents are often encouraged by their mentors to present their work at retreats and societal meetings, thereby providing additional opportunities for networking, exploring research as a possible career option, and developing valuable presentation skills.

Obtaining a Research Position

The first step to securing a research position is to identify an area of interest and contact a mentor to arrange a meeting. Almost all research faculty members have websites summarizing their research, and it is important to have a fundamental understanding of the major research aims of a particular laboratory. A meeting should be arranged in-person to discuss possible projects and roles. This also provides an opportunity to meet other lab members and to get a general feel for how a particular laboratory is organized and run. Attending lab meetings and journal clubs with other lab members is often encouraged and can be quite helpful. If the mentor agrees to a personal meeting, this is often an indicator that he or she does have the funds to support students or residents during their time in the laboratory. If funding is not available, it should be incumbent upon the principal investigator to disclose that early in the dialogue, but the applicant should also inquire about funding during the initial meeting if no mention about it is made.

Table 16.1 Programs of study for MSTP candidates

- Biochemistry
- Bioengineering
- Bioethics
- Biophysics
- Cell and development biology
- Chemical and physical sciences
- Computational biology and bioinformatics
- Immunology
- Molecular biology and genetics
- Microbiology and infectious disease
- Neuroscience
- Pathology and mechanisms of disease
- Pharmacology
- Public health
- Physiology
- Social and behavioral sciences

Before starting medical school, some students with significant research experience have made the determination that academic research will comprise a significant portion of their careers. To that end, some of these individuals will matriculate into combined degree M.D./Ph.D. training programs, otherwise known as physician-scientist training programs, or, when federally funded by the NIH, Medical Scientist Training Programs (MSTP). Prior to the inception of these programs dedicated to the training of physician-scientists, a small percentage of physicians with M.D. degrees entered postdoctoral training in basic science laboratories, sometimes after additional subspecialty fellowship training, in order to begin their careers in academia. Faced with medical school debt in the setting of a career choice that is already less lucrative than alternative career paths (private practice, e.g.,), individuals who otherwise would have chosen to do research were being deterred from becoming physician-scientists by sheer financial burden. The NIH recognized these obstacles and began funding medical/graduate schools in the 1960s to establish MSTPs that not only covered tuition expenses but also provided graduate student stipends for the duration of their training. There are now hundreds of MSTPs throughout the United States that are affiliated with accredited medical schools, offering Ph.D. graduate training in a wide variety of disciplines. Such disciplines include but are not limited to those listed in Table 16.1.

The objective of these programs is to train physicians to become versatile clinicians, researchers, mentors, inventors, and leaders in their respective academic field. With both clinical and research training, physician-scientists are uniquely positioned to approach basic science problems framed within a clinical context of human disease processes, thus ultimately achieving synergies in the academic setting that otherwise would not be possible. Although physician-scientists spend most of their professional time doing research relating traditionally to human biology and pathophysiology, many also maintain clinical responsibilities. Most physician-scientists work at university medical centers and research institutes, although some also work in industrial settings.

The M.D./Ph.D. curriculum typically spans 7–9 years, which is a shorter course relative to separate M.D. and Ph.D. training. This is largely due to the fact that many of these programs have streamlined the curriculum, allowing overlapping coursework to count simultaneously toward medical and graduate school credit. Traditionally, M.D./Ph.D. students start with the preclinical medical curriculum during the first 2 years, and when third-year medical students progress onto clinical clerkship rotations, these students will commence the Ph.D. portion of their training in a thesis laboratory. Students are often encouraged to do research rotations to find their thesis laboratory in the summers between (and sometimes before) medical school. After completing the thesis dissertation and defense (the duration is variable depending on the individual project, but usually spans 3–5 years), the student then returns to complete the clinical clerkship rotations. One of the advantages of having dual-degree training is the flexibility in post-graduate career options that are offered to these trainees. While most students do enter residency training after graduation, some individuals choose to enter postdoctoral research training or begin working in consulting or industry without further clinical training.

Currently, some residencies also have research-track programs designed to facilitate and encourage the development of academic physician-scientists. These programs offer stipend enhancement, additional funds for research materials, travel expenses for conferences, and sometimes guaranteed fellowship training of the individual's choosing at that institution. This is due to the fact that trainees with M.D. and Ph.D. degrees are highly sought-after and comprise a promising pool of junior faculty candidates with the potential to fill academic positions at the institution. In particular, some internal medicine residency programs affiliated with large academic research centers have developed research-track residencies that shorten the duration of residency training by 1 year in order to allow for an additional year in fellowship training. These "short-track" programs provide fellows with additional time to develop their research and compete for funding in anticipation of becoming junior faculty after completion of their postdoctoral training.

Other Dual-Degree Programs

In addition to M.D./Ph.D. training programs, some institutions offer other dual-degree programs, such as M.D./M.A., M.D./J.D., M.D./M.B.A., and D.O./Ph.D. The M.D./M.A. programs are relatively more common, and, even if combined programs are not officially offered, medical students electing to take a temporary leave of absence from their training can often pursue research in a laboratory for 1–2 years and obtain a Master's degree at the end of their research. However, due to the more intensive research training offered by MST programs that are tailored toward training academic physician-scientists, M.D./Ph.D. applicants have a perceived advantage over those with M.D./M.A. candidates for residency, fellowship, and faculty positions. Nonetheless, M.D./M.A. trainees with an interest in continuing their research careers in academia are eligible to apply to many research-track residency programs.

How to Apply

MSTP/PSTP

Undergraduate applicants for M.D./Ph.D. programs should have a strong academic record with a solid science GPA and MCAT scores (note: some programs also require GRE scores) as well as extensive research experience with evidence of independence in the laboratory. Applicants should also have a record demonstrating a commitment to medicine and compassionate care. In addition, medical students pursuing M.D.-only training who later develop an interest in pursuing Ph.D. training after a research experience can also apply. Many MST programs welcome M.D. student applications for admission.

While some applicants can have multiple research experiences in different labs, others can have more continuity in their research projects if they remain in a laboratory for a longer period of time. Candidates who are invited for interviews are often assessed by their ability to discuss their research projects intelligently and coherently. Although coauthorship on publications and attendance at societal meetings are not required, these attributes can considerably strengthen a candidate's application. A research mentor's letter of recommendation can also have significant bearing on the applicant's competitiveness.

Pursuing Research From An Established Career

There are few structured programs for established practitioners seeking to become involved in research. However, once a practitioner has identified a mentor, the mentor can assist in obtaining or providing funding. Most investigators involved in translational research welcome clinicians due to their insight into disease processes, and clinicians derive great satisfaction from participating in a project related to their clinical interests.

A listing of the various research career pathways which one may take is shown in Fig. 16.1.

Mentorship

The most crucial component of pursuing a research career is identifying the appropriate mentor. Individuals seeking a research experience have a broad array of goals and expectations for their time in the laboratory. Some students may have limited experience in "wet-bench" research and are only looking for basic exposure to common laboratory techniques and how day-to-day operations of academic research function. On the contrary, other physician-scientists near the end of their postdoctoral training may be looking for a supportive mentor who will facilitate his

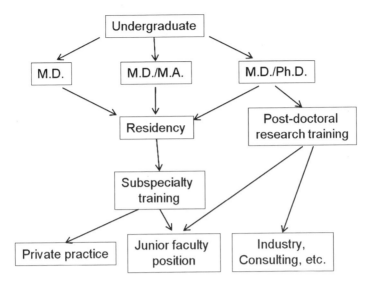

Fig. 16.1 Research career pathways

or her transition to a career as an independent principal investigator. It is absolutely critical that individuals seeking a research experience ensure that their goals and expectations align with those of the mentor.

First, general research interests must be shared between the mentor and the mentee. If the individual seeking a research experience is particularly interested in gastrointestinal disorders, there may be little benefit for him or her to enter a cardiology research lab. However, it is important that the mentee not be too narrow in scope, as this myopic view can quickly limit the number of potential mentors. For example, there may be only one laboratory at a given institution that studies the biochemistry of malarial infections, which may or may not be well suited for the mentee. Keeping an open mind about research projects, and focusing more on the quality of the mentor–mentee relationship and the laboratory environment can result in more fruitful research experiences.

Second, the laboratory environment is also an important consideration. A large, "high-powered" laboratory with 35 graduate students, technicians, and postdocs can easily overwhelm a mentee who needs more day-to-day guidance and interaction with the principal investigator. However, such an expansive lab with strong funding and technical resources could be an ideal environment for an independently minded senior postdoc planning on becoming an independent investigator. A junior faculty investigator with a small lab of 5–6 members may be better suited to a mentee looking for more hands-on instruction from the mentor.

Other considerations – does the mentor foster a sense of competition within the lab to drive productivity? How willing is the mentor to allow for senior postdocs to take away a particular project or valuable reagents with them to begin their own careers? How much support from other lab staff (animal husbandry, technical assistance, core laboratories) is provided? Depending on the level of expertise of the mentee seeking the research experience, all of these should be factored into determining the suitability of a particular lab for that individual.

Funding

As discussed previously, funding for research during residency training is readily available. In many programs, research is integrated into the program, and trainees continue to receive their residency stipend during their research years. If funding is not provided by residency programs, many professional societies, such as the American Medical Association, the American Academy of Pediatrics, and the American College of Surgeons, offer funding for qualified applicants.

For postdoctoral fellows who have completed residency training, there are additional funding opportunities provided by the NIH. The NIH offers a variety of Career Development Awards, also known as K awards as well as postdoctoral fellowships. Depending on the particular field of research (clinical or basic science research), different K awards are available. For example, the K12 award is a Mentored Clinical Scientist Developmental Program grant. The K08 award is a Mentored Clinical Scientist Developmental award for research in areas that do not involve human subjects, and the K23 award is for Mentored Patient-Oriented Research which involves human subjects. Senior fellows who have completed a substantial portion of their research training and have the support of their mentors apply for these funds that will allow them to transition into junior faculty positions.

Fundings in specific fields of research for postdoctoral fellows and junior faculty are available from private organizations such as the American Cancer Society, American Heart Association, etc. Several clinical societies offer funding for clinical as well as translational science including the Society of Surgical Oncology, American College of Surgeons, American Society of Clinical Oncology, etc.

Once a student/clinician has results of their research, it is important to present the findings at scientific meetings and to publish the work. Attending meetings and presenting data foster interactions with other investigators in the field which can lead to not only constructive criticism and new ideas, but also new collaborations. Publications in reputable journals demonstrate productivity and will help with obtaining future funding. Leadership in a research field arises, in part, from demonstrated expertise in a specific area.

Summary

A representative pathway that might lead to an academic career in medicine is demonstrated in the case vignette in Fig. 16.2.

Katharine received a B.S. degree in biology. During 2 summers in college, she worked in a laboratory as a Howard Hughes Undergraduate Research Fellow, where she studied cell cycle progression in yeast. She then matriculated in an M.D./Ph.D. program. For her thesis in the immunology program, she focused on the role of chemokine receptor signaling in neutrophil homeostatis. She then entered residency training, "short-tracking" in the internal medicine, followed by a fellowship in hematology/oncology. During the research years of her fellowship, she developed a mouse model to study graft-versus-host disease and anti-tumor immune responses. She was awarded a K08 career development grant, after which she became Assistant Professor of Medicine and Immunology.

Fig. 16.2 Case vignette

Medical students and physician trainees can benefit from research experiences during their education, even if they do not intend to pursue a career in academic research. Research experiences teach valuable skills and provide important networking opportunities that otherwise could not be attained in standard curricula. For those individuals who are interested in pursuing a career with some component of academic research, either in basic science "wet-bench" research or clinical research, there are multiple training pathways that can facilitate career development in these areas. One of the most widely recognized training pathways is the dual-degree M.D./Ph.D. program. MSTP students demonstrate a strong interest in both clinical medicine and research, and they can choose to pursue Ph.D. graduate work in a broad array of disciplines. After graduating from these programs, these individuals are highly sought-after by academic programs, and they have considerable flexibility in career options. Most pursue research in an academic setting with some clinical responsibilities, while others seek to work in industry or other fields. Regardless of the niche occupied by these physician-scientists, the training they receive allows them to be uniquely prepared for the challenges encountered across the full spectrum of medical subspecialties and scientific fields.

Additional Resources

http://www.nigms.nih.gov/Training/InstPredoc/PredocOverview-MSTP.htm. A general overview of Medical Scientist Training Programs provided by the National Institute of General Medical Sciences.

http://www.aamc.org/students/considering/research/mdphd/programs.htm. A comprehensive list of M.D./Ph.D. training programs, including those funded independently of the NIH.

http://www.mdphds.org/. Guidebook written by students for prospective M.D./Ph.D. students.

http://www.physicianscientists.org/. American Physician Scientists Association.

http://www.hhmi.org/grants/office/. Research opportunities offered by the prestigious Howard Hughes Medical Institute.

http://homepage.uab.edu/paik/rr.html. A list of research-track residency programs in internal medicine.

Ley TJ, Rosenberg LE. The physician-scientist career pipeline in 2005: build it, and they will come. JAMA. 2005;294(11):1343–51. An excellent overview on trends and issues relevant to physician-scientist career development.

http://www.mudphudder.com/funding-opportunities/residents/. A thorough list of competitive research grants that are awarded to residents and fellows. Many of these grants are provided by professional medical societies, such as the American Medical Association, the American Academy of Pediatrics, and surgical subspeciality societies.

http://www.ama-assn.org/ama/pub/about-ama/ama-foundation/our-programs/medical-education/seed-grant-research.shtml. The AMA Foundation established the Seed Grant Research Program in 2000 to encourage medical students, physician residents and fellows to enter the research field. The program provides $2,500 grants to help them conduct small basic science, applied, or clinical research projects.

http://www.ddcf.org/Medical-Research/Program-Strategies/Clinical-Research/. The Doris Duke Charitable Foundation seeks to provide funding opportunities for medical students, junior faculty, and senior faculty to advance translational and clinical research.

Chapter 17
Careers in Medical Education

Simona F. Shaitelman

Key Points

- Working in medical education will make you a better doctor and enable you to serve better a number of key constituencies (patients, institutions, and the public at large).
- There are numerous roles – formal and informal – for you to play if you are interested in medical education.
- You can obtain a background in medical education with or without a formal graduate degree in education.

Introduction

There is a growing community of physicians interested in medical education. Indeed, more academic medical centers are acknowledging the importance of education and are creating clinician educator tracks that acknowledge that time spent teaching is as worthwhile as time spent in the laboratory. This makes sense. As our knowledge of the human body expands, there are increasing amounts of information that physicians are required to learn and process.

Until recently, however, there has been little discussion – and even less consensus – about the best methods and techniques to use in training the physicians of tomorrow. The lack of discussion and agreement reflects, in part, the difficulty of the issues involved. There is no easy answer about how to tailor medical education to

---

S.F. Shaitelman, MD, EdM (✉)
Department of Radiation Oncology, Division of Radiation Oncology, The University of Texas
MD Anderson Cancer Center, 1515 Holcombe Blvd, Unit 1202, Houston, TX 77030, USA
e-mail: SFShaitelman@mdanderson.org

R.D. Urman and J.M. Ehrenfeld (eds.), *Physicians' Pathways to Non-Traditional
Careers and Leadership Opportunities*, DOI 10.1007/978-1-4614-0551-1_17,
© Springer Science+Business Media, LLC 2012

a variety of personalities and specialties within medicine. Also, teaching physicians how to be educators and to think thoughtfully about how to educate others requires innovation, as well as institutional support. In these difficult economic times, resources are often used for other purposes.

Despite these hurdles, it is clear that theories of pedagogy are tremendously valuable in shaping how medicine is taught to physicians. The purpose of this chapter is not to discuss the various theories that can be used in medical education. Rather, the primary aim is to highlight the benefits of medical education itself. Even if there is little agreement at the present time about the best ways to educate physicians, it is clear that having a cadre of physicians dedicated to medical education offers major benefits to a variety of interested parties – to physicians, to patients, and to institutions. This chapter will also provide a brief discussion about the various roles that an individual can play should he or she desire to work in the field of medical education and about the resources available to obtain the necessary credentials.

The Benefits of Working in Medical Education

The first, and perhaps simplest, reason to pursue an interest in medical education is that it will make you a better doctor. There is an old Roman adage attributed to the author Seneca – *qui docet, discit* ("He who teaches, learns") – that contains a great deal of truth. In thinking about how best to transmit information to students, you are provided with an opportunity to refresh your own skills and keep those skills sharp. You are also provided with a personal space that enables you to reflect on your own experiences and to think about alternative modalities of treatment. And the transmission of information is not a one-way street. As a teacher, you will listen to and learn from your students as well. In so doing, you will also be exposed to new perspectives flowing from those students – some of whom have extraordinary stories and experiences of their own – and these perspectives may reshape how you view a particular disease or its treatment.

It should go without saying that you will accrue many of these same benefits in your interactions with patients. And with patient care, specialized training in medical education will offer you an additional weapon in your arsenal to combat illness – it will allow you to apply the tools of pedagogy toward impacting the practices of your patients. This applies not only to a pediatric population just starting to learn good health practices but also to an adult population that may need to unlearn habits that are harmful to health. An understanding of learning theory and cognition can help to guide you as a clinician in changing the behavior of individual patients. On a larger scale, such an understanding can be useful in shaping the health practices of entire populations, through public health campaigns. The public benefits tremendously from the development of a well educated, thoughtful cohort of young physicians.

Second, immersing yourself in medical education provides you with a pivotal role in the transmission of medical knowledge from past to future. In June 2004,

Table 17.1 Summary of the benefits of working in medical education

Working in medical education will…

- Enable you to hone your skills
- Give you space to consider alternative modalities of treatment
- Provide you with additional tools to influence patient health practices
- Provide you with a role in the transmission of medical knowledge
- Enable you to shape future physicians and the field of medicine
- Give you an opportunity to become involved in administration within a medical school

New York Times columnist Abigail Zuger, M.D. wrote a terrific piece entitled "Paying Homage to the Wisdom of Voices From Medicine's Past," in which she described her own experience of being able to diagnose subacute bacterial endocarditis due to an article published in 1942 that contained the diary entries of a third-year Harvard medical student who had suffered from the disease himself and had described the subjective experience of the illness. Two other emergency room physicians had completely missed the diagnosis, Zuger suggests, because they had not been privy to this sort of information. As a clinician educator, you serve as a bridge between past and future in passing along the valuable lessons of the past. As Zuger so aptly puts it, "one might make the case that those who study the past in medicine are not so much condemned to repeat it as, occasionally, privileged to do so." Table 17.1 provides a list of some of the benefits you may experience by working in medical education.

Third, and related to the subject of the future in particular, becoming involved in medical education will allow you to take an active role in shaping the future of the field of medicine. Teaching students, mentoring them, and helping them in their professional (and personal) development allow you to shape both individuals and the physicians and researchers of tomorrow, and this is often a source of pride among physicians. Simply put, it is personally rewarding to the physician to be an educator.

Fourth, if you are interested in becoming involved in the higher levels of administration within a medical school, then a background in medical education is helpful. As medical schools are fundamentally educational institutions, they seek out those who have specialized training in education to support their mission of training future physicians. (And it bears mention that medical schools benefit greatly in other ways from having trained educators on their faculties; as discussed below, they are often the best doctors and leaders in their fields. The presence of these individuals on staff in turn often draws patients and research dollars to the institution). Specialized training in medical education will also serve you well in becoming involved with residency training programs. Serving as a dean of a medical school or as program director of a residency program will enable you to have a large impact on the career development of many future physicians.

Last, but not least, many of the best physicians are those who are involved in medical education. This makes sense, given all of the benefits articulated above. Those physicians who are savvy enough to recognize these benefits are usually the ones who are similarly savvy in practicing their own particular specialties. And as a physician, it is a wonderful experience to be surrounded by such people – thoughtful people with similar interests who are motivated to excel.

Roles for Physicians to Play in Medical Education

In light of all of the benefits cited above, it is worthwhile to discuss several roles that a physician can play should he or she desire to become involved in medical education. A summary of these career options is provided in Table 17.2.

First, as already mentioned, physicians can adopt formal administrative roles within academic medical institutions, such as becoming deans or residency program directors. Although these roles are prestigious and provide physicians with great influence over young physicians and medical students, they often have a number of limitations that deserve mention. For instance, the time spent advising residents or medical students may limit the number of hours that can be spent in the clinic. This in turn requires flexibility from the other physicians and administrators in the practice group. Also, administrative positions are often limited to those individuals who have many years of experience at the institution, thereby excluding it as a possibility for those who seek to participate in medical education either during or immediately following medical school.

Second, many academic institutions have created formal, nonadministrative positions to acknowledge the importance of education to their missions. This position is frequently known as a "clinician educator," with some variation across institutions. Working as a clinician educator allows one to combine work as a clinician with work teaching medical students and residents. The clinician educator track enables faculty at large academic centers to work toward tenure through dedication to educating young clinicians. Clinician educators are often given protected time in their schedules to dedicate toward teaching. Promotions take into account the work devoted to medical education, and this work is elevated to comparable prestige as that of working in the clinic or laboratory. Grants may be available to fund medical education projects, thus helping to secure additional protected time for this work.

A third possibility is that the physician retains no formal title to acknowledge his participation in the education of residents and medical students, yet the physician attempts to work with trainees as much as possible. This, for example, can be the role of a staff physician in a medical center or private practice that has no residents

Table 17.2 Possible career options in medical education

- Dean
- Residency program director
- Clinician educator
- Physician who has no formal educational title yet allows trainees to rotate through his/her practice or shadow him/her

or medical students on a regular basis yet allows those individuals to rotate through their practices or shadow them on an occasional basis. This educator "track" is no less valuable, as it often allows trainees to be exposed to new areas of medicine and different kinds of practices that might not be seen in a typical academic medical center.

How to Obtain a Background in Medical Education

Deciding on a formal role to play as a medical educator is only part of what should be considered by interested physicians. They should also consider obtaining a graduate degree in education. This grants the physician an extra certification (or "badge") in the field of medical education. Although the majority of people actively involved in medical education do not have such a degree, an increasing number of medical schools and graduate schools of education do offer dual degree programs combining both degrees. As these degree programs expand and become more commonly attended, it may be expected for academic employers to require applicants to have such training, especially given the avowed educational mission of their institutions.

No matter whether this development comes to pass, the certification granted by a degree in education at a minimum demonstrates to future employers a certain dedication to the field. Also, as medical schools look to choose people to promote to positions of leadership, the extra degree may provide you with an advantage when different candidates are considered.

If a graduate degree in education is the course decided upon, it bears mention that many graduate schools in education still do not have a particular curriculum dedicated to medical education (notwithstanding the fact that a dual degree program may formally exist). A listing of some of the current programs is shown in Table 17.3. Therefore, if you choose this path, you will have to work with faculty both in the schools of medicine and education to find appropriate mentors and to

Table 17.3 Graduate programs in medical education

Vanderbilt University: MD/M.Ed. http://peabody.vanderbilt.edu/MDMEd_Joint_Degree_ Program.xml
Harvard Graduate School of Education: http://gseweb.harvard.edu/
Columbia University Teachers College: http://www.tc.columbia.edu/
Stanford University School of Education: http://ed.stanford.edu/
Masters in Medical Education Leadership, University of New England: http://www.une.edu/com/ mmel/
University of Iowa Masters in Medical Education: Office of Consultation and Research in Medical Education: http://www.medicine.uiowa.edu/ocrme/masters/programoverview.html
University of Southern California, Keck School of Medicine, Master of Academic Medicine: http://mededonline.usc.edu/
University of Pittsburgh, Institute for Clinical Research Education, Master of Science in Medical Education: http://www.icre.pitt.edu/degrees/ms_meded.html

tailor coursework to your particular needs. When asked, many academics in the field of education welcome the opportunity to work with physicians. There is a wide breadth of knowledge in the fields of learning theory, organizational leadership, and education outreach, among others – knowledge that is just starting to be applied to the field of medical education. An increasing number of clinician educators are incorporating these academic subdisciplines into their practices.

An alternative to pursuing a formal graduate degree in education is conducting concerted research in the field of medical education. This can be done under the mentorship of a clinician educator or a faculty member in either a graduate school of education or a medical school. Through designing, implementing, and writing up research projects relating to medical education, you can learn much about the various subdisciplines within medical education. In addition, a published paper serves as another credential of expertise in the field.

Similarly, attending conferences where medical education issues are discussed can provide you with excellent opportunities to meet many people in the field working in a variety of healthcare settings. You will obtain not only innumerable networking opportunities but also the ability to collaborate on different projects.

Additional Resources

Josiah Macy, Jr. Foundation: Provides grants to fund projects in medical education http://www.josiahmacyfoundation.org/index.php?section=home
Accreditation Council for Graduate Medical Education ("ACGME"): Academic Medicine, Journal of the Association of American Medical Colleges: http://journals.lww.com/academicmedicine/pages/default.aspx
Medical Teacher, An International Journal of Education in the Health Sciences: http://www.medical-teacher.org/MEDTEACH_wip/pages/home.html
Medical Education Online: http://med-ed-online.net/index.php/meo

Chapter 18
Medical School Deans and Other Senior Administrative Officers

Kathleen Franco

Key Points

- Transitioning from research, clinical practice, and frontline teaching to becoming a senior administrative officer in a medical school requires careful planning and preparation.
- Create a personalized plan to succeed as a leader in medical education, including gaining educational and administrative experiences.
- Find suitable mentors and take advantage of a local and national network of leaders in education and administration.

Introduction

Perhaps there is a seed planted during medical school or later as a junior faculty member that leads one to consider the dream of achieving a leadership position in medical education. There is a growing body of literature and multiple training programs that point the way. This chapter will offer considerations when making the choice to pursue a senior leadership position. The responsibility of the medical school is to train future physicians. The responsibility of the dean extends over the entire process, including faculty management, financial operations, student performance, and maintenance of educational values. Although this chapter will primarily refer to the dean, there are many other important senior medical positions for consideration and much of the information in this chapter will be helpful to individuals

K. Franco, MD (✉)
Cleveland Clinic Lerner College of Medicine of Case Western Reserve University,
9500 Euclid Ave. Na 2-21, Cleveland, OH 44185, USA
e-mail: francok@ccf.org

R.D. Urman and J.M. Ehrenfeld (eds.), *Physicians' Pathways to Non-Traditional Careers and Leadership Opportunities*, DOI 10.1007/978-1-4614-0551-1_18,
© Springer Science+Business Media, LLC 2012

considering these transitions. For example, there may be a variety of associate and assistant deanships available in an institution. A senior associate dean or vice dean may organize the medical education provided to trainees. An associate dean may be assigned to student affairs while another may take on the admission process. There is often a dean of curricular affairs as well as one for faculty development. Additional deans may include assessment and evaluation, graduate medical education, continuing medical education, diversity, and others, if helpful to a particular medical school's mission. There may be one senior medical leader in charge of clinical education while another encompasses basic sciences. Schools with an emphasis on research may have an individual assigned in that area.

There are also key players within the department such as a chair, vice chairs, residency program director, clerkship director, and research director. As medical schools usually are part of a large Medical Center, the hospital will have a chief executive officer, chief of staff, chief financial officer, and other officials. Brater [1] offers a brief description to compare and contrast these roles. For some positions, particular committee experiences are invaluable. If one has participated on the admissions committee for medical students or residency selection and enjoy recruitment, they may want to consider becoming an associate dean of admissions. Residency program directors, clerkship directors, and those involved with student counseling may be drawn more to student affairs. Likewise physicians who have participated in curriculum design in multiple arenas might explore an associate deanship of medical education or curriculum. Volunteering early for these various committee assignments will strategically allow the individual to throw their hat in the ring when the position opens. Building strong communication skills and keeping an eye out for opportunities are invaluable to the physician looking for these transitions.

Why Pursue a Senior Administrative Role and How Can I Benefit?

Pangaro [2] interviewed 15 leaders in medical education. Reading their individual stories demonstrates a wide variety of reasons physicians may desire academic leadership positions. The ripples of your work can spread far beyond your patients and include your junior faculty, residents, students, and many of the patients they will treat. Many physicians have the wish to make things better than how they found them. Taking a leadership role gives one the opportunity to find better solutions and to truly make a difference. Physicians report more personal satisfaction after gaining greater control over the daily schedule and activities at work. Taking charge of one's life again and the happiness that evolves from that eases the transition into a leadership role. Some may fear that giving up patient care is unthinkable but in truth many continue a small portion of their practice, even as a dean. One aspect of caring for others is replaced by the multitude of mentoring opportunities that arise. Seeing your protégé blossom and flourish is sometimes more exciting than having done that yourself in earlier years. Spending time with young, enthusiastic trainees keeps you young, inspired, and hopeful about the future.

Likely the physicians best suited for these roles are also those individuals who cherish the patient–doctor relationship, but in addition have always had a passion for teaching. Now you can impact selection of the best teachers and the best teaching styles. Beyond that is the ability to look at the entire institution and explore what can be done to improve the overall education of medical students. For those who love financial planning and seeking out donations for a good cause, serving can benefit a multitude of future lives in the years to come.

How Can I Benefit My Patients?

This may seem like a very strange question to include in this chapter but in my opinion is very appropriate. Certainly, you will not be able to see as many patients as you once did, now that you have taken on a leadership role. However, you will never know how many patient lives you actually have touched through your impact on others in training and on the faculty. For example, helping define a patient-centered mission for the medical school and modeling that through your own behavior leaves an important legacy. Leading discussions at faculty and training meetings about putting the patient first, and professionalism reaffirms that that is a commitment of all who work at the Medical Center. Leaders can also impact who gets admitted or hired, seeking those who have humanitarian values that follow the mission.

General Considerations Before Creating a Personal Plan

Leadership roles offer exciting extensions or transitions from the care of patients to the care of individuals on a team. There are likely as many ways to achieve one of these roles as there are physicians who hold them. This chapter aims to discuss various paths that leaders have chosen, as well as qualities they have had prior to taking the position or have developed since accepting the role. There are courses offered by the American College of Physician Executives, the multiple graduate schools of public health, the Executive Leadership in Academic Medicine (ELAM) for women, and many others that offer executive training. In addition many institutions like Harvard, McGill, the Cleveland Clinic, the University of Texas, the University of Nebraska, Beth Israel Deaconess Medical Center, and many more have developed their own programs to grow leaders from within as well as outside the institution. In the past it was clear that being a good clinician and a good researcher, in addition to having an interest in education, were perhaps at the top of the qualifications to become a dean. The current status of medical schools and medicine in general now requires a separate set of skills and attributes. Nonetheless, excellence in clinical work and research is required for credibility among the faculty. So in truth most deans in this era will fulfill the old criteria, as well as the new proficiencies and personal characteristics.

Current courses often focus on various leadership styles, management, and negotiation. There has been an increasingly rapid turnover in medical school deans, chairs, and other senior administrators. In part this may be due to rapid changes in current finances and some leaders feeling unable to make needed adaptations. Today, the image of a full-time faculty member reading journal articles for hours on end in their offices is essentially dead. Deans are faced with frustrated faculty trying to balance extremely heavy clinical loads, weekly teaching sessions, and less protected time for scholarship and research. Those who have devoted their energy to research find a more competitive funding environment, along with heavy teaching responsibility.

The dean, who must remain enthusiastic about change, finds him or himself in an empathic position with faculty while trying to urge them to increase productivity. As one reviews this advice, it is clear that the serving leader model has much to offer. [3] The servant leader will assist faculty reporting to them to become their very best. Many authors' papers discussing leadership describe the necessity of surrounding oneself with bright energetic individuals on the team. Empowering team members and giving them ownership of specific projects increases their contentment with the job while making the leader more effective. This style of leadership does not just happen after one becomes a dean, but should be cultivated in prior areas of responsibility. More often than not, good team leaders will have favored status among candidates for these top positions in medical schools. As is often said, "there is no *I* in team." One's competitive spirit should be directed toward the outside where clinical or grants competition may be intense, while the medical school team needs the leader's encouragement for group success.

Longnecker et al. [4] surveyed 340 physician leaders in 281 AAMC member institutions. They reported "keys to job success included personal stature and relationships, clear definition of responsibilities, and the commitments of the Senior administration to the position." Although many of these physicians were chief medical officers, it is clear that the same qualities are helpful in almost any senior leadership position in medical schools. There is often a period of transition and conflict as one moves from being a faculty member to an administrative role. Changes in responsibility, stressful boundaries, and second guessing are challenges for the new leader [5]. Whether that is a chair, dean, or chief medical officer, there are multiple expectations from diverse directions. Faculty peers will not want their special relationships with the new leader to change and may struggle with ambiguity and allegiances. Maintaining and building on mutual respect for one's values, competence, and interpersonal communication are all invaluable to the new leader.

Forecasting and managing fiscal crises requires precious time and creativity. If one's approach is to see opportunity and effect timely structural change in policy or the administrative table, then the leader may successfully weather the storm. Communication with faculty is essential. Banta et al. [6] note the importance of long-range planning enhanced by the successful use of stakeholders. Deans and other medical officers are far more successful when they have received education on how to plan and manage these changes.

In the past, interim leaders were often chosen to be place holders acceptable to the administration and some were given the opportunity to try out for the leadership role. Grigsby et al. [7] report interim leadership is increasing, due to the more frequent turnover of deans, chairs, and other leadership positions. They urged that interim leadership receive formal training and mentorship. They describe the competencies needed by interim leaders to include the following: knowledge of the business of medicine; interpersonal communication skills; conflict resolution; ability to build and work with teams; and succession planning.

Duda [8] offers six principles that cultivate leadership in medicine beyond research and clinical expertise. She urges developing a vision, cultivating a plan, focusing on priorities, seeking counsel, coaching or mentoring, periodically reassessing, and finally enjoying the journey. Honest self-reflection is critically important to determine what one has to do to become strong leadership material. She also described various leadership styles including affiliated leadership, democratic leadership, pacesetting leadership, and coaching leadership. Duda believes the most successful leaders are those who can shift from one style to another style when the situation requires.

Many authors, including Duda [8], recognize the need for soul searching before making a decision to enter senior leadership. Examining likes, dislikes, strengths, and weaknesses is necessary. Questions to ask one's self before making a transition from the clinic to a senior administrative office include such points as the following: Can I think of mission globally, instead of department centered? Do I have the traits and skills needed for the position or am I willing to learn them even if that would make a dramatic reduction in my time at home? Am I willing to make the sacrifices needed to risk change and the possibility of it failing? Can I set aside past struggles with others in the institution? Do I really have a passion for education that would lead to improvements in the education process and lives of future patients? Am I ready to accept giving up a large portion of my patient practice? Can I be clinically competent with a small practice?

After Deciding to Take the Leap, How Do I Create a Plan?

One of the most helpful readings I found was written by Coleman et al. [9] as they followed two imaginary faculty members developing their careers in academic medicine. One had a clear plan and made decisions based on the plan that would enhance her likelihood of becoming a leader in the Medical Center. Although the other had terrific teaching skills and patient care, her decisions were much more random and circuitous. Clearly the earlier the plan is developed, the more likely the physician is to achieve his or her goal. Initially, the physician will want to make certain that they have a well-structured curriculum vita, begin an educator's portfolio, and reflect on the selection of an excellent mentor. Over the course of a career, the desired position may change as the individual moves up the ladder. At each stop there will be short-term and long-term goals that can be met by pursuing activities

Table 18.1 Leadership plan #1

	Volunteer to teach	Assist the person currently in that role	Volunteer to do a needs assessment or develop plan of improvement	Participate in national meetings (e.g., AAMC)	Help write a new curriculum or program information review	Publish and collaborate in area
Course director	✓	✓	✓	✓	✓	✓
Clerkship director	✓	✓	✓	✓	✓	✓
Residency program director (or fellowship)	✓	✓	✓	✓	✓	✓

Adapted from Coleman et al. [9]

locally and nationally. When to volunteer and accept new responsibilities must be given a great deal of thought to produce the desired outcomes. Coleman et al. [9] give many specific tips from designing your plan early and knowing expectations for promotion to establishing yourself as both a local and national leader (Tables 18.1 and 18.2). The why and how of finding successful mentors are emphasized.

Education Programs

A good way to begin is to investigate offerings at your own institution. Most large institutions now offer a host of faculty development sessions about teaching and curriculum design. In addition, courses are offered on organizational and leadership skills, communication and negotiation, and reviews of ways physicians can become more involved in their medical school. For example, looking at my own institution, current options include exploring innovative opportunities, engaging leaders to set goals, collaborative problem-solving, intellectual property, competence in patient care and working relationships, diversity leadership, hottest new IT trends, and improving communication among the generations. Many institutions, like ours, have offerings weekly and require patient care coverage and the department chair's permission. Those to ask what is available include officials in the curriculum office, graduate medical education, academy, or continuing medical education. In addition, some institutions finance doctors who may want additional formal education at another local university. The dean can also select persons to attend other more extended training and coaching, to be discussed in sections below.

Some programs are designed for specific specialties, although they may include factors important to any leader. Specialties have national organizations for residency program directors and most have developed a closely linked organization for clerkship directors. These are frequent next steps after one has been actively teaching and developing curriculum. Besides these specialty education organizations offering

Table 18.2 Leadership plan #2

	Achieve leadership role in department or division	Recruitment and selection experience	Participate in key institutional committees (education)	Publish in education	National leadership in educational committees	Business and financial training	Curricular design training
Dean	✓	✓	✓	✓	✓	✓	
Associate dean	✓	✓	✓	✓			
Admissions	✓	✓	✓	✓			
Student affairs	✓		✓	✓	✓		
Curriculum	✓		✓	✓			
Vice chair of education	✓						✓

Adapted from Coleman et al. [9]

classes, there are many other national opportunities in leadership training sponsored by colleges, universities, and professional societies [9].

The Harvard Macy Institute Fellowship program has been highly successful is promoting a variety of innovative improvements in medical education. Leaders are nominated to go from their home institutions to learn how to develop a needed plan for change in their own institution. Under the tutelage of skilled and experienced trainers, they learn about program implementation and outcome evaluation. Leadership, motivating others for change, and informational technology are also part of the program.

The Executive Leadership in Academic Medicine (ELAM) is another extended program that brings national leaders together to coach women in academics on leadership skills, strategic career planning, and management techniques that allow them to lead departments or organizations [10, 11]. Once again these physicians are nominated to attend. This is another organization that has a good track record for producing and mentoring leaders with many alums continuing to participate in the organization.

The Robert Woods Johnson Clinical Scholars Program provides two solid years of training in health service research, policy development, and preparation for academic careers.

Family Practice and Internal Medicine have developed outstanding training opportunities. Leadership Enhancement and Development or LEAD was established by the American College of Physicians. Plan development, leadership skills, and shared materials from other schools can be invaluable to the young academic. Likewise, the National Institute for Program Director Development (NIPDD) was the brain child of family physician educators who knew that learning about accreditation, developing skills to communicate with difficult residents, and encouraging teachers and trainees to approach patient care with the right attitude did not always come naturally. Their successful track record testifies to why leaders in other specialties may have been inspired to develop programs of their own.

Additional organizations that offer executive training helpful to future deans include the American College of Physician Executives and the American Management Association. The former provides assessment to build a customized program and executive coaching. There are general courses on negotiation, influence, informatics, presentation and interpersonal skills, running effective meetings, and facilitating team dynamics. Both organizations offer courses online and in many diverse cities.

Many business schools offer physician executive training that can be helpful in preparation for an academic administrative role. Wharton at the University of Pennsylvania, Weatherhead at Case Western Reserve University, Columbia, Booth at the University of Chicago and Duke offer courses to improve negotiation skills, enhance strategic planning, and provide financial awareness in the current healthcare economy. Although not specific for deans or academic executives, the training can enhance the physician's skill set. These are only a few of the universities offering such programs. Many are online as well as on site. Asking Google for dean

Table 18.3 Plan of action

Volunteer to teach
Develop excellence in teaching
Set career goals
Find a good mentor
Plan how to gain promotion
Network locally, regionally, nationally
Publish in education
Ask to assist in position you desire
Learn about skills needed
Proactively seek opportunities

Adapted from Coleman et al. [9]

training brought up over a thousand possibilities but one should look at the quality in addition to the convenience when making selections.

In summary, transitioning from research, clinical practice, and frontline teaching to becoming a senior administrative officer in a medical school can be immensely rewarding. It is not unusual to hear these individuals say this was the best job they ever had. Creating a plan that outlines helpful committee and organizational experiences is a first step (Table 18.3) [9]. A local and national network can be very beneficial when used effectively. Finding a great mentor or mentors and selecting needed course work add greatly to what you can offer. If you are already well prepared at the time an opportunity presents, you will have a much better chance to land your dream job.

References

1. Brater DC. The organization of medical education: a brief guide. In: Pangaro L, editor. Leadership careers in medical education. Philadelphia: ACP Press; 2010. p. 31–50.
2. Pangaro L. Profiles of leaders in medical education. In: Pangaro L, editor. Leadership careers in medical education. Philadelphia: ACP Press; 2010. p. 199–284.
3. Jennings K, Stahl-Wert J. The serving leader. Pittsburgh: Third River Partners; 2003.
4. Longnecker D, Patton M, Dickler RM. Roles and responsibilities of Chief Medical Officers in Member Organizations of the Association of American Medical Colleges. Acad Med. 2007;82(3):258–63.
5. Petersdorg RG. Deans and deaning in a changing world. Acad Med. 1997;72(11):953–8.
6. Banta TW, Busby AK, Kahn S, Black KE, Johnson JN. Responding to a fiscal crisis a data – driven approach. Assess Eval High Educ. 2007;32(2):183–94.
7. Grigsby RK, Aber RC, Quillen DA. Commentary: interim leadership of academic departments at U.S. medical schools. Acad Med. 2009;84:1328–9.
8. Duda RB. Physician and scientist leadership in academic medicine: strategic planning for a successful academic leadership career. Curr Surg. 2004;61(2):175–7.
9. Coleman T, Buckley P, Fincher R-M. Developing a career in academic medicine. In: Pangaro L, editor. Leadership careers in medical education. Philadelphia: ACP Press; 2010. p. 73–100; 98–9.

10. Dannels S, McLaughlin J, Gleason KA, McDade SA, Richman R, Morahan PS. Medical school deans' perceptions of organizational climate: useful indicators for advancement of women faculty and evaluation of a leadership program's impact. Acad Med. 2009;84(1): 67–79.
11. Richman RC, Morahan PS, Cohen DW, McDade SA. Advancing women and closing the leadership gap: the Executive Leadership in Academic Medicine (ELAM) program experience. J Womens Health Gend Based Med. 2001;10(3):271–7.

Suggested Reading

Banta TW, Busby AK, Kahn S, Black KE, Johnson JN. Responding to a fiscal crisis: a data-driven approach. Assess Eval High Educ. 2007;32(2):183–94.

Bordage G, Foley R, Goldyn S. Skills and attributes of directors or educational programmes. Med Educ. 2000;34:206–10.

Coller BS. Reflections on being a chair of medicine, 1993 to 2001 – part 1. Am J Med. 2004;116(1):68–72.

Coller BS. Reflections on being a chair of medicine, 1993 to 2001 – part 2. Am J Med. 2004;116(2):141–4.

Cuff P, Vanselow N, Neal A, Carr J. Prescription for the relief of curriculum constipation. (Review). PsychCRITIQUES. 2005;50(2). Electronic connection 2004-21484-001; www.apa.org/pubs/databases/index.aspx ISSN 1554-0138

Editorial. Enabling women in medicine to reach the top. Lancet. 2009;374(9699):1394.

Eisen JG. The role of the department chair in departmental decision-making. Diss Abstr Int. 1997;57(7A):2893.

Haden NK, Chaddock M, Hoffsis GF, Lloyd JW, Reed WM, Ranney RR, et al. Knowledge, skills, and attitudes of veterinary college deans: AAVMC survey of deans in 2010. J Vet Med Educ. 2010;37(3):210–9.

Lee A, Hoyle E. Who would become a successful Dean of Faculty of Medicine: academic or clinician or administrator? Med Teach. 2002;24(6):637–41.

Lobas JG. Leadership in academic medicine: capabilities and conditions for organizational success. Am J Med. 2006;119(7):617–21.

McCurdy FA, Beck G, Maroon A, Gomes H, Lane PH. The administrative colloquium: developing management and leadership skills for faculty. Ambul Pediatr. 2004;4(1):124–8.

Pangaro L, Bachicha J, Brodkey A, Chumley-Jones H, Fincher RM, Gelb D, et al. Alliance for clinical education: expectations of and for clerkship directors: a collaborative statement from the alliance for clinical education. Teach Learn Med. 2003;15(3):217–22.

Rayburn WF, Alexander H, Lang J, Scott JL. First-time department chairs at U.S. medical schools: a 29-year perspective on recruitment and retention. Acad Med. 2009;84(10):1336–41.

Rich EC, Magrane D, Kirch DG. Qualities of the medical school dean: insights from the literature. Acad Med. 2008;83(5):483–7.

Schuster B, Pangaro L. Understanding system of education: what to expect of, and for, each faculty member. In: Pangaro L, editor. Leadership careers in medical education. Philadelphia: ACP Press; 2010. p. 51–72.

Steinert Y, Nasmith L, Daigle N. Executive skills for medical faculty: a workshop description and evaluation. Med Teach. 2003;25(6):666–8.

Tarpley JL, Tarpley MJ. Tarp's baker's dozen: instructions to beginning program directors and some lessons learned. J Surg Educ. 2009;66(5):285–7.

Verrier ED. Becoming a division chief. J Thorac Cardiovasc Surg. 2001;121:S19–24.

Selected Educational Opportunities

American College of Physician Executives. www.acpe.org

Association of American Medical Colleges. www.aamc.org

Columbia Business School. www.columbia.edu

Duke Fuqua School of Business. www.fuqua.duke.edu

Executive Leadership in Academic Medicine ELAM (Women's Leadership Resources). www.mephu.edu/ELAM

Harvard Macy Institute. www.harvardmacy.org/programs/overview.aspx

University of Chicago Booth School of Business. www.chicagoexec.net

University of Pennsylvania Wharton School of Business. www.executiveeducation.wharton.upenn.edu

Cleveland Clinic Academy Leadership Track. www.academy.clevelandclinic.org

Selected Specialty Groups Offering Resources

American College of Physicians. www.acponline.org

American Association of Family Practice. www.aafp.org

Association of Directors for Medical Student Education in Psychiatry. www.admsep.org

Association of Professors of Gynecology and Obstetrics. www.apgo.org/home

Association of Program Directors in Internal Medicine. www.im.org/About/AllianceSites/APDIM

Consortium of Neurology Course Directors. www.aan.com/go/education/clerkship/consortium

Council on Medical Student Education in Pediatrics. www.comsep.org

Society of Teachers of Family Medicine. www.stfm.org

Part V
Law, Advocacy, and Public Service

Chapter 19
Legal Careers in Medicine

Key Points

- Health law and public health law are two legal fields where a medical background is beneficial.
- There are many exciting practice settings for a lawyer interested in healthcare: nonprofit organizations, law firms, government, and industry.
- Law can be a powerful tool in addressing social determinants of health and health rights.

Introduction

On the first day of my contracts class in law school, my professor warned that our medical school friends would be nervous to know that our first case, *Hawkins v. McGee*, involved medical malpractice. Law and medicine, doctors and lawyers, have often seemed to be on opposing sides. Yet law and medicine intersect in interesting ways. There are many practice areas in law for which a medical background is an asset, such as medical malpractice and patent law. There are also many ways in which the law can be used to promote health, through policy and litigation.

Law plays a powerful role in addressing social determinants of health. There is growing recognition that some of the largest gains in health can be achieved by addressing social determinants of health, which the World Health Organization

D. Gaskin (✉)
Student at Harvard Law and Harvard School of Public Health, 677 Huntington Avenue,
Kresge Building, Floor G, Mailbox 398 Boston, MA 02115, USA
e-mail: dgaskin@jd12.law.harvard.edu

R.D. Urman and J.M. Ehrenfeld (eds.), *Physicians' Pathways to Non-Traditional Careers and Leadership Opportunities*, DOI 10.1007/978-1-4614-0551-1_19,
© Springer Science+Business Media, LLC 2012

defines as "the circumstances in which people are born, grow up, live, work and age, and the systems put in place to deal with illness. These circumstances are in turn shaped by a wider set of forces: economics, social policies, and politics" [1].

Attorneys can help improve living and working conditions through litigation and advocacy by addressing low wages, occupational hazards, lead in homes, medical negligence, and access to social programs, such as food stamps and Medicaid.

These aforementioned areas are some of the multiple ways in which the law affects health and healthcare. Consequently, there are many different legal practice settings for which a medical background is helpful – nonprofit organizations and corporations, law firms, government, and industry.

Why Law? A Personal Story

I had always gone to college thinking I'd be a doctor. I was a pre-med, but also a government major. I was struggling to figure out which of these disciplines I liked more. [I went to medical school and] I thought that I could find ways to use my M.D. beyond clinical practice. There were many people who viewed the M.D. as a way to learn something about the field [of medicine], but also as a tool to do something else. That really interested me.

[Going to law school] was useful for sharpening my skill sets. [In both law and medicine I learned about] the importance of taking data and getting to an endpoint that is defensible. But in science, you are trying to rule out the gray areas…[whereas] law focuses much more on the gray areas [and] exploring their limits to make a case.

Ultimately, I thought that patent litigation was a good way to use my M.D. When you are reading through a patent, you find details regarding the scientific background that led to the invention…and being able to read that as a natural second language without having to look everything up, makes me a better and more effective lawyer. A lot of what I did in medicine has a payout on a daily basis… [it's] a living, breathing background with real utility for me as a lawyer.

-Dr. Hassen Sayeed, M.D., J.D.

Practice Settings

There are a variety of practice settings in which one might leverage a medical and legal degree. These include nonprofit organizations, law firms, government, and industry (see Fig. 19.1).

Nonprofit Organizations and Non-profit Corporations

An individual interested in public health can work for a nonprofit organization as a lawyer. Lawyers at nonprofit organizations often represent clients and help them receive social services. Other lawyers at nonprofits advocate for policy changes,

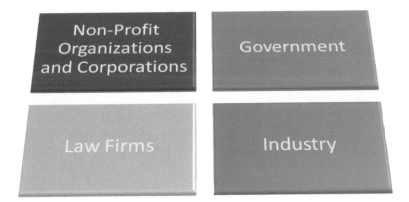

Fig. 19.1 Categories of legal practice settings

through research, lobbying, and testimony. And some lawyers work toward recognition of a right to health.

Nonprofit organizations often focus on specific health issues, such as HIV/AIDS, and in specific geographic areas. Some non-profit organizations work on domestic health issues and represent clients in the United States, while other nonprofit organizations work on global public health issues.

Additionally, lawyers who work for nonprofit organizations can help promote the mission of these organizations by providing legal support as in-house counsel. An in-house attorney might deal with many different legal areas – such as administrative law, contract law, employment law, patent law, and trusts and estates – that are important for a nonprofit organization.

Examples of nonprofit organizations involved in healthcare or public health include AIDS Action Committee, American Medical Association, EarthJustice, Healthcare for All, Médecins Sans Frontières, New York Lawyers for the Public Interest, Partners in Health, Physicians for Human Rights, Unite for Sight, the Whitman Walker Legal Services Program, and World Vision Foundation.

Hospitals are a type of nonprofit corporation where lawyers work. Lawyers who work for hospitals might do different types of work than a lawyer at a health issue-oriented nonprofit organization. In-house attorneys at hospitals work on general compliance and reimbursement issues, patient consent and confidentiality, and issues related to human subjects research.

Law Firms

Attorneys with a medical background who work for law firms frequently focus on intellectual property law, food and drug law, and/or health law. An attorney practicing in intellectual property law might focus on patent litigation. A medical background is particularly helpful in patent litigation because patents are commonly complex and based on fairly intricate science.

Health lawyers focus on antitrust, fraud, Medicaid and Medicare reimbursement issues and defend against medical malpractice. Health lawyers may also advise clients on regulatory issues, such as Health Insurance Portability and Accountability Act (HIPPA). Clients can include hospitals, pharmaceutical companies, health IT companies, biotechnology companies, medical groups and research institutions.

Public interest law firms are for-profit firms that advance missions through litigation and some public interest law firms focus on health. One example is the National Health Law Program. Public interest law firms do many types of legal work. A public interest law firm may try to improve health access and health services for racial minorities, immigrants, the elderly, the disabled, and the uninsured. A public interest law firm may also advocate for changes to health policy.

Plaintiff's firms are for-profit law firms that represent plaintiffs, often in large class-action cases. A plaintiff's firm might represent an individual who has faced unsafe work conditions or employment discrimination. Additionally, a plaintiff's firm could help a client who has been exposed to harmful chemicals, or who has been harmed by pharmaceuticals, medical devices, or medical negligence. A medical degree is advantageous in these tort actions. For example, in medical malpractice cases, a medical background enables an attorney to look at a potential client's patient records and determine if there has been a deviation from the reasonable standard of care.

Government

Government is another practice setting in which lawyers with medical backgrounds often work. The United States Department of Health and Human Services (HHS) has an Office of the General Counsel that advises the Secretary of HHS. The Office of the General Counsel is involved in many different areas important to our healthcare system, such as federal contracting, administrative law and high-level freedom of information requests (FOIA). HHS encompasses agencies such as the Food and Drug Administration (FDA), the National Institutes of Health (NIH), the Centers for Disease Control and Prevention (CDC), the Center for Medicare and Medicaid Services (CMS), the Indian Health Service (IHS), and the Agency for Healthcare Research and Quality (AHRQ). The Office of the General Counsel houses attorneys who advise these specific agencies. Some health areas that attorneys work on specifically include drug approvals, food safety, vaccine safety, bio-terrorism preparedness, and patient privacy.

State government also provides numerous opportunities in health law and public health law. For example, a Department of Public Health lawyer sometimes tackles serious ethical issues, such as whether and if an individual with multidrug resistant tuberculosis should be quarantined. Lawyers for a Department of Public Health also deal with administrative hearings. At an Attorney General's Office, a lawyer, commonly called an Assistant Attorney General, defends the state's health agencies, such as the Department of Public Health and the Department of Social Services, in state and federal litigation. In addition, an Assistant Attorney General sometimes is involved with compliance issues, defends the state against class-action lawsuits and represents state hospitals.

Another practice setting is intergovernmental organizations, such as the United Nations and the World Bank. These organizations often promote health by providing funding for public health projects. Lawyers at these and similar intergovernmental organizations often deal with contract dispute litigation, compliance issues, and corruption and fraud related to specific projects.

Industry

A medical background can be advantageous for work in the healthcare industry as well. An individual with a medical background can provide nuanced advice and creative solutions. Furthermore, a lawyer with a medical background might understand the culture better and have more credibility with industry professionals.

Insurance companies, managed care organizations and pharmaceutical companies all have in-house counsel. Attorneys who are in-house counsel for insurance and managed care companies handle general legal issues such as compliance, reporting requirements, and rate payment agreements. At an insurance company or a managed care company, a medical background would be helpful in determining what medical procedures should be reimbursed and covered. Lawyers for pharmaceutical companies help file patents, enforce patents, challenge patents and defend patents. Lawyers at pharmaceutical companies also deal with the drug approval processes, compliance issues, and reporting requirements.

Requirements

To work as an attorney in a nonprofit organization or corporation, a private, public interest, or plaintiff's law firm, a governmental agency or in an industry, a Juris Doctorate (J.D.) is required. It takes 2–3 years to get a J.D. and afterward graduates must pass a bar exam to gain admission to a state bar and practice.

To gain admission into law school, students usually must take the L.S.A.T. Applicants interested in medicine or health may apply to law school after graduation from college, after the completion of a medical degree, or concurrently during medical school as an increasing number of universities have established J.D.-M.D. dual degree programs (see Fig. 19.2). Many of these programs allow students to earn a J.D. and M.D. in less time than it would take to earn both degrees separately. Some programs allow students to complete a J.D.-M.D. dual degree program in 6 years.

Prospective applicants need not decide whether they will do a combined degree program before entering medical school or law school as some schools allow

Baylor College of Medicine
Case Western Reserve University School of Medicine
Duke University School of Medicine
Mayo Medical School
Ohio State University College of Medicine
Southern Illinois University School of Medicine
Texas Tech University School of Medicine
University of Arizona College of Medicine
University of Arkansas College of Medicine
University of Chicago Pritzker School of Medicine
University of Florida College of Medicine
Vanderbilt University School of Medicine
Yale University School of Medicine

Fig. 19.2 Medical schools with combined J.D.-M.D. programs

current first or second year medical students or law students to apply to the joint J.D.-M.D. program after the first year or two of medical school or law school. Students must meet the independent entrance requirements for both the medical school and the law school to participate in a university's combined J.D.-M.D. program.

In addition, many law schools have loan repayment assistance programs to help law students who go into public interest careers (which includes nonprofit organizations, government and public interest law firms) or who make less than a designated amount of money to repay their loans.

A J.D. is not required for all job opportunities within law. Physicians are in high demand to work with law firms as "experts," particularly in medical malpractice cases. Physicians also consult to help law firms with specific projects, such as developing a doctor and hospital rating system. To explore legal careers, consider speaking to current lawyers and volunteering at a health-focused nonprofit organization, law firm or legal services center.

Conclusions

Health law and public health law are exciting, dynamic areas of the law. A medical background can be beneficial for the practice of these areas of law. Yet attaining both a medical degree and law degree requires a huge investment in time, energy, and money. Have a good idea about how your medical and law degree can complement each other and advance your career. Consider reaching out to professionals who work in health law or public health law to learn more about the type of work they do and their specific backgrounds.

There is truly a need for more individuals with interdisciplinary backgrounds to become involved in public health and medicine. If you do decide to pursue an M.D. and J.D., don't be dissuaded by what seems to be a daunting and less-travelled path.

Acknowledgments Many thanks to Catherine Pattanayak , Hassen Sayeed, and Devesh Tiwary for their comments and help with this chapter.

Reference

1. World Health Organization. Social determinants of health: key concepts. http://www.who.int/social_determinants/thecommission/finalreport/key_concepts/en/index.html. Accessed 14 Oct 2010.

Additional Resources

To explore the intersection of law and medicine, visit the American College of Legal Medicine's website at http://www.aclm.org/

For more information about the field of public health law, consider Larry O. Gostin's Public Health Law: Power, Duty, Restraint. 2nd ed. Los Angeles: University of California Press; 2008.

For further information about corporate and business law firms with healthcare and intellectual property practices, some useful websites include the Vault http://www.vault.com, the NALP Directory of Legal Employers http://www.nalpdirectory.com/, the American Bar Association's Health Law Section, http://www.abanet.org/health/, the American Bar Association's Intellectual Property Section, http://www.abanet.org/intelprop/, and the American Health Lawyer's Association, http://www.healthlawyers.org/

To learn more about public interest law firms and plaintiff's firms, consult the Bernard Koteen Office of Public Interest Advising at Harvard Law School's (OPIA) Private Public Interest and Plaintiff's Firm Guide at http://www.law.harvard.edu/current/careers/opia/planning/career-resources/docs/privatepiguide2010.pdf

For additional information on universities with J.D.-M.D. combined degree programs, please visit http://services.aamc.org/currdir/

For general information about law schools and law school requirements, go to the Law School Admission Council's (LSAC) website at http://lsac.org/

Chapter 20
Additional Opportunities in the Legal Field and Applying to Law School

Gregory Dolin

Key Points

- Opportunities in the legal arena include organized medicine, teaching, patents, healthcare law, business, among others.
- Career path includes taking the LSAT, getting admitted into a law school, passing the bar exam, and doing a judicial clerkship.
- While one can hold both a medical and a law degree, both professions require a great deal of time commitment and continuing education.

Introduction

One of the most versatile graduate degrees is the *Juris Doctor* (JD). Although commonly thought of as only leading to the practice of law, the law degree allows the individual to work and be competitive in a number of industries, including (as should be apparent to the reader of this book) medicine. That said, it would be surprising if a doctor or a future doctor did not ask why he would need a law degree. After all, doctors and lawyers are often portrayed as sworn enemies. The reality, however, is more complicated. A doctor with a law degree is becoming more and more common with every passing law school graduation. In this chapter, I will describe several opportunities that are available to physicians with law degrees.

G. Dolin, MD, JD (✉)
University of Baltimore School of Law/Johns Hopkins University School of Medicine,
Baltimore, MD 21201, USA
e-mail: greg.dolin@gmail.com

R.D. Urman and J.M. Ehrenfeld (eds.), *Physicians' Pathways to Non-Traditional Careers and Leadership Opportunities*, DOI 10.1007/978-1-4614-0551-1_20,
© Springer Science+Business Media, LLC 2012

Afterwards, I will explain what is necessary to obtain such a degree and offer a few notes of caution about law school in general.

Organized Medicine

A law degree may serve a physician well if he wishes to dedicate his time to organized medicine, be it the American Medical Association, the State Society, or a specialty organization. By their nature, all of these organizations deal with legal issues that impact the practice of medicine. Whether it is the new Medicare fraud and abuse rules, or proposal to adjust the scope of practice for various medical professions, doctors need to know whether and how to respond. To be sure, most of these organizations have sophisticated in-house and outside attorneys who advise them on these matters. However, having a fuller understanding of the legal landscape would allow a member physician to more fully engage with the issue both inside the organization and during lobbying activities.

By way of an example, consider the AMA's Council on Legislation. The Council is charged, amongst other things, with evaluating pending legislative and administrative proposals that will impact the practice of medicine. Although the Council is advised by the AMA's attorneys, ultimately the voting power and the responsibility for the decisions made resides with the physician members of the Council. Imagine how much more convincing and authoritative is the voice of someone who understands not just the generalities and broad strokes of policy, but the minute details as well. A person with such an understanding could be a lead voice in the body, and could better represent the decisions made to the membership at large. By the same token, a person with a legal education would be a better external spokesman to the non-physician policy-makers (whether in the legislative or executive branches). Such an education would allow its holder to engage the policy makers in a more precise and detailed discussion of almost any proposed bill or rule. In short, a legal education can be an invaluable asset in organized medicine.

Teaching

Another opportunity for doctors with legal education is teaching either in law school or in medical school. More and more law schools educate their students on the very basic concepts of law and legal duties of physicians. Concepts such as malpractice, informed consent, duty of disclosure, patient's rights and physician's legal duties are introduced to medical students – often during their first year of school. Therefore, someone knowledgeable ought to teach these concepts. It is hard to imagine a person better suited to the task than someone who has both legal and medical education. To be sure, because the courses of this type are relatively short, it is not likely that this can be sole employment. However, such an opportunity can be combined with active clinical or research practice. It would also allow a physician practicing in a specialty where student rotations are few to interact with medical students on a regular basis.

An alternative to teaching in medical schools is teaching in law schools. This opportunity comes in two varieties – an adjunct professor and a permanent faculty member. The former option is in many ways similar to the medical school teaching opportunity. It allows one to teach a usually small course every year that focuses on some discrete issue at the intersection of law and medicine or science. Generally, and unsurprisingly, the course would be more legally-focused than a similar arrangement in medical school. Thus, anyone undertaking such an endeavor would not only need to have a law degree, but will have to keep up with current developments in the law. On the other hand, because adjuncts usually do not teach core courses, but rather elective seminars, they can choose when and how often they are willing to teach. The elective offerings in law school that could benefit from being taught by a doctor-lawyer are vast and varied. Courses on alternative and complementary medicine, medical malpractice, and healthcare delivery, just to name a few, would profit from being taught by someone who has a medical education and practices (or previously practiced) medicine as his primary profession.

The other career option is that of a permanent member of a law school faculty. This is radically different from the previous two teaching options. Whereas the other two options presuppose that one would continue to engage in medicine as primary occupation, becoming a permanent member of a law school faculty presupposes just the opposite. A permanent member of a law school faculty is expected to engage in serious legal scholarship in addition to teaching students. The scholarship, of course, can be related to the medical or scientific field, but the scholarship has to be legal in nature. This means that there will be little time for other professional endeavors, and certainly not enough to remain a *good* doctor.

While one can hold both a medical and a law degree, both professions require too much time commitment and too much continuing education to be able to do both at the highest level. Therefore, to the extent that excellence is the goal, one of the two professions has to be chosen to the exclusion of another.

Should one choose law over medicine and within that choice choose legal academia, one would most likely begin making steps towards that career fairly soon out of law school. While there may be a number of pathways to legal academia, the most common involve clerking for a (usually federal) judge right after law school, publishing one or more law review articles prior to applying for a position, and often completing an academic fellowship in one of the law schools. Although a number of people made the transition to legal academia later in their careers, there is a palpable preference on the part of law schools to hire younger promising intellectuals rather than former practitioners.

A legal academic with a medical degree may be well suited to teaching Torts (as that class often draws on issues from medical malpractice); Professional Responsibility and Ethics (as that course would allow for interesting comparisons between doctors' and lawyers' duties to their clients), as well as more specialized courses such as Healthcare Law, Law and Psychology, Law and Science, etc. Additionally, as medical school and pre-medical curriculum would have provided significant scientific training, teaching patent law courses (especially courses on biotechnology and patents) would seem to be a natural fit. The same is true of the research part of the job.

All of the aforementioned areas would likely be a good fit and should generally be of interest to someone who wishes to utilize medical knowledge in legal academia.

The Practicing Attorney

Obtaining a law degree of course presents one with an opportunity to enter practice of law full-time. Lawyers who are also trained physicians are quite sought after. While there is no restriction on which field of law one can practice (once one is admitted to the bar), there are certain fields that are a natural fit for an individual with medical and/ or scientific training and background. The most obvious ones are patent law, healthcare law, and medical malpractice law. I will briefly discuss each of these.

Patent law deals with obtaining patents on various inventions and then litigating over the patents obtained. Because patents are complex documents that are drafted at the intersection of law and science, attorneys who deal with patents usually have a scientific background. Indeed, it is not uncommon for patent attorneys to have Master of Science or PhD degrees. When the technology involves medical devices, instruments, or pharmaceutical products, knowledge and perspective of someone who is a trained physician is often invaluable. Not only can a competent physician-cum-lawyer understand the technology quickly, and build legal strategy accordingly, he can be extraordinarily useful in communicating with inventors and expert witnesses, both of whom are usually scientists and not lawyers.

In addition to patent litigation, one can practice "patent prosecution." This area of practice involves "prosecuting" patent applications in the US Patent and Trademark Office (USPTO). In other words, the practice involves filing the applications and attempting to convince the Patent Office that patents should ultimately issue. In order to be licensed to work before the USPTO, it is not enough to merely be an attorney. The Office requires that anyone seeking to represent clients in the patent proceedings possess either scientific or engineering education. This is so because the representative needs to understand not only the legal standards, but also the state of the art of the relevant technology. The attorney needs to be able to differentiate the invention on which the patent is sought from that which has been invented and disclosed previously. This may be an impossible task in disciplines such as medicine, pharmaceuticals, and the like, unless the attorney is educated in those or related areas. For this reason, having a medical degree is highly useful to those who seek employment as patent prosecutors.

Another area of law that could be of interest to a trained physician is healthcare law. This area is too broad and varied and the space allocated to this chapter is too short to fully discuss all that is subsumed under the heading of "healthcare law," but the more obvious and popular areas should be mentioned. First, the practice in the area of Food and Drug law (usually in front of the Food and Drug Administration) would be a prime target for lawyers with medical degrees. Same is true for practice in the area of healthcare fraud and abuse (either on the prosecuting or defense side). One who has spent time practicing medicine can ferret out the fraud or, conversely, the weaknesses in government's case, than one without medical practice experience. Healthcare financing law is yet another area where first-hand experience provides competitive advantage to the attorney practicing in this field. These are just examples of a very broad, varied, and exciting area of law. What is also interesting is that one can specialize in healthcare law not only by being a "practicing attorney" – i.e., working for a law firm, but also by working for a lobbying firm, or for an administrative agency, or as a staff member in the legislative branch. Furthermore, one can move with relative ease between these employments and use experience gained in one job to excel in the other.

The third area of legal practice where the combination of medical and legal degrees provides an advantage to the holder is medical malpractice. This is true irrespective of whether one chooses the plaintiff or defense bar. In either circumstance, and for obvious reasons, the medical expertise is extremely useful for an attorney. Should one become a plaintiffs' attorney, that expertise can be used to separate meritorious cases from the frivolous ones fairly quickly. If one is more inclined to work on defense's side, then the expertise can be used to better advise clients whether their actions were indeed negligent and whether settlement rather than trial is appropriate.

Other Options

By any means, the above-list should not be thought of as exhaustive. There are many other opportunities a physician with a legal education (or a lawyer with a medical education) can pursue. Possibilities are varied and can include everything from lobbying to investment banking to consulting to running for public office. Ultimately, no matter what path is taken, what will be important to figure out is how the acquired education and knowledge can be melded to yield maximum benefits in the chosen career.

The Path to and Through Law School

Admission to law school is dependent mostly, if not exclusively, on two criteria: undergraduate GPA and the score on the Law School Admission Test (LSAT). While some law schools will take other measures of ability (such as graduate degree, prior work experience, etc.) into account, the admission process is overwhelmingly governed by the combination of the GPA and LSAT. The LSAT is administered four times a year: in June, September/October, December, and February. Although many schools, including the top ones, have rolling deadlines, the February administration is oftentimes too late to seek admission for the following September. The LSAT is a multiple choice exam that tests logical reasoning, reading comprehension and analytical reasoning. Doing well on the LSAT is absolutely crucial to getting into a highly ranked school.

It is also important to point out that law schools are not like medical schools in terms of quality of education and post-graduation career options. Whereas medical schools all follow the same basic curriculum and provide the same basic exposure to variety of diseases and patients, the quality of education in law schools is much more varied. Furthermore, unlike medical schools, where one's choice of residency is significantly determined by the performance on the USMLE exam and not necessarily the name or type of school attended, the choice of law school is highly influential if not determinative in the career choices. For these reasons, one should think long and hard before accepting an offer of enrollment from a not highly ranked school, especially if the offer is not accompanied by a significant scholarship. Simply put, it is hard to justify an investment of over $100,000 when the return may never materialize. In short, in choosing a law school, one must be cautious and inquire into the placement of recent graduates. At the same time, this is not to say that only graduates of top law schools get good and interesting legal jobs. Every year, graduates of law schools that are not in the top ten get prestigious judicial clerkships (including those with the Supreme Court), jobs in large law firms, interesting government employment, and so on. The chances of landing those jobs, however, are directly related to the prestige of the law school.

After graduating from law school, an aspiring attorney must take the bar exam in the state where he wishes to practice. Unlike the USMLE, the bar exam must be taken in each state where license is sought (though some states will waive the exam for attorneys who have been licensed in another state and in practice for over 5 years). In most states, the bar exam is administered twice a year – in July and February. One should sit for the bar, even if one plans to continue practicing medicine rather than law. Being admitted to the bar gives added weight to the law degree credential. Most law graduates take bar review courses in preparation for the bar. Despite the high anxiety associated with the exam, graduates of top law schools almost uniformly pass the exam, and graduates of other US schools do so by overwhelming numbers. Once the bar exam is passed (the results usually come out 4–5 months later), one's legal education is complete, and upon satisfying the character and fitness requirements, one is admitted to the practice of law and can embark on any of the careers previously described.

Additional Information

American College of Legal Medicine: www.aclm.org
Law School Admission Council: www.lsac.org
United States Patent and Trademark Office: www.uspto.gov
American Intellectual Property Law Association: www.aipla.org
American Association for Justice, also known as the Association of Trial Lawyers of America: www.justice.org
American Medical Association: www.ama-assn.org
Association of American Law Schools: www.aals.org

Chapter 21
Politics and Legislative Advocacy

Alexander Ding

Key Points

- Physicians should be active in civic engagement and can have an active political life.
- Multiple routes of political involvement can range from small tasks to large career changes.
- Physicians can have high impact in advocacy because they are well-respected; however, learning the art of politics can make them even more effective.

Introduction

Physicians are frequently seen as public servants, selflessly caring for the ill masses, the frail, and the vulnerable. Yet, too often physicians are hesitant or even loath to participate in public service and engage with, or serve as, politicians. Many physicians believe, as does much of the general public, that politics is a dirty game. Doctors feel because of the social status of their profession that we are above politics and above the fray. We would instead encourage and urge you to involve yourself in this realm.

Doctors often fail to recognize the role that they can play in the public discourse. As the government assumes a larger role in healthcare systems and financing, physicians will likely take more interest in politics, as decisions made not at the bedside, but rather in Washington or state capitals begin to affect patient care, physician livelihood, and professional autonomy. A common Washington insider saying goes as follows: "if you are not at the table, you are on the menu."

A. Ding, MD, MS (✉)
Department of Radiology, Massachusetts General Hospital/Harvard Medical School,
55 Fruit Street, Boston, MA 02114, USA
e-mail: adingl@partners.org

R.D. Urman and J.M. Ehrenfeld (eds.), *Physicians' Pathways to Non-Traditional
Careers and Leadership Opportunities*, DOI 10.1007/978-1-4614-0551-1_21,
© Springer Science+Business Media, LLC 2012

Table 21.1 Public confidence in each group to recommend the right thing for healthcare reform

% Confidence	All	Democrats	Independents	Republicans
Doctors	77	78	74	79
Hospitals	64	62	63	65
Academics	61	76	61	43
US President	49	83	44	13
Pharmaceuticals	30	29	27	33
Health insurers	26	25	25	28

Physicians also fail to recognize the skills and knowledge that they have to translate well into public service. Not only are physicians well versed members of the healthcare delivery system who can provide expertise on myriad aspects of the clinical, organizational, and economic aspects of healthcare, but they are also looked toward for leadership. Doctors are by profession and training leaders of clinical teams, medical homes, medical staffs, and hospitals. We are staunch patient advocates who know how to stand up for our patients, and we know how to speak for others when they cannot speak themselves. The thinking process in which we are trained emphasizes differential diagnoses and cost-benefit analysis, thereby allowing us to consider multiple solutions to a problem and to deliberatively consider both pros and cons of each. We recognize the importance of evidence-based practices, surely something that would serve well as the foundations of legislation.

The esteem in which we are held by the general public also means we are looked upon by the people for guidance and leadership. A Gallup poll from March 2010 [1] found that over three-quarters (77%) of Americans had confidence in physicians to reform the healthcare system (see Table 21.1). This was 13% more than the next highest group (hospitals), and more than 28% higher than the President of the United States. Physicians also commanded the top bipartisan support and confidence. This level of support is an invitation to lead and the following discussion will provide you with more practical information and resources for you to get more involved.

Physicians are busy professionals, and the juggling of clinical practice, family life, administrative duties, and sometimes research seems daunting in and of itself. However, participation in the political arena is not an all-or-none game. Multiple avenues for involvement exist from marginal involvement to new career paths. In this chapter, we will discuss the various ways to become more involved in the political process and perhaps even to run for elected office, which physicians are increasingly interested in doing.

Elected Office

Running for political office is a challenging endeavor and many physician-politicians have stated that the race for office is even tougher than medical school and residency training. However, serving the public in this way is a great honor and privilege.

Multiple levels of elected office exist, including local, state, and federal positions. Opportunities primarily start in the legislature or other special jurisdictions, such as the school board. Executive and constitutional offices are difficult to get your start in without prior legislative experience or large financial backing, and some locales which have elected judicial offices are likely out of reach for most physicians.

Generally, physicians are viewed as trustworthy, caring, and intellectually capable by the public, which are traits noted to be important for officeholders to possess and serve as a great foundation for physician candidacies. A national study from the American Medical Association Political Action Committee [2] from 2008 reported the public perception of physician-candidates. Respondents stated that physicians' perceived traits most helpful for a role in office are their ability to effectively research complex issues and the ability to make sound decisions in stressful situations.

Surprisingly, medical doctors were not seen as the best qualified individuals to serve in the public office because of their perceived limited expertise in the health-care field. At the time, respondents noted the economy to be the most important issue facing the country, with healthcare as a distant second. Respondents also did not believe physicians were able to manage the rough nature of politics. Therefore, physician-candidates would be wise to establish early credibility in a wide variety of social issues, and to focus their campaign on issues most important to voters. While establishing an expertise in the healthcare system is important, "perseverating" on healthcare is not likely to appeal to a winning base of voters. Nevertheless, as the economy revitalizes and the broad national health system reform legislation passed in 2010 rolls into effect, more physicians will run for office and use their expertise in healthcare to their advantage.

In fact, at the time of this writing 47 physicians were running for national office, in addition to the 16 physician-politicians already in office. This number has been steadily increasing in this century, with 22 physician-candidates in 2006 and 30 in 2008 [3]. However interestingly, this current count of physician members of Congress and Senate is not at its peak. During the first century of the American Congress, up to 5% of all elected officials were physicians.

Even individuals who are interested in running for office are often at a loss for where to start. Having roots in your home district, familiarity with the community and civic engagement are a near must for a credible start. While physicians are used to formal training programs before practice, politics does not have such a requirement. Therefore, the challenges of being a candidate are often underestimated and not well understood or addressed. For example, physicians rarely have much experience in fundraising. Increasingly, candidates are required to raise more and more money to be seen as a viable candidate, to afford experienced staff, and to pay for expensive media campaigns. In 2006, the average national Senate candidate raised $3.3 million and the average House candidate raised over $650,000 [4, 5]. This was an approximately 33% increase compared with just two election cycles prior.

Campaigns require well-thought-out planning, including addressing campaign strategy and formulating a message. Dealing with the media, driving fundraising, managing public appearances, and voter contact are all unfamiliar territory for most

Table 21.2 Campaign
considerations

Personal qualifications and attributes
Local and national political environment
Message formulation
Media buys
Campaign strategy
Staff management
Fundraising and contribution reporting
Public appearances, speeches, and debates
Voter contact and get-out-the-vote
Opposition research

physicians and can scare many potential candidates from even starting. These and other considerations are listed in Table 21.2. Fatal miscalculation and misunderstanding of these important components for a successful campaign have led many candidates to lose a race much before it has even started.

The American Medical Association Political Action Committee is well aware of this overwhelming nature of campaigns and runs an annual campaign school and a candidate workshop for physicians interested in running for office and for those helping other candidates with their races. The school focuses on pedagogy related to all of the issues addressed above and also runs a mock-campaign for a more nuanced understanding of all the moving parts in a campaign. The school's success has seen the election of multiple members of Congress, Senate, and local physician-politicians, including nearly half of the physician members of the 111th Congress. If you are considering running for office or helping in a campaign, the school is free of charge and with the mission to educate more physician-candidates.

Appointed/Selected Positions

If putting yourself in front of people for elections disagrees with your personality or goals, seeking appointed positions can be another avenue for political involvement. In government, at all levels, there are numbers of positions that require technical expertise in healthcare. Certainly, there are high level and high profile appointments that include well-known positions such as Surgeon General, Secretary of Health and Human Services, and Commissioner of the Food and Drug Administration. These positions do generally go to people who are well connected politically or have high-caliber academic names behind them. As the new health system reform legislation is implemented, more government commissions and committees will be formed, and the need for appointed leaders will increase.

Numerous appointed positions exist at all levels of government requiring those with healthcare expertise (see Table 21.3). The overwhelming majority are not high profile, and the approval process is generally without much fanfare or contention.

Table 21.3 Examples of appointed positions at various governmental levels

Local (county or city)	State	Federal
Medical Examiner–Coroner	Board of Registration in Medicine	Secretary of Health and Human Services
Director of Health Services	Commissioner of Public Health	Surgeon General
Commissioner of Mental Health	Director of Medicaid	Commissioner of the Food and Drug Administration

For example, there are local health and/or public health boards, which often seek members with a background in healthcare. The appointment process is often opaque and it can be difficult to figure out how to apply or be considered for one of these positions. Some places have formal applications, which are available on their websites, however, more often they are offered to those more politically involved. Therefore, a relationship with your government official and their staff can be quite helpful in identifying these opportunities. The time commitment for these opportunities can vary widely from full-time job to occasional meetings after hours. The Federal government does have a listing of all available Federal appointed positions in a book known as the Plum Book, which is published every 4 years just after the Presidential election.

If you have an interest in really experiencing and working in the day-to-day affairs of running the government, consider a staff position with a member of the legislature, an executive office, or with a legislative committee. While this would require that you take a hiatus from your clinical duties, a lot can be gleaned from these opportunities. A number of physicians took the opportunity during the recent federal health overhaul legislative session to work for the President's White House Office for Health Reform, the Senate Committee on Health, Education, Labor, and Pensions, and in the officers of multiple legislators as Legislative Directors for Health.

There are a number of opportunities for medical students and residents, in particular, for staff positions in legislators' offices and within organized medicine. Nearly every legislator offers internships, in which medical students would be able to bring a significant advantage of health system understanding that undergraduate college grads simply cannot grasp. The American Medical Association offers positions for medical students and residents to spend a defined amount of time in their government relations offices, which includes training on interacting with Congress and may present with an opportunity to testify before a Congressional hearing. Other specialty organizations have similar offerings, including the American College of Radiology and the American Society of Anesthesiology. Young physicians and junior staff may consider the ultimate public service and leadership opportunity to work in the White House as a fellow, which is a highly prestigious and competitive program, where young professionals work at the highest levels of the federal executive branch. Government and professional organization websites will have more information on these opportunities.

Legislative Advocacy

Taking part in the political process does not always require a formal position in government. In fact, many practicing physicians across the country engage their government officials on a regular basis and in doing so provide legislators and governors' perspective and insight into the challenges and problems faced by actual patients and physicians in the trenches. These relationships with legislators are mutually beneficial as physicians have the ear of an influential person, and legislators gain a better understanding of the results and consequences of their proposals.

Many physicians take part in engaging their elected officials through organized medical groups. Virtually all of your professional organizations, including the American Medical Association, state and local medical societies, and specialty professional associations have departments dedicated to legislative advocacy and government relations. These organizations hire professional lobbyists to represent you, the practicing physician, when working with legislators. While the term "lobbyist" may have negative connotations, they are vital members of your professional organizations' staff who are your eyes, ears, and voice in interactions with the government. It would be impossible to be a practicing physician trying to manage all of the day-to-day workings and proposals in government along with your daily clinical schedule. Lobbyists, sometimes known as government relations staff, have established relationships with government officials and their staffs and leverage these relationships to educate members of the legislature on issues important to your practice.

Nevertheless, just because your professional organization has professional staff speaking on your behalf, it does not mean that your engagement with your elected officials is not important. Generally speaking, elected officials are more interested in hearing from the practicing physician and a constituent than the lobbyist. You, as a physician, see and understand the day-to-day practice of medicine and how the government's laws and regulations are actually affecting patient care. You tell the story of your practice, your staff, and your patients and how government is either helping or hurting your efforts in taking care of your patients who may also be your legislator's constituents.

There are several tips that can make you more effective when speaking with elected officials. First, you have to figure out what the message is that you are trying to convey. This can be figured out simply by thinking this through and being organized before you start your session or it is often helpful to touch base with your professional organization that can help you focus. Second, once you know what your message is going to be, staying on message is vital. It is easy to ramble, take tangents, and be diverted from your message. But, if you really want to make sure your official hears what you are trying to say, don't stray too far from your intended line.

Legislation and regulation is a complex task, as is medicine and the healthcare system; sometimes it seems as if both sides of the table are speaking different languages. Therefore, it is important for you to explain your ideas simply, minimizing jargon and technical speak. You should also try to do a little education and give a

Table 21.4 Tips for speaking with your elected official

Call or email your official's office to schedule a meeting

An in-person visit is always most effective

If you can only call, write or email, personalize it with your own experience

Come up with a coherent message and stay on message

Use layman's terms and avoid medical or policy jargon

Leverage your own experience and use anecdotes

Highlight how proposed policies will affect your practice and your patients

Encourage your representative to take a stance or a leadership role on the issue

Always be respectful

broad overview on complex issues that you simply cannot expect someone outside of your profession or field to fully grasp. While you may be frustrated that others don't understand your issues, there is no better opportunity than now to fill an empty vessel. The use of anecdotes is especially helpful. Politicians both understand and are trained to leverage emotions. Therefore, if you can use this skill in your anecdote telling, it is bound to be more effective than citing statistics and facts (which is how physicians understand and are trained).

Remember, you are having a discussion with your representative in government. This is not a lecture where you do all the talking and the end of the meeting is when you are done delivering your message. Be concise and clear. Give the legislator and staff a chance to ask for clarification or for questions. Also, don't be hesitant to ask them for their position and their support on your issue. Just be cognizant that they may not yet have decided or may disagree with your position.

The most important piece of advice, however, is to be respectful to both elected officials and their staff for obvious reasons. Remember that you represent yourself, other physicians, and your patients. Certainly, there may be times where you disagree with their position, but there is never an excuse for acting badly. In politics there are no permanent enemies, and it is important that you maintain relationships and not burn any bridges.

For example, information on practical ways to more effectively communicate with your government leaders and for a better understanding of the legislative process may be found in your State Medical Society's Legislative Handbook, which is full of useful advice and information for how to more effectively advocate for your issues. These may be available if you contact your Medical Society, and similar resources may be available from your own professional organization. A summary of points to keep in mind when speaking with elected officials is listed in Table 21.4.

Other (Easier) Ways to Get Involved

Beyond the ways to get involved described above, there are a number of other ways to whet your appetite for politics. It is vital that physicians take part in their communities, as leaders and mentors, and even a little contribution can go a long way.

In a robust democracy such as ours, there is an endless cycle of campaigns and elections. An old political adage states that "all politics is local." Therefore, a great way to get involved in community and politics is to help out a local politician's campaign.

Monetary donations are always important for a successful campaign, and contributing funds to your preferred candidate or political action committee (PAC) can be very helpful in supporting a person or organization with their goals. You could even take it further and offer to hold a fundraiser for a candidate at your home or set up your own "Physicians for XXX candidate" group.

Despite the necessity of money in campaigns, a more hands-on approach is to actually volunteer and to donate your time. This arguably is more vital for the success of a candidate. You might offer to make phone calls, walk precincts, become one of the campaign staff, or really use your technical expertise in medicine and offer to serve on a candidate's health advisory committee.

No matter what you decide is the right role for you, should maintain an active political life whether it is for a cause, a candidate, an organization, or an ideal. You can call and write your elected officials and you can extend your hand and offer them more, perhaps some of your expertise in healthcare. Always do what you feel is the right thing for your colleagues and your patients. And don't forget to VOTE!

Acknowledgment The author would like to acknowledge and thank Jim Wilson, PhD. from the American Medical Association for many of the resources and references used in writing this chapter.

References

1. Gallup Poll. 5 Mar 2010. http://www.gallup.com/poll/126338/obama-retains-trust-congress-healthcare.aspx. Accessed 20 Jul 2010.
2. AMPAC/Marketscope Research on Physician-Candidates. Internal documents from American Medical Association. 3 Jun 2008.
3. Fritze J. Doctors pursue House, Senate seats. USA Today. 20 Apr 2010. http://www.usatoday.com/news/washington/2010-04-19-doctors_N.htm. Accessed 20 Jul 2010.
4. OpenSecrets.org. http://www.opensecrets.org/industries/indus.php?ind=H01. Accessed 22 Apr 2011.
5. Federal Elections Commission. http://www.fec.gov/finance/disclosure/disclosure_data_search.shtml. Accessed 22 Apr 2011.

Suggested Resources

American Medical Association. http://www.ama-assn.org.
American Medical Association Political Action Committee. http://www.ampaconline.org.
Massachusetts Medical Society. http://www.mms.org.
The Plum Book (for appointed Federal positions). http://www.gpoaccess.gov/plumbook/.

Chapter 22
Organized Medicine

Samantha Rosman and David A. Rosman

Key Points

- Decisions are being made every day that affect the health of your patients and the way you practice medicine. Organized medicine is *your* vehicle to have a say in these decisions on behalf of your patients and your profession. Use it.
- While there are a vast array of different state and specialty medical societies, there is no "one" society or "best" way to be involved. While they may have different areas of focus they all share a common overall goal – to improve the profession of medicine, the healthcare system in which we practice, and the health of our patients.
- Despite how complex and daunting it may seem, getting involved in organized medicine is easy – the organizations are welcoming and need you to participate. If you have an idea, get involved and share it, it may end up as a headline in the news, or changing laws or health policies.

S. Rosman, MD (✉)
Department of Pediatrics, Division of Emergency Medicine, Harvard Medical School,
Children's Hospital Boston, Boston, MA, USA
e-mail: Samantha.rosman@gmail.com

D.A. Rosman, MD, MBA
Department of Imaging, Massachusetts General Hospital, Boston, MA, USA

R.D. Urman and J.M. Ehrenfeld (eds.), *Physicians' Pathways to Non-Traditional Careers and Leadership Opportunities*, DOI 10.1007/978-1-4614-0551-1_22, © Springer Science+Business Media, LLC 2012

Introduction

Samantha's Story

My career in organized medicine began somewhat accidentally during my first year of medical school. Little did I know what a large part of my career in medicine it would become. I was interested in care for the uninsured and, at the time, working to start up a student-organized free clinic in New York City. A friend who knew of my interests said to me "You should come to the American Medical Association (AMA) meeting this December." Not knowing too much about it, but being an enthusiastic first year medical student, I soon found myself in Orlando at my first AMA meeting. As I listened to debates on everything from care for the uninsured to smoking in public places to the clinical skills assessment exam I was fascinated and instantly hooked. There were so many issues that affect our profession, how we practice medicine, and the health of our patients that I couldn't imagine not being involved.

So, at the next few meetings I applied to serve on convention committees for the AMA Medical Student Section (MSS), then ran for a regional position and eventually for a national MSS position. At the same time, I got involved with my state medical society and my specialty society delegation to the AMA. At the end of my intern year I ran for and was elected to a position on the AMA Board of Trustees, a position I held for two 2-year terms. During my 4 years on the Board of Trustees I traveled across the country speaking to physicians and patients alike about the critical problem of the 45 million uninsured in this country, who are living sicker and dying younger, and the importance of health system reform that provides access to healthcare all Americans (Fig. 22.1).

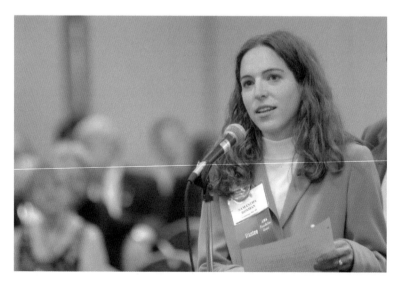

Fig. 22.1 Dr. Samantha Rosman at the AMA House of Delegates

David's Story

My career in organized medicine started eerily similarly to Samantha's. I was a first year medical student, and was at lunch discussing care for the uninsured with a fellow first year. He recognized my interest in improving our health system and suggested I go to a Mass Medical Society (MMS) MSS meeting. I went and, never shy, engaged in a debate with the chair of the section regarding a resolution that he had written and wanted to send to the MMS House of Delegates (with all the voting physicians of the organization) so it could become MMS policy. After a long debate, I felt satisfied with the result and declared, "Ok, I am ready to vote." The chair turned somewhat affectionately and said "Actually Dave, you don't have a vote." However, my voice had been heard, and starting at the next meeting I did have a vote. I learned that I had become a part of an incredibly fair and democratic organization.

I've never looked back. I've served in many capacities – with the MMS, my specialty society (the American College of Radiology) and the AMA including as Trustee of both MMS and AMA. Through all of these experiences, I have been consistently impressed with how effective one voice can be at moving an organization for the betterment of our profession and to the benefit of our patients. I am proud of physicians – for creating such organizations and moving them so forcefully for the benefit of our profession and most importantly, our patients.

A Map of Organized Medicine

The map of involvement in organized medicine is incredibly complex and can be drawn from many perspectives. Basically, there are state societies (and county societies within most states) and specialty societies, most of which then send representatives to the American Medical Association.

Depending on which specialty you practice, your choice of specialty society may be simple or more complex. The subspecialization of specialty societies is becoming as complex as the subspecialization of medicine itself. For example if you are a surgeon you likely belong to the American College of Surgeons, but if you are a neurosurgeon you may also want to belong to the American Association of Neurological Surgeons and/or the Congress of Neurological Surgeons. If you practice pediatric neurosurgery you may also consider the American Society of Pediatric Neurosurgeons. For some, the subspecialization may go even further than this. You will likely let your area of interest guide you in choosing to be a member and/or active in some or all of your potential specialty societies. Most specialty societies also have state and/or local chapters. Table 22.1 demonstrates the ten largest specialty societies. There are many ways to count members. Some of these societies allow medical students and others do not. Further some release their member count and others do not. This list is in alphabetical order with inclusion defined by size of delegation to the AMA.

Table 22.1 Ten largest specialty societies

- American Academy of Orthopedic Surgeons
- American Academy of Pediatrics
- American Association of Family Practitioners
- American College of Obstetricians and Gynecologists
- American College of Physicians
- American College of Radiology
- American College of Surgeons
- American Psychiatric Association
- American Society of Anesthesiologists
- American College of Emergency Physicians

Table 22.2 Standing AMA councils

- Council on Medical Service
  Addresses socioeconomic factors that influence the practice of medicine
- Council on Medical Education
  Addresses medical education by recommending educational policies for both graduate and
    continuing medical education
- Council on Legislation
  Assists in the interpretation of legislation pending before Congress
- Council on Ethical and Judicial Affairs
  Maintains and updates the AMA Code of Medical Ethics. Analyzes timely issues confronting
    physicians and the medical profession
- Council on Science and Public Health
  Reports on medical, public health, and scientific issues that affect the practice of medicine,
    the public health system, the quality of patient care, and the translation of scientific
    research into patient treatment
- Council on Constitution and Bylaws
  Fact-finding and advisory committee on matters pertaining to the AMA Constitution and Bylaws
- Council on Long Range Planning and Development
  Makes recommendations to the AMA Board of Trustees regarding important strategic issues
    and directions related to the AMA's vision, goals, and priorities

Your county and state medical societies are determined by where you live and/or practice. In most states you will join your county society through your state and the county sends representatives to the state society.

The American Medical Association is a national physician organization whose policy is set by a House of Delegates made up of representatives from the specialty and state medical societies. The AMA House of Delegates currently convenes twice a year to consider and set policy for the AMA.

The breadth of issues tackled by these organizations is large and thus the AMA and almost all state and specialty societies, elect or appoint members to councils and committees on various topics such as legislation, science and public health, ethics, medical education, and more. A list of standing AMA councils is shown in Table 22.2. These councils and committees may report to the Board of Trustees of the society, to the policy making body of the society or even directly to the membership.

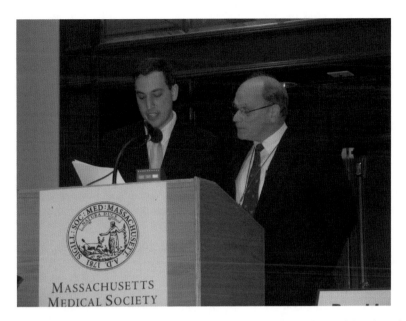

Fig. 22.2 Drs. Jesse M. Ehrenfeld and Richard S. Pieters, Vice Speaker and Speaker of the Massachusetts Medical Society

Furthermore, because one can easily feel lost and/or underrepresented in a large organization, the AMA and many state and specialty societies also have sections to represent minority interests. Some of these sections have votes within the larger policy making body of the organization while some serve more in an advisory capacity. Examples of such sections or groups include: medical students, resident/fellows, young physicians, senior physicians, women physicians, minority physicians, organized medical staff, LGBT (lesbian, gay, bisexual, and transgender) physicians, etc. Many of these sections have their own committees and leadership structures that not only are easy to get involved in, but can also serve as training grounds for more senior leadership positions.

Though it may seem that the map of organized medicine is fact rather than interpretation, the links between societies are sometimes less clear than one might think. The state and specialty societies are independent organizations that are not "members" of the AMA. However, AMA policies are made by its House of Delegates, which is comprised of representatives from the states and specialties on a proportional basis – i.e., we are a radiologist (David) and a pediatrician (Samantha) from Massachusetts and are both members of our state and specialty societies as well as the AMA. So, Massachusetts gets to count us both in their delegate count and the ACR and AAP each count one of us. So if you are not a member of the AMA, you are costing your state and/or specialty votes within the AMA HOD. Join all three (or more) – be counted and be heard! But we digress. Below in Fig. 22.2 is our take on the relationships of the organizations.

How to Get Involved

There are a number of ways to get involved in organized medicine. Often students and physicians choose to involve themselves along more than one path simultaneously.

In medical school generally you are not eligible for membership to a specialty society, (though there are a few exceptions to this and once you are a fourth year student you can often join the society of your soon-to-be specialty) so your involvement can be at the county, state, and national level. Generally, most students get involved in either the American Medical Association or the American Medical Student Association (AMSA), or both. While these two organizations are often seen (and see themselves) as diametrically opposed, I (Samantha) joined and participated in both throughout medical school and gained a great deal from my participation in each.

AMSA and the AMA have different goals and provide different resources and opportunities. AMSA, as the name implies, is a student-governed organization. The AMA, in contrast, has a MSS (as well as a resident fellow section and a young physician section) but encompasses members from the full life cycle of medical training and practice. When the AMA speaks, it is representing all physicians, rather than students alone. As a result, AMSA has the ability to speak more freely on issues it cares about than does the MSS of the AMA because when any section of the AMA speaks it is speaking on behalf of all physicians in the house of medicine. I believe that this, in large part, is responsible for the view that AMSA is liberal and the AMA is conservative. However, if you look into AMA policy further you will find that the AMA passes a substantial amount of progressive policies on issues such as LGBT rights, work hours reform, and the uninsured. In fact, it has been our experience that benefit to the profession and our patients is the ultimate arbiter on what will become AMA policy and that Red versus Blue has little role to play.

AMSA offers incredible workshops on student leadership, humanism, and online resources on international electives, humanities, and career development, in addition to blogs and online exchanges to allow networking with other students around the globe. The AMA has the breadth of the federation of medicine to call upon and thus has unparalleled mentorship as well as avenues into every part of the medical world. We would advocate joining both. Both the AMA-MSS and AMSA have councils and committees that you can participate in for either a single meeting alone or over the course of a year or more. At the AMA you can also be elected or appointed to a slotted seat (reserved specifically for a medical student) on a full AMA council or even the Board of Trustees and serve along with physicians from across the country.

As a student, generally the easiest way to begin your involvement is to seek out the AMSA or AMA chapter at your medical school. They often host meet and greets, lectures, debates, community service activities, and more. Seek out your chapter leadership and get involved. They will likely help you get involved at the state and national level if you are interested as well. Your state medical association likely has a student section and councils or committees with slotted seats for students

Table 22.3 Typical committees of a state medical society

- Public health
- Global medicine
- Ethics and professional standards
- Communications
- Emergency preparedness
- Lesbian, gay, bisexual, and transgender health
- Legislation
- Finance
- Diversity in medicine
- Environmental and occupational health
- Information technology
- The list goes on and on!

as well (see Table 22.3). If you find yourself at a medical school without an AMA chapter contact the AMA-MSS and/or your state medical society and they will be more than happy to help you get a chapter started at your school. Similarly, national AMSA is happy to help if you are lacking an AMSA chapter.

As a resident/fellow, you may find yourself a bit more on your own as you don't have a ready-made chapter to guide you into involvement. Don't be discouraged though – there are still plenty of local and national opportunities. You are probably already a member of your specialty society as many are free for resident/fellow members and for those that are not, many programs pay for membership for their trainees. Most specialty societies have state chapters and committees that would welcome your involvement and some have resident/fellow sections as well. You may not easily hear about these though, so contact your specialty society and ask – they will be more than happy to point you in the right direction. In addition to your specialty, you should consider involvement in your county and state medical associations as well as the AMA. Most of these societies have resident/fellow sections, slotted resident/fellow seats on councils or committees, and governing bodies that would welcome your involvement. On the state level contact your state medical association (or their RFS section) and they will help you get involved and on the national level you can contact the AMA-RFS.

BONUS TIP

At least one AMA meeting a year has a poster symposium for students and residents/fellows. Presenting a poster is a great way to get your dean or program director enthusiastic about sending you to the AMA meeting. Then, you can not only add the poster to your resume, but get to see the rest of the AMA meeting – perhaps make contacts for fellowship and make a little policy all at the same time!

Table 22.4 How to get involved in organized medicine

Medical student
- First, know that it is easy! There are many ways to be involved!
- Seek out the AMSA or AMA chapter at your medical school
- If your medical school has no AMA or AMSA chapter, contact the AMA-MSS, the National AMSA, and/or your state medical society and they will be more than happy to help you get a chapter started at your school
- Find a senior student or staff mentor. People like to be admired and like others who want to be involved!
- Check out the bonus tip above. A poster helps smooth bridges

Resident/Fellow
- Fewer Residents/Fellows than students are involved. If you want in at this stage, you are a valuable commodity and can get important positions quickly!
- See if you have staff at your hospital who is involved. Ask them!
- If your Specialty Society has a state chapter, call them and ask if they have a Resident/Fellows Section and who you can contact
- If not, call your National Specialty Society and ask for the Resident/Fellows Section
- Call your state society and ask if they have an Resident/Fellows Section and who you can talk to to get involved
- Check out the bonus tip above. A poster will make your program director happy and supportive

Young physician
- See if you have more senior staff colleagues who are involved. Ask them to hook you in
- Call your state society or the state chapter of your specialty society and see if there is a committee that you can be involved in. These groups are usually desperate for help!

As a practicing physician you may not find the slotted seats or sections that help ease the transition into organized medicine for students and residents/fellows but we assure you that your state and specialty will do everything they can to help you get involved. If you are a young physician (generally under age 40 or in your first 8 years of practice) many societies will have a section for you as well and may have slotted committee seats for you. Often finding a committee or council to participate in that coincides with your areas of interest or expertise is a good way to get involved and begin to network.

An overview of ways to get involved in organized medicine is shown in Table 22.4.

Why Pursue Organized Medicine?

There are innumerable national, state, and specialty medical societies all with slightly different focuses and emphases – but all with a similar overall goal – to improve the profession of medicine, the healthcare system in which we practice, and the health of our patients.

Decisions are made every day that affect the practice of medicine – by Congress, by the alphabet soup of governmental agencies and independent agencies such as

HHS (Health and Human Services), FDA (Food and Drug Administration), CMS (Centers for Medicare and Medicaid Services), AHRQ (Agency for Healthcare Research and Quality), ACGME (Accreditation Council for Graduate Medical Education), RRC (Residency Review Committees), FSMB (Federation of State Medical Boards), ABMS (American Board of Medical Specialties), JCAHO (actually now renamed "The Joint Commission"), IOM (Institute of Medicine), by insurance companies, and by hospitals just to name a few. Yet, as physicians, we are the ones who have devoted the majority of our lives to studying medicine, who spend our days practicing medicine within the healthcare system, who see, firsthand, how each and every decision effects our patients. We see how Medicare cuts force our colleagues out of practice and leave our seniors unable to find primary care physicians. We see a broken liability system lead us to practice defensive medicine – to order that extra lab or get the CT scan we don't think is necessary – and see baseless lawsuits devastate our colleagues' families and lives. We see skyrocketing liability premiums force our Ob/Gyn colleagues to give up the practice of obstetrics, or neurosurgeons to move out of the state. We see uninsured patients wait and let simple problems turn into life-threatening conditions because they are afraid they can't afford a doctor's visit. We see the effects of public health crises like obesity and smoking – the teenager in our office suffering from type 2 diabetes, and the mother dying in the hospital of lung cancer from a lifetime of smoking.

Organized medicine ensures that the voice of physicians is represented at the many tables at which critical decisions effecting healthcare practice and public health are made. It ensures that physicians are the ones making the recommendations on quality improvement and education within their specialties. Standards for medical schools are maintained by the Liaison Committee for Medical Education (LCME), which is appointed by the AMA and the AAMC (Association of American Medical Colleges). Similarly, the ACGME (Accreditation Council for Graduation Medical Education) and its RRCs (Residency Review Committees) maintain standards for and accredit residencies. Their members are appointed by the AMA and the relevant specialty societies. Often when State Medical Boards are making decisions about whether a physician has acted rightly or wrongly after a complaint has been filed, they will look to the AMA's CEJA (Council on Ethical and Judicial Affairs) Code of Medical Ethics. As you can see, organized medicine works to have physicians' voices making the decisions about our training, practice, and ethics. If a void were left, someone else would fill it and likely not with the knowledge necessary to do justice for our profession and our patients (Fig. 22.3).

How Can I Benefit from My Involvement in Organized Medicine?

Involvement in organized medicine provides countless unique opportunities that physicians generally don't have in their everyday lives. First, at the most basic level of membership and involvement, organized medicine affords an incredible

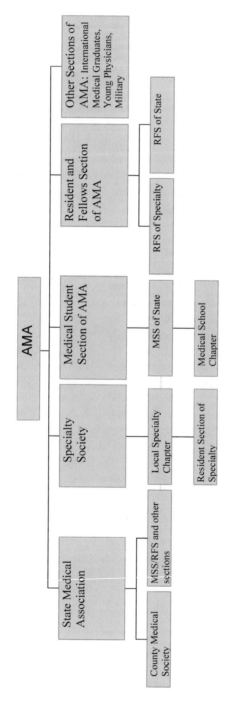

Fig. 22.3 Overview of organized medicine

opportunity to stay up to date on the issues that are critical to your state, specialty, or nationally to physicians – on everything from bills in Congress or the legislature to highlights of published journal articles to tips on maintaining certification or dealing with insurers. This level of involvement is important for every physician and given a busy practice, is all that most desire. Also, by being involved at this level, you ensure that you are being counted as your state, specialty, and AMA lobby on your behalf to ensure those laws and regulations are in your and your patients' best interest.

However, say you have an issue that you believe is important but is not being addressed by your societies or worse – your societies are, in your opinion, representing the wrong side on the issue. The societies offer ample opportunity to be heard. You can write a resolution (if that sounds foreign, it is easy to call up the society and say that you want to do so and they will happily guide you through the process), argue for its passage and see how your idea becomes a new lobbying priority for the organization. If you think the AMA, state, or specialty society has gotten it totally wrong on a topic, don't quit! Argue your point! If you wish to be heard and can make a compelling argument, you can often turn the organization to advocate for your belief! The worst way to make your point is to leave the organization because it means one less person with your point of view will be heard.

If you choose to get involved in a council or committee for a medical society, you will undoubtedly learn a great deal from your fellow committee members, from the talented medical society staff, and often from political and healthcare leaders with whom your committee interacts. We have seen for many physicians how serving on a committee or council can lead to further opportunities both within organized medicine as well as at a healthcare leadership or political level.

The networking that takes place within organized medicine is a benefit most don't recognize when they join but many find to be one of the most rewarding parts of their involvement. We know and are friends with hundreds of physicians across the country of all ages and specialties as a result of our involvement. As a student and resident/fellow this access to mentors and colleagues is unrivaled, though we would argue it is no less incredible or important as you continue along your medical career. Seasoned physicians who have dedicated much of their careers to organized medicine are usually ecstatic to find young people who are similarly enthusiastic. The connections you make can help shape your career.

Further, as noted above, the AMA appoints members to many decision-making bodies such as the ACGME, The Joint Commission, LCME, and RRCs. Specialty societies also often appoint members to decision-making bodies as well such as the specialty board or RRC. State societies may appoint representatives to state committees and medical boards. As a result, involvement in organized medicine can mean not only an incredible networking opportunity but also an opportunity to be appointed into the leadership of these groups yourself.

In addition to the direct leadership, networking and mentorship opportunities, the financial returns of being involved in organized medicine are also incredible. In addition to the small things like discounts on books, CME, insurance products, and resources needed to run your practice (coding books and practice management guides), you get larger returns such as a proportional share when the AMA or your state society sues an insurance company on your behalf or the AMA and your state and specialty societies protect your ability to see senior citizens by lobbying against cuts in Medicare (the most recent was a 21% cut that was thwarted – multiply your future income by 21% and decide if that is worth the membership fee which keeps these organizations strong and doing such work for you).

While the AMA is lobbying nationally for all physicians, your state and specialty societies are doing things for you as an individual on a more local or specialty-specific level. Local political issues can be dealt with only by your state society and can mean tremendous benefits for your practice – such as fighting the trial lawyers to get tort reform in your state. Your specialty society avails you of CME opportunities as well as looks out for your specialty in ways that a larger organization like the AMA cannot. Although membership to all of these can be costly, it is nowhere near the cost of allowing any of them to fail. Their direct and indirect benefits to you are hundreds of times more valuable than their membership dues.

How Can I Benefit My Patients?

The advocacy detailed above should never be thought of as for physicians only. We entered this profession to make sick people well and to give comfort when our healing efforts fail. The first line of AMSA's mission statement is: The AMSA is committed to improving healthcare and healthcare delivery to all people. Similarly, the AMA's mission, since 1847 has been: To promote the art and science of medicine and the betterment of public health. Organized medicine exists, in large part, to help doctors help their patients. Year after year we come to meetings and listen and participate as doctors vociferously advocate on behalf of their patients.

The accomplishments of organized medicine on behalf of our patients are too many to enumerate. Over the past 100 years, organized medicine has refined a code of medical ethics, improved the quality of medical training, worked to ensure patient safety, and fought for critical public health measures such as seat belts, polio vaccination, and opposition to tobacco. Our healthcare system and our patients are far better off today thanks to the advocacy of these organizations and physicians like you.

How Much Education and Other Background Do I Need?

This all may seem too grandiose or perhaps daunting. It doesn't need to be. The wonderful thing about organized medicine is that you don't need any additional education or background. What organized medicine most needs from you is your experience as a student, resident, or practicing physician. It needs your perspective on what is working well and what the challenges are for you, your colleagues, and your patients.

If you have additional background, it can, and will come in useful. The world of organized medicine is full of a variety of different experts on everything from ethics, to public health, to health insurers and health systems, to medical education. It is this diversity of perspectives and expertise that allows organized medicine to do the work and advocacy it does.

So to get involved all you need is to become a member and participate. Your interest may be in global issues such as advocacy for health system reform, medical liability reform, or Medicare payment reform. Or your issue may be more focused; you may be frustrated that you couldn't access the flu vaccines your patients needed this past year because of problems in the distribution, or that your medical school enacted a mid-year retroactive tuition increase, or that you aren't getting enough education on talking to families of dying patients in residency. All of these issues and more have been and will continue to be debated in organized medicine and, as a result, let organized medicine advocate for an improved healthcare system on your behalf. The world of organized medicine is large and it has every day effects on your practice and your patients – the choice is to be involved in making the rules or to be subject to them without having had input.

Additional Resources

The AMA: http://www.ama-assn.org/
The AMA Medical Student Section: http://www.ama-assn.org/ama/pub/medical-students/medical-students.shtml.
AMA-Resident Fellow Section: http://www.ama-assn.org/ama/pub/about-ama/our-people/member-groups-sections/resident-fellow-section.shtml.
AMA Young Physician Section: http://www.ama-assn.org/ama/pub/about-ama/our-people/member-groups-sections/young-physicians-section.shtml.
Links to State Medical Societies: http://www.ama-assn.org/ama/pub/about-ama/our-people/the-federation-medicine/state-medical-society-websites.shtml.
Links to National Medical Specialty Societies: http://www.ama-assn.org/ama/pub/about-ama/our-people/the-federation-medicine/national-medical-specialty-society-websites.shtml.
AMSA: www.amsa.org.
Accreditation Council for Graduate Medical Education (AGME) www.acgme.org.
The Joint Commission (Formerly JCAHO).

Chapter 23
Physician Opportunities in the United States Uniformed/Military Services

Jeremy M. Huff and D. Kiley Mortensen

> **Key Points**
>
> - Medical practice in the various military services offers unique experiences often not replicable in standard medical practice.
> - Numerous opportunities for educational financial support are available throughout the stages of one's career.
> - Opportunities for development of leadership skills are integral to the mission of the military services.

Introduction

One of the most unique practice opportunities currently available to many physicians in the United States can be found in the United States uniformed services. The uniformed services that currently offer commissions to physicians include the United States Army, United States Navy, United States Air Force, and the United States Public Health Service Commissioned Corps. Physicians in the military/armed services (Air Force, Navy, and Army) are managed under the direction of the Department of Defense (DOD). The Department of Health and Human Services manages physicians in a uniformed service, the Public Health Service Commissioned Corps, and a non-uniformed service, the National Health Service Corps (NHSC).

J.M. Huff, DO, CAPT, USAF Medical Corps (✉)
Department of Anesthesia, Wright-Patterson Medical Center, Wright-Patterson AFB, OH 45431, USA
e-mail: Jeremy.huff@wpafb.af.mil

D.K. Mortensen, DO, CAPT, USAF Medical Corps
Department of Anesthesia, Wilford Hall Medical Center, Lackland AFB, TX, USA

R.D. Urman and J.M. Ehrenfeld (eds.), *Physicians' Pathways to Non-Traditional Careers and Leadership Opportunities*, DOI 10.1007/978-1-4614-0551-1_23, © Springer Science+Business Media, LLC 2012

Physicians in the uniformed services are employees of their respective government departments. Each uniformed service has its own distinct mission, requiring medical support personnel to be flexible within the scope of that mission. Despite particular mission related differences, there are many similarities. Professionals interested in a career in one of these government agencies are afforded a number of opportunities. These options are available at various career milestones ranging from undergraduate studies, medical school, residency/fellowship, and ultimately clinical practice.

Clinical Practice

Clinical practice in the military setting can be extremely similar to that practiced in the civilian community. Standards of care are the same as those established in civilian practices by civilian association and organizations. For much of one's career, clinical responsibilities and practice patterns may be indistinguishable from civilian practice.

One of the medical corps missions is to provide support for the local communities wherein they reside. There are oftentimes opportunities to extend services into the community, as is seen with military trauma centers providing care for nonmilitary patients. Some civilian institutions will have affiliation agreements with their local military training installations where active duty residents and physicians may provide medical services in the civilian location.

Military physicians treat active duty personnel, their immediate family members, DOD beneficiaries and retired servicemen and women. Within this group are patients of almost every demographic. An added benefit is the honor and opportunity to treat those in active duty service. Active duty men and women are typically athletic with health conscious lifestyles due to the rigorous fitness requirements.

Military clinics and hospitals offer services comparable to those offered in similar sized civilian hospitals, including significant subspecialty support. The government invests in state of the art equipment to insure that its beneficiaries have access to world class healthcare. Military physicians are often at the forefront of directing the standard of care for trauma and medicine as they treat the wounded in conflict areas.

Leadership/Management Opportunity

While there are many components of military clinical practice that are similar to civilian practice, military practice does offer the potential for variety unseen in standard practice. As both physicians and officers, professionals serving in the armed forces often have administrative and supervisory responsibilities beyond that which their equivalent civilian counterparts might have. As physicians and officers' progress

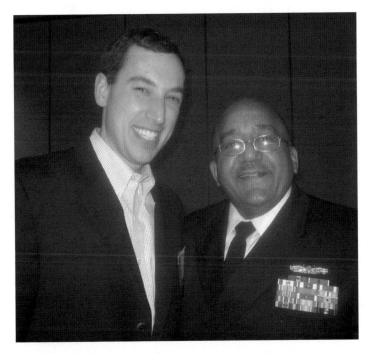

Fig. 23.1 Vice Admiral Adam M. Robinson Jr., M.D., Surgeon General of the US Navy (*right*) with Lieutenant Commander Jesse M. Ehrenfeld M.D. (*left*) after receiving the American Medical Association's Nathan Davis Award for Outstanding Government Service

in time and rank they will often see increases in these administrative responsibilities. This often provides unique challenges and immense learning opportunities. Those in command, such as the Vice Admiral Robinson – Surgeon General of the Navy – pictured in Fig. 23.1, are responsible for the oversight of large numbers of personnel, equipment, and financial assets. Lessons learned from these on-the-job experiences combined with professional military education (PME) courses centered in leadership and ethics can be applicable throughout one's personal and professional career.

Educational Opportunity

Military institutions have a unique emphasis on continued education and training. Due to the chance and often inevitability of deployment into foreign areas, military units tend to train constantly on the various scenarios that could be encountered in the wartime setting. Team familiarity and stable knowledge of policies and procedures help military physicians maintain high quality medical care in atypical environments.

Many military institutions train medical residents, advanced practice and registered nurses, and technicians of many varieties. Physicians willing to impart quality lessons/ skills on a host of eager learners will find the military learning environment a rich opportunity. Often new graduates of residency programs will find themselves in teaching situations much sooner than in the civilian community.

Deployment/Humanitarian Missions

Deployment to conflict zones is a possibility and even probability as a military physician. This responsibility offers an opportunity for medical practice in a unique and often austere environment. While deployed during wartime, the medical corps mission includes not only providing care for members of the armed services, but also members of the immediate and surrounding communities. A large part of deployment missions are, in fact, humanitarian in nature. Deployment offers the ability for persons to come in contact with diverse cultures, alternate medical systems, be involved in training scenarios with allies from other countries, and experience medical situations only found in wartime activities.

Military physicians have the occasional opportunity to be involved in humanitarian missions, unlinked to areas of combat, in diverse areas of the world. Missions to areas of central and South America, the Caribbean, and Southeast Asia are periodically undertaken. The military will respond to natural disasters as seen in the recent hurricane Katrina and earthquake in Haiti. These opportunities permit the military physician to have the potential for a practice that is much more far reaching than the average civilian counterpart.

Unique Practice Opportunities

For physicians who are undecided on their career path or are unable to initially secure a residency program, the opportunity to serve as a General Medical Officer (GMO) exists. GMO's are typically physicians who have completed medical school, their first postgraduate year (internship) and some, who have completed residency training. All GMO's must have secured active, current medical licensure in the state of their choice. These physicians often are involved in primary care activities and practice occupational and safety medicine. Many will undergo additional training courses in aerospace medicine (flight surgeons) and dive medicine (dive officers) in support of their particular assignment.

Those with specialty training such as flight surgeons, for example, will typically be responsible to maintain the safety environment and medical readiness of pilots. They constantly train, in peace or wartime, with their designated units. As the situations arise, as in wartime, they will deploy to personally oversee the health and safety of those units. As in the case of flight surgeons, an added benefit is that many receive firsthand instruction in flight operations, with many accruing hundreds of hours of flight time.

Another unique opportunity that is relatively new for select physicians serving in the Air Force is involvement in the Critical Care Air Transport Teams (CCATT). CCATT is a highly trained unit, consisting of a physician with critical care experience (anesthesiologist, internist/pulmonologist, and surgeon), critical care nurse, and respiratory technician. These teams function to provide high quality, aeromedical evacuation services to victims of combat casualties, natural disasters, or other situation necessitating critical care transport.

Career Path

The opportunity to complete a military career is one that many physicians find appealing. Routes to entering government service as a physician are numerous and will hereafter be outlined. Those in the uniformed services are promoted based on time and performance factors. A specific amount of time is generally required for promotion, however, there are slight pay increases given yearly and at specified intervals. Initially, an officer will tend to have their clinical responsibilities occupy the majority of their time with small amounts devoted to administrative and leadership roles. As one advances in rank, however, the administrative aspect to their practice will increase. As one reaches the upper ranks (O5 and O6) he or she will tend to have significant amounts of time devoted to not only administrating their clinical practice, but potentially a number of specialties. Following 20 years of service, career officers are given the opportunity to retire from their government positions. At this time they are also eligible for the collection of a monthly retirement benefit and medical benefits. The retirement benefits are based on grade, number of qualifying years and applicable taxes. A list of rank and rank equivalency among the US Military is shown in Table 23.1.

Undergraduate Education

There are a number of financial assistance programs (FAPs) available for students pursuing or wishing to pursue an undergraduate degree. These programs are available to applicants who meet each agency's individual eligibility criteria which include: citizenship requirements, physical exam/fitness standards, a security check, and academic achievement. Undergraduate assistance programs are strictly for undergraduate academic majors. Each service will forecast its needs for certain academic majors and then offer competitive scholarships to fill those forecasted needs. Selection into an undergraduate assistance program does not ensure selection into medical programs, or the opportunity to immediately pursue medical education following undergraduate training. Once selected, applicants will receive scholarship

Table 23.1 United States military rank chart

Rank	Army	Navy Coast guard	Marines	Air Force
Enlisted ranks				
W1	Warrant Officer 1 (WO1)	USN Warrant Officer 1 – WO1	Warrant Officer 1 (WO)	No warrant
W2	Chief Warrant Officer 2 (CW2)	USN Chief Warrant Officer 2 – CWO2 USCG	Chief Warrant Officer 2 (CWO2)	No warrant
W3	Chief Warrant Officer 3 (CW3)	USN Chief Warrant Officer 3 – CWO3 USCG	Chief Warrant Officer 3 (CWO3)	No warrant
W4	Chief Warrant Officer 4 (CW4)	USN Chief Warrant officer 4 – CWO4 USCG	Chief Warrant Officer 4 (CWO4)	No warrant
W5	Chief Warrant Officer CW5)	USN Chief Warrant Officer (CWO5)	Chief Warrant Officer 5 (CWO5)	No warrant
Officer ranks				
O1	Second Lieutenant (2LT)	Ensign (ENS)	Second Lieutenant (2nd Lt.)	Second Lieutenant (2nd Lt.)
O2	First Lieutenant (1LT)	Lieutenant Junior Grade (LTJG)	First Lieutenant (1st Lt.)	First Lieutenant (1st Lt.)
O3	Captain (CPT)	Lieutenant (LT)	Captain (Capt.)	Captain (Capt.)
O4	Major (MAJ)	Lieutenant Commander (LCDR)	Major (Maj.)	Major (Maj.)
O5	Lieutenant Colonel (LTC)	Commander (CDR)	Lieutenant Colonel (Lt. Col.)	Lieutenant Colonel (Lt. Col.)
O6	Colonel (COL)	Captain (CAPT)	Colonel (Col.)	Colonel (Col.)
O7	Brigadier General (BG)	Rear Admiral Lower Half (RDML)	Brigadier General (Brig. Gen.)	Brigadier General (Brig. Gen.)
O8	Major General (MG)	Rear Admiral Upper Half (RADM)	Major General (Maj. Gen.)	Major General (Maj. Gen.)
O9	Lieutenant General (LTG)	Vice Admiral (VADM)	Lieutenant General (Lt. Gen.)	Lieutenant General (Lt. Gen.)
O10	General (GEN)	Admiral (ADM)	General (Gen.)	General (Gen.)
	Army Chief of Staff	Chief of Naval Operations and Commandant of the Coast Guard	Commandant of the Marine Corps	Air Force Chief of Staff
	General of the Army (reserved for wartime only)	Fleet Admiral (reserved for wartime only)		General of the Air Force (reserved for wartime only)

support for tuition and books. All applicants will assume an active duty service obligation after their training. Active duty obligations can vary; however, typically amount to a year of obligated service for each year of financial support (average of 4 years).

Reserve Officer Training Corps

The Reserve Officer Training Corps (ROTC) is a commonly identified program on the campuses of many high schools and colleges. This program encompasses multiple scholarship types ranging from high school scholarships, in-college scholarships, and scholarships for individuals who are already enlisted in military service. As the number, types, and eligibility of each scholarship are varied, interested undergraduate students should contact a recruiter from each service to have options specifically outlined.

Uniformed Service Academies

The United States Air Force Academy, United States Naval Academy, and the United States Military Academy (West Point) options are available to motivated students wishing to complete their undergraduate educations in the most unique of military training environments. The application process for each of these institutions is extremely selective. Applicants must demonstrate excellence in academic, extracurricular/leadership, physical fitness, and other areas to be competitive. All applicants must obtain a nomination from a member of Congress or the Vice-President of the United States.

Those who matriculate will simultaneously receive training in military/leadership studies as well as courses towards their respective undergraduate academic degrees. All tuition, related fees, room and board, as well as a nontaxable monthly stipend are provided. Following their graduation, they will receive active duty commissions into their respective services and assume a minimum active duty service commitment (5 years).

Medical Education Opportunities

There are a number of opportunities in which one can receive their medical education in or through the uniformed services. These programs exist to provide educational support to prospective physicians and thereby securing trained assets for future active duty service. Currently, there are three predominant pathways in which future physicians can enter into active duty service and receive financial assistance.

Uniformed Services University School of Medicine

The Uniformed Services University (USUHS) located in Bethesda, MD is one of the premiere institutions for the training of physicians who will ultimately practice medicine in the military or public health setting. The Navy, Air Force, Army, and the Public Health Service are represented. Prospective medical students must submit applications and are interviewed similar to the application processes found in any civilian institution. As part of the acceptance process, however, applicants must undergo a physical examination and security check. Each service has its own forecasted needs and, therefore, a limited number of positions available. Once accepted, a student will have the opportunity to choose from the available scholarship positions. Only the agencies with scholarships remaining will then be able to present acceptance offers, so students who desire selection by a particular service should apply early.

Students who choose to matriculate into the Uniformed Services University must accept an active duty commission as an officer in the particular service whose scholarship they accepted. Once commissioned as an active duty officer (Navy Ensign, USAF/Army second Lieutenant), students receive benefits including salary, medical benefits, and tax-free food and housing allowances. See the section "Benefits" for specific information. All costs of medical training are paid for by the service which offered the scholarship.

As a condition of the scholarship awarded, a student incurs an active duty obligation in their chosen service for 7 years. Following medical training, students are required to complete an internship in a military training program. Most will complete their residency training in a military program with a few being granted deferment for training in civilian institutions. Once physicians are no longer in a training role, they begin to fulfill their active duty service obligation, typically serving in the specialty in which they trained.

Armed Forces Health Professions Scholarship Program

Another opportunity to enter military medical practice is through the Armed Forces Health Professions Scholarship Program (HPSP). This program is individually administered by each of the military services. Prospective medical students who are applying to medical (MD) or osteopathic (DO) schools may, at the same time, apply for the scholarship in their desired service. Three and four year scholarships are available in limited quantity. The scholarship application is complete once all application materials, a physical examination, and a civilian medical school acceptance has been secured. Local recruiters aid and give directions to the students throughout this process. Students who are awarded the scholarship accept a commission into the inactive reserve component of the service whose scholarship they accepted. They remain in this inactive reserve capacity throughout their civilian medical school training.

In return for their future commitment, students receive a living stipend (approximately $2,000/month) plus payment of tuition, fees, and required supplies. Occasionally, an additional signing bonus is offered. While being a student, they will be required to spend one month each year, typically during the summer months, on active duty. One of these months, during the first or second year of medical school, is spent at the service-specific commissioned officer training course. During this intense course, students receive an abbreviated military education with concentrated training on how to be an effective officer. In the 3rd and 4th years of medical school, active duty months are routinely spent in a military hospital performing a standard third or fourth year clerkship. This time is typically utilized in an audition capacity in a program that the student would consider for residency. Following graduation from medical school, those who enrolled in the HPSP will either matriculate into a military or civilian residency program.

Financial Assistance Program

Those physicians who have completed their medical school training and are either in or have completed their residency training have the opportunity to receive commissions and practice within the specialty in which they are trained. This program is known as the Armed Forces Financial Assistance Program (FAP). Providing that one of the military services has a forecasted need for a particular specialty and the applicant meets all the application criteria (citizenship, security check, practice history, medical/physical fitness qualifications) an opportunity may exist to join through this program. Trained physicians sign a contract either during or after residency training.

Physicians in residency who sign on under this program are offered a living stipend (around $2,000/month in 2010) and a yearly bonus (approximately $45,000 in 2010). They are commissioned into the reserve component of their chosen service and promoted to a rank commensurate with their level of experience (usually a Captain in the USAF and Army, Lieutenant in the Navy). By accepting this compensation they assume an active duty service commitment equal to the number of years funded. Once their residency training is complete, they are recommissioned into the active duty force, attend the officer training course and will typically practice medicine in the specialty in which they are trained.

Physicians who are already residency trained and who wish to enter military service may also be able to do so through the FAP. They are commissioned directly into active duty service and promoted to a rank and pay level commensurate with their level of training and experience. They will receive the standard military benefits package and are usually eligible for specialty incentive bonuses each year. Additionally, they may be, and are typically, eligible for incentive signing bonuses based on the number of years that they agree to serve.

United States Public Health Service Commissioned Corps

The Public Health Service (UHPHS) Commissioned Corps is the uniformed service funded through the Department of Health and Human Services under the direction of the US Surgeon General. This organization is charged with addressing the host of public health and safety related issues in the United States. The Corps are also integral in responding to both domestic and international disasters as part of its humanitarian mission. Officers in the USPHS are assigned to work in any number of possible locations, depending on their specialty and experience. Physicians may work in underserved communities like Native American reservations, urban environments or even in positions in government agencies like the Centers for Disease Control (CDC).

Those serving in the commissioned corps must meet many of the same eligibility requirements found in the other uniformed services. Benefits packages are also similar and include access to all the amenities found on military facilities. Rank and pay are determined by education and experience. The Commissioned Corps accepts applications of individuals who have already completed at minimum 1 year of an accredited internship program and have an active, current state medical license. Bonus and incentive pays may be available.

National Health Service Corps Scholarship and Loan Repayment Program

These programs, also administered through the Department of Health and Human Services, provide financial incentives to students and physicians willing to pursue careers in primary care medicine for underserved populations. Primary care specialties are specifically defined as Family Medicine, Internal Medicine, Pediatrics, Obstetrics and Gynecology, and Psychiatry. Physicians and students who accept financial support through the NHSC must agree to serve a specified period of time in designated healthcare shortage areas defined by the National Health Service (available on the NHSC website). Unlike the military where physicians are assigned practice locations, the NHSC scholarship allows physicians to choose from the vast number of available positions and sites in order to repay their contract obligation.

Students who accept this scholarship *must* be certain of their intent to pursue a primary care specialty as they face penalties equaling 3 times the cost of the scholarship plus interest if they choose to violate the terms of their contract. Students receive tuition, required fees, reimbursement of specified reasonable costs, and a living stipend (approximately $1,300/month in 2010) while in medical school. Service obligations are typically 1 year of service in a designated underserved area per year of financial support.

Postgraduate Training Opportunities

Residency Training Opportunities

Medical students entering residency following either accession through the Uniformed Services University Medical School program or the HPSP may then be selected for training in a military administered residency training program. As there are limited numbers of positions available, some students will be required to pursue their postgraduate training in accredited civilian institutions in lieu of military directed-programs. Military programs are accredited by the Accreditation Counsel for Graduate Medical Education (ACGME) and as such, have educational programs administered by board certified physicians in that particular area of study.

The military programs have a diverse number of residency programs available; however, only a limited number of positions are available for each specialty. All graduating medical students on military scholarships are required to apply through the Joint Service Graduate Medical Education Selection Board (JSGMESB). This board consists of the specialty consultants for each medical specialty in each of the three military services. All members of this committee score applicants for their particular specialty and then applicants are ranked by their respective military branch. Scoring includes evaluation of the preclinical and clinical years of medical school, board scores, interview results, and letters of recommendation, prior military service, and publication history.

Once scored, applicants are distributed into the available forecasted residency positions. If the service has a need above their capacity to train in military programs, then a "deferment" for civilian training is often approved. Those chosen for military service will be recommissioned into active duty following medical school graduation and complete their residency training in the military program. Individuals in chosen to complete their desired specialty in a military program will be required to complete that training in any of the various training sites. They may not have much control on the location of their training program. Students who are granted deferred positions remain in the inactive, obligated reserve component of their service, and are free to compete for a position in their civilian residency and location of choice. Deferred officers may only accept positions in the specialty that has been approved by their military service.

Occasionally, the numbers of applications for both deferred and military positions is above the numbers of available positions. In this case, students not selected for training may be offered only a military or deferred civilian internship. Graduates of the Uniformed Services University Program are typically required to complete their internship year in a military program. All applicants will complete an internship as it is required for medical licensure in most states. Once completed, they may reapply for their desired residency program or practice as a GMO and repay their accrued commitment prior to completing residency. Although no individual will be required to train in an undesired specialty, they may not be initially guaranteed a military residency or civilian residency deferment but will repay their commitment as a GMO.

Fellowship Training Opportunities

Similar in many ways to the residency application and selection process, those who have military commitments can choose to apply for fellowship selection through the JSGMESB. The board, based on forecasted needs, will approve residents for training in military fellowship programs, as civilian deferments, or as a civilian sponsored status.

As with residency programs those in military programs will train in an active duty capacity at a military facility. Salaries and benefits of those in military fellowships are covered by the military service. Additionally, those in military fellowship are eligible for primary certification specialty bonuses following graduation from residency. For example, a critical care fellow is eligible for the specialty bonuses of his/her primary certification (surgery/anesthesiology) while completing their fellowship. Physicians in military fellowship programs generally accrue additional active duty obligation at the rate of approximately 1-2 years/year of training.

Deferred fellows are free to secure a civilian fellowship in whatever specialty was approved. They are placed in inactive, reserve status for the duration of their approved fellowship program. Deferred fellows, like deferred residents, receive their pay and benefits from their civilian institution, not their military branch. They accrue no additional active duty obligation for their fellowship training time.

A civilian sponsored fellow remains on active duty status for the duration of their fellowship training. Civilian sponsored fellows complete their fellowships in civilian programs that typically have prearranged agreements with the particular service. Sponsored fellows receive their active duty pay, benefits, and bonuses from their respective service, not the civilian institution in which they train. For their sponsorship they accrue additional service commitments typically at the rate of 2 years per year of sponsorship/training. They are eligible, like those fellows in military institutions, for their primary certification specialty bonuses. This generally amounts to military fellows receiving considerably more compensation than their civilian colleagues. A civilian sponsored fellow is highly desired by many fellowships across the nation as they are of little financial burden on the partnering institution. This can be a great opportunity to train at a highly respected institution-a position that might otherwise be difficult to obtain.

Professional Military Education (PME)

PME is designed to improve the leadership and organizational skills of military officers. Each branch of the military has distinct courses organized in various intervals throughout the rank structure. Courses are typically graduate level and eligible for master's degree credit. The core curriculum for the various PME courses includes leadership skills, ethics, and military strategy and organization courses. PME is required at various intervals for career/rank advancement in the military.

For those physicians desiring continued promotion through the ranks of the medical corps, they must secure the appropriate PME at various intervals in their career. This can often be completed as part of a self study/distance learning curriculum or in residence at a particular training site, although in residence is typically preferred. Costs associated with such PME are covered through the respective military branch. Skills and understanding acquired from these courses are vital to the demands of the unique military organization and leadership structure.

Benefits

Officers in the Armed Forces receive a complete benefits package including competitive salary and a tax-free food and housing allowance. Additional amenities include: 30 days of paid vacation, paid sick days, maternity and paternity leave, paid federal holidays, no cost dental care and healthcare, and low-cost personal insurance. Low-cost medical healthcare is available for immediate family members. Servicemen who serve a sufficient period of time (20 years) may be eligible to receive a substantial retirement benefit, qualification for Veteran's Affairs home loans, and medical and educational benefits offered under the Montgomery GI Bill. Physicians in the Armed Forces receive additional yearly physician incentive bonuses, bonuses based on specialty certification, a board certification bonus, as well as bonuses for assuming additional service obligation above that which is assumed during training. In many specialties, compensation is comparable to that seen by those in civilian practice.

Resources/Additional Resources

United States Military Academies. http://www.usna.edu/homepage.php, http://www.usafa.af.mil/, http://www.usma.edu/.
Medical Education Information. http://www.usuhs.mil/, http://www.airforce.com/opportunities/healthcare/, http://www.goarmy.com/amedd.html, http://www.navy.com/navy/careers/healthcare/?campaign=van_healthcare.
US Public Health Service Commissioned Corps Information. http://www.usphs.gov/default.aspx.
National Health Service Corps Information. http://nhsc.hrsa.gov/.
US Navy Professional Military Education. http://www.usnwc.edu/, http://www.usnwc.edu/, http://www.ndu.edu/.
US Air Force Professional Military Education. http://acsc.maxwell.af.mil/aboutACSC.asp, http://www.au.af.mil/au/awc/awchome.htm, http://sos.maxwell.af.mil/sos.html, http://sos.maxwell.af.mil/asbc.html.
US Army Professional Military Education. http://www.carlisle.army.mil/, http://www.cgsc.edu/, http://www-tradoc.army.mil/.
Military Benefits Information. http://www.dfas.mil/, http://www.gibill.va.gov/, http://www.va.gov/.

Part VI
Social Sciences, Journalism, Architecture, and the Arts

Chapter 24
MD-PhD in the Social Sciences

Erica Seiguer Shenoy

Key Points

- The doctoral degree is primarily a research degree.
- Consider the time trade-off carefully.
- Think ahead: an MD-PhD program is a major commitment and you need to consider your career objectives in this context.

Introduction

Most are familiar with the route of the MD-PhD, where the PhD training is in the biological sciences. It is only relatively recently, however, that combined programs offering doctoral training in the social sciences have been developed. Research ranging from health economics and health policy to anthropology and the history of medicine are now available to physicians in training who are committed to pairing clinical and research careers in the social sciences.

The purpose of doctoral studies – whether focused in immunology or economics – is to train students to become independent researchers. That is to say to have the necessary skill set to develop relevant research questions and design studies to answer those questions. The goal of this chapter is to help the reader navigate the decision to pursue joint studies in medicine and the social sciences.

E.S. Shenoy, MD, PhD (✉)
Division of Infectious Diseases, Department of Medicine, Massachusetts
General Hospital, Boston, MA 02114, USA
e-mail: eseiguershenoy@partners.org

R.D. Urman and J.M. Ehrenfeld (eds.), *Physicians' Pathways to Non-Traditional Careers and Leadership Opportunities*, DOI 10.1007/978-1-4614-0551-1_24, © Springer Science+Business Media, LLC 2012

Making the Decision to Pursue a Doctorate in the Social Sciences

Similar to the decision to go to medical school to become a physician, the decision to pursue a doctorate in the social sciences is one to consider carefully. It goes without saying that you should have a strong interest in the field. But further, what do you want to accomplish that requires a PhD? If your dream is to become a physician and work on public health projects, or to work in an administrative role as an adjunct to practicing medicine, a research degree is likely not necessary. If you imagine developing and implementing a research project, mentoring graduate students and postdocs, then a PhD may be useful.

Doctoral studies and the process of completing a dissertation will develop skills that are essential for a career in research. First, coursework in your field of choice will provide a framework for developing a dissertation topic. Depending on your area of interest, you may need training in statistics, including hands-on practice with a variety of statistical software packages, or decision analysis or a variety of other areas. Coursework will also provide a deep grounding in the literature of your chosen field, thus helping you to determine what areas may benefit from further research. These pursuits may result in dissertation opportunities. In a doctoral program, you will also likely begin to learn about teaching – through teaching assistant positions. This is another important component of your education as most clinician-researchers are also teachers. As a teaching assistant, you may learn about development of the course syllabus, you may teach sessions and grade papers, and may discover that one of the best ways to know a subject in depth is to teach it to someone else. As you work towards developing your dissertation, you will likely work as a research assistant to potential mentors. Such opportunities are an important aspect of doctoral studies because they not only provide you with potential research ideas, but allow you to work with more experienced researchers at developing a project, which is good preparation for your dissertation.

Doctoral studies require a significant investment of time that will likely delay your advancement in the medical profession (at least in the early stages). While your medical school classmates are finishing residency, pursuing fellowships, or advancing to attending-level positions, you will be at least several years behind in the medical hierarchy. This is not to say you won't "catch up" to your medical school peers but there should be no doubt that the time required to complete graduate studies may slow your advancement.

One way to think about whether or not what you want to do in your professional life is to identify individuals who are currently doing the kind of work you imagine yourself doing 10–15 years from now. Then, review their training path and career trajectory. Contacting and speaking with these professionals is also a good idea because often they may have advice on the kind of training they feel is essential to the work they do. Important questions to ask are: why did you choose training program X? Given the work you are currently pursuing, would you have elected another program/path in retrospect? What skill set do you feel is necessary to be successful in your research? Gathering data on several individuals you consider role models may help to focus your thoughts on whether or not the MD-PhD route is appropriate for you and your career objectives.

Choosing a Program

There are many different programs out there. The first distinction to be made among these is how formalized the combined program truly is. While MD-PhD programs in the biological sciences have been around for decades, are generally well-funded, and importantly, well-accepted within the academic community, those in the social sciences are more recent and thus issues surrounding funding and peer-acceptance may be more salient.

Formal programs exist at many institutions. The existence of the program does not necessarily guarantee the opportunity of funding through the Medical Scientist Training Program (MSTP – the common NIH-supported training mechanism for MD-PhDs). It is critical for you to understand how funding is structured (if at all) prior to applying or enrolling in such a program. Formal programs may also offer other benefits besides funding, including structured mentorship, the availability of alumni who can provide advice and serve as role models, and a clear path to combining your medical and graduate school studies.

If a formal program does not exist at the medical school or graduate school where you hope to enroll, there is always the option of working with the medical school and a mentor in a graduate school to craft a personalized, de-novo program. This route may be riskier than enrolling in a well-established combined program, but there are great rewards if it is the right fit for you. As opposed to medical education, where your success does not rely on one or a few individuals, doctoral level training in many ways does rely on just a few individuals – those with whom you will develop your dissertation research – that is, the chair and other members of your dissertation committee. While it is often impossible to know who will eventually become your mentor, it is riskier to attend an institution where there is only one or a few options as opposed to an institution with both numbers and variety of potential mentors.

Combining a Medical and Research Career

Starting from the time you apply and interview for a combined program going forward, you will ask yourself and others will ask of you (often in an interview situation!) about how you plan to combine a medical and research career.

The first thing to understand is that there is no single right way. There are plenty of models of physician-scientists out there who are successful in both arenas, but there is no magic to how this comes about.

Fig. 24.1 Considerations when
contemplating a research and
clinical career

Considerations When Contemplating a Research and Clinical Career

- Think about the potential research time / clinical time ratio.

- Think about the financial trade-offs between research and clinical practice.

Fig. 24.1 Considerations when contemplating a research and clinical career

There are, however, some clear constraints or what be considered "reality checks" as outlined in Fig. 24.1.

1. Most quote a rule of thumb for the divide between research and clinical work as 70/30. That is, to have a successful research career (i.e. be awarded prestigious grants from the National Institutes of Health–NIH– among others, publish in top journals, and develop a successful group of other researchers led by you), a commitment of at least 70% of your time to research is required. Thus, you first should consider whether practicing medicine 30% of the time (or less) is appealing to you. You should also consider, when choosing your medical specialty, whether the specialty is conducive to such limitations in clinical practice. As might be imagined, a career in neurosurgery may not thrive with such limited clinical experience.

2. There are financial consequences to focusing the majority of time and effort in research and not in clinical practice. This is not to be underestimated in terms of importance and requires you to think ahead to the possibility of starting and supporting a family (if you have not already done so at this point) as well as servicing undergraduate, professional and graduate school debt, if applicable.

That said, these rules are most applicable in the arena of academic medicine and may not apply should you decide at some point to leave academic or clinical medicine altogether, perhaps to focus entirely on research in the academic sector, government or private industry. In fact, the MD-PhD training will likely open up so many career opportunities for you that choosing from among them will be an enviable challenge.

While the role of clinician-scientist at an academic medical center is the most well-known and well-tread path, other opportunities abound. In the private, non-profit sector, MD-PhDs in the social sciences can work in both administrative and research capacities. The ability to integrate clinical care into your career in such a scenario is likely very much organization-specific. The same is true for positions in the Federal government, either at the National Institutes of Health, the Food and Drug Administration, the Centers for Medicare and Medicaid Services, or other health-related government entities. Again, how to integrate clinical work in these organizations is individual and organization-specific. The pharmaceutical, biotechnology, or medical device industries is another possible career trajectory. While one may think of individuals with PhDs in the biological sciences as more typical candidates, these industries also value skills developed in the study of social sciences such as economics, decision analysis, biostatistics, ethics, and communications, among many disciplines.

Perhaps most importantly, individuals who are flexible and driven will do the best with combined MD-PhD training in the social sciences. By virtue of having such diverse interests, and with the goal of combining them into a career, these individuals are most likely to be comfortable in uncharted territory, developing a career that may not be traditional, but will most likely be well-rewarded.

Personal Experience

My own personal experience is reflected in this chapter. I knew from very early on in life that I wanted to be a physician – that decision was solidified before I finished high school. At the same time, I had a wide range of interests in politics and policy. In college, I majored in molecular biology and did a significant amount of coursework in public policy. By the time I was deciding on applying to medical school, I knew I wanted additional training in health economics. At the time, however, there were few formal programs out there. Several mentors encouraged me to pursue my interests.

I searched for individuals who were working in a capacity I could see for myself in the future. I emailed them, out of the blue, explaining my interests and asking the same questions I describe above. I learned a great deal from these interactions and their advice led me to apply to several programs, ranging from those without a formal combined program to those with a formal established paths.

In the end, I chose the MD-PhD program at Harvard University, with the PhD program in health policy. Within this program I was admitted to the economics track, and completed both the MD and the PhD in a total of 8 years. Combining both medical school and graduate studies in health economics was a challenge, but as I went through the program, I noticed a cultural shift in how the training was perceived. As I started my training and would explain to medical colleagues what I was studying, I might get quizzical, though interested responses. But towards the end of the program, the reaction became one of great interest and excitement of having two very unique skill sets that could be very synergistic, especially in a time in which health policy and economics was on the front pages of the newspapers and on the minds of the majority of Americans. Suddenly, combining these two disciplines seemed to make perfect sense!

I was fortunate to have wonderful mentors throughout medical school and graduate school. I was a teaching assistant for college and graduate students and worked on a variety of research projects in many disciplines, including public health, business administration, healthcare quality, healthcare financing, and economics. After graduating, I went on to complete a residency in internal medicine and am now in an Infectious Disease fellowship program. Infectious diseases, which has been an interest of mine for many years, provides numerous avenues to apply my doctoral training.

The path I have chosen is one path of many. Many of my colleagues have chosen alternative paths, completing the PhD prior to medical school, or even after residency as a part of fellowship training, and everything in between. This is to emphasize that there is no "right" way to go about completing your training. Understanding why you want to pursue a combined career, and determining that a doctorate is the right training for you, however, is a fundamental aspect of creating your own path to success.

Additional Resources

American Association of Medical Colleges (AAMC) MD-PhD. http://www.aamc.org/students/considering/research/mdphd/.

American Physician Scientists Association (APSA) MD-PhD. http://www.physicianscientists.org/careers/training/md-phd.

MD-PhD Applicant Q & A page from University of Pennsylvania.

Chapter 25
Journalism, Publishing, and Writing

Michael Axley

Key Points

- When pitching a story, prepare beforehand. Research the story idea before presenting it – it is more effective than simply asking for an opportunity.
- Find an angle on the story that makes it original and reflects your significant insight.
- Don't save the best for last. Get right to the point of your article, starting it in the first paragraph.

Introduction

The bandwidth of medical information, for consumers and professionals, expanded exponentially with the advent of the Internet.

As a result, the opportunities for physicians to participate in journalism, writing, and publishing are fundamentally changed and increased. There are now a bewildering number of choices for doctors who want see their work published in areas outside of scientific journals.

Ten years ago, roughly, an individual seeking to learn to work as a reporter had two options: (1) start from the bottom up at a newspaper or television station; (2) obtain a journalism degree, and then look for a job. Medical reporting itself, as well as science journalism as a whole, was a specialty of sorts – like sports journalism, or legislative journalism – a type of beat, that one started looking into after applying oneself to more general topics, such as courts, police, suburban municipalities, and so on.

M. Axley, MD, MA (✉)
Department of Anesthesia and Perioperative Medicine, Oregon Health
and Science University, Portland, OR 97239, USA
e-mail: msaxley@gmail.com

R.D. Urman and J.M. Ehrenfeld (eds.), *Physicians' Pathways to Non-Traditional Careers and Leadership Opportunities*, DOI 10.1007/978-1-4614-0551-1_25, © Springer Science+Business Media, LLC 2012

That framework changed abruptly around the turn of the century. In the space of two or three years, journalistic web sites sprung up. We understand now they would come to dominate the business of journalism; at the time it was not so clear.

Even so, the training that the traditional (print and television) modes of reporting instilled remains important today, and it is worth the time to familiarize yourself with some of those principles if you desire to be published or appear on a public screen. I'm going to emphasize print journalism, because that's my background.

Why Pursue Journalism?

When considering what type of media is most appropriate for a given piece, probably the first item of business would be figuring out the goal of the article at hand (let's for a minute assume that we are talking about a simple article, as opposed to a multiplatform media event). In pursuit of this goal, it is worth reflecting on why you want to write this article in the first place. Let's look at a few possible reasons why people might want to undertake writing about medicine.

"I want to make some money." An admirable goal. If you are reading this chapter, odds are you are pursuing a medical career, either as a medical student, a resident, or a practicing physician. To be blunt, there is no way that pursuing a career in journalism will offer greater compensation than that which you already have or will shortly command.

"I'd like to supplement my income writing about something I find interesting." An excellent idea, and one well within the reach of most time-starved medical professionals. Keep in mind, however, that freelancing or part-time employment in the field of journalism in general, and medical journalism specifically, is no gold mine. A moonlighting shift spent in the emergency room of your local public hospital will yield at least three times more than a longer article (let's say 1,000 words). That's because the days of editors paying a dollar a word are gone – now we're talking 25 cents a word, if that. Conceiving, researching, talking to sources, and writing that 1,000 word article is going to take longer than a moonlighting shift, by a fairly decent margin.

"I want to enrich my life by writing and helping to educate my patients." Outstanding! Here are some suggestions by way of getting started.

How Can My Patients Benefit?

Where to turn as an aspiring journalist? Websites, health specific or general news sites. Blogs. Newspapers, industry sites, encyclopedic sites, self-help forums, self-publishing sites, patient-to-patient forums, personal web domains, to name a few. To winnow these possibilities down, it may help to reflect on the goal of a given article – who are the readers of this information and what does one hope to achieve? Define the audience, and then think about the forum best suited to reaching this audience.

Patients, and the public at large, have a vast appetite for medical information and reporting. The medical industry, its products, and its oversight, generate some of the biggest stories of our times. From the big news and media sites to the local community newspaper, news data is broken down, reorganized, produced, and sent out in all of its various forms to be consumed.

Every story has a place in this network of information, sometimes many places, each with a corresponding readership.

So, for example, what type of outlet, and audience, are appropriate for an article about the epidemic of obesity? There are some caveats. Obesity itself, as a topic, is too large. How can it be narrowed down to a manageable article, one that recognized experts can comment on quickly? It is also important to think about your audience so that when the piece is complete, they will actually be able to comprehend the subject matter. Consumer articles, for instance, should be written so that they can be understood by a 14 year old.

One Place to Start Would Be Locally

All hospitals, large and small, have a media department. This hospital may be a facility that employs residents, or staff physicians. It may be a facility where one has privileges, while also being a partner or employee in a practice of some sort. In this media department, there will be folks whose job it is to manage the hospital website, including the production of articles. There will also be, depending on the size of the hospital, editors, writers, public relations specialists, photographers, and graphic designers. In addition to the website, these professionals may also produce newsletters, magazines, video productions, special exhibitions, and so on.

In short, almost every medical center already has in place a media outlet. And the media they produce, more than likely, is well suited to the audience for basic, consumer-oriented reporting, if one is writing for the public, or for medical professionals, if one is looking to specialize.

Is this really a good place to start? How much of an audience will they really have, anyway? How is publishing in my hospital newsletter going to burnish my street credibility?

First, dollars to doughnuts the reach of a local hospital media department is broader than one might think. Second, they likely have people in-house who will be able to help with ideas about possible avenues for your writing, perhaps even assign topics or help with editing. A quick phone call will yield dividends: "Say, can you tell me who is in charge of editing the hospital newsletter?" "I wonder, can you tell me how I can get an article on the hospital website? Is there someone I could talk to?" The person you want to talk to has a name, and the receptionist knows what it is. Might even be the receptionist, who knows? Just ask.

The other issue, of course, is the eternal conundrum: "I want to write and get myself published, but I haven't been published yet." Hmm. The first question out of any editor's mouth, after listening to a pitch, assuming one gets to make a pitch, will be a request for clips. A clip is a copy of a previously published article, which they will then use to judge a reporter's ability to write the article proposed. At the top of that clip, or preferably clips, will be a byline. Your byline, signifying that you researched, wrote, and published said article. No bylines, no clips. No clips, maybe call back when you get some.

Even if the article on increasing numbers of pediatric patients with slipped epiphyseal plates is only published on the orthopedic subsection of your local hospital website, it will still come with a byline and the page can be printed and copied or sent as a link in an e-mail. Now, it's a clip. Once you have accumulated some clips to buttress your credentials, you are in a position to start looking somewhat farther afield for publication opportunities.

What Type of Training or Education Is Required?

Part of the fun of participating in the field of journalism is the real fact that it is egalitarian – there aren't really ranks of reporters, just some who have better access. Good writing will eventually find an outlet. And if you cannot write and cannot be coached, that too will be out there, for all to see.

Back in the day, training for a career as a reporter meant working your way up through the ranks, until by means of writing skill, political manipulation, or sheer good luck you landed in front of a typewriter with a deadline coming up fast.

Not that there weren't journalism schools – there were, and they were busily producing graduates. These graduates would then find their way to newspapers, or television stations, where they would be assigned to the same remote, low-level bureaus and given the same enthusiastic hazing they would have received had they not paid for that fancy degree.

As media outlets expanded, however, filling up new media as well as increasing numbers of hours in the day, it simply started to be more efficient to receive at least some training by way of a formal journalism program. Graduates of these programs had more choices, but these choices still looked pretty similar to the newspaper and the television channel – maybe writing feature length news stories for MSNBC, for example, or a cable channel instead of network.

Now, it's almost as though all bets are off again. But the journalism programs still do a decent job communicating the basic skills of the field. Most of these programs are 2 years long (the graduate programs). Most of them will run in the mid-five figures for tuition. They are still helpful, but not necessary, to the practice of journalism.

Medical journalism (the print variety) spans the gap from two paragraph Wikipedia entries entreating the reader to add adequate sourcing to expansive, well-written, and thought-provoking articles in the New Yorker.

Take the New Yorker piece vs. the Wikipedia entry. The polish of the one compared to the other is obvious. What may not be so evident is – the time spent writing, rewriting, editing, and writing again. Not the one article, but the article before that, and the series of articles before that as well. This is a way of saying that while anyone can write, it takes time spent writing to be involved as a cogent player.

That, if anything, is the takeaway point of this chapter. If you have the desire to write, publish, or participate in medical journalism, at any level, the first and most important task is to start writing.

Which Raises the Question: What Should I Write About?

The answer: whatever you like. Whatever interests you. If you are interested in a topic, likely it is fascinating and will make a great story. Particularly if there's a human angle – there are people involved. Remember, however, that other smart and talented people are out there, some of whom enjoy writing, and they probably thought this same idea would make a great story too.

That is to say, what's your angle on the story? Quick, think of an idea, something you think would be interesting to read about. Now, do a quick search on the web. Good lord, who knew there were hundreds of stories on obesity in teenagers, or water births, or adult vaccination? Maybe that isn't such a fine idea after all.

Nope, it's still a great idea, and you still have a contribution to make. But in order to make that contribution, one needs to figure out what it is about that idea that really makes it stand out above the background noise. Detail, so important in medicine, is no less important in journalism. How does adolescent obesity affect bone structure? Are certain types of fracture more common among obese adolescents? Is surgery more complicated? How?

With an idea in mind and basic research performed, one can start to look for sources who can shed more light on a story and verify the accuracy of the reporting. These are experts who, on the basis of their personal experience, can discuss a given topic with expertise and without rambling. The idea is that when called upon, these sources will yield pithy, entertaining quotes, about five sentences or less in length, that will illustrate an important point in a story.

> There are kids out there who are going to be crippled because we don't pay enough attention to their weight," said Dr. Ilene Veritas, chair of orthopedic surgery at North Sound General Hospital. "This problem is not going to go away.

Dr. Veritas, of note, has a keen and fundamental interest in this topic, and can assist you by providing relevant journal articles. She also knows other experts and will be happy to provide you with their phone numbers. She might even know a patient who would be willing to be interviewed. Be sure to present proper identification, in the form of: "I'm a reporter writing for the Mid-State Courier. I was given your name a possible source for an article about childhood obesity." Don't talk to kids without their parent's permission.

Stories are made or broken by the quality of reporting, and in part that means the quality, and number, of sources. Sources are dug up by research on the story topic itself. Who in the area has published scientific articles on a particular topic? Is anyone in the region particularly active on a newsworthy health initiative? Who heads up the local nonprofit clinics – what are their concerns? Who chairs the foundation for the recent all-city half-marathon?

By the way, I recommend taping interviews. Make verbal note of that point before taping your subject. Most of us cannot type accurately enough, quickly enough, to capture a source's statements exactly, nor can we write in shorthand. If a source's comments cannot be reproduced exactly, they cannot be placed in an article as a direct quote from that person; instead, they need to be paraphased, or placed outside of quotation marks. For example: Dr. Veritas went on to say that obese children face much greater risks to their health because of their weight. Paraphrase weakens the impact of a story – used too frequently, it also weakens credibility. Quotations read better and send the message that a reporter has a professional edge.

Since this is not a chapter on writing technique, I won't spend too much time discussing the organization of a written piece. I do want to address two parts and one principle of the general news article: *the "lede," the nut, and the inverted pyramid*.

The lede is the first paragraph of the story. In this paragraph, the reporter either leads into the reason for the article or piques the reader's curiosity sufficiently to allow them to continue reading on.

The second paragraph is called the nut. In the nut, the reporter informs the reader of the reason for the article and either outlines the article's structure or informs the reader of certain important facts (i.e., who, what, when, how, why, and where).

The lede and the nut are the most important parts of any news story, because conventional wisdom suggests most readers will not make it past these two paragraphs. That finely tuned and meticulously written story on the health hazards of a particular car seat will inevitably founder on the reefs of the Red Sox versus Yankees box score. Every time, or at least nine times out of ten. And that's even among women, who will be the predominant audience for most types of health reporting.

Keeping this generality in mind results in the use of a story structure called the inverted pyramid. This is a story structured so that the most important material, including the facts of the matter at hand, are in the starting paragraphs. Do not back into a story. Do not save the best for last. In that position, the best will not be seen by its intended audience. Instead, consider throwing out a short hook and then getting right to the heart of the matter. Better yet, dispense with the hook – they usually don't read as well as they write. Just go right at the story, from the first paragraph onward. Once the core of the article is presented there will be time to get into the details.

As an aside, another reason for use of the inverted pyramid is the speed with which it allows an article to be produced. Think reporters on deadline with 30 min to churn out an accurate 500–1,000 words. What strategy best suits this scenario? Get the important stuff out first, check your facts, then start adding quotes and color. Least important stuff at the bottom, because that's where the editors are going to start cutting as they shorten your piece. Still works that way today.

The mechanical structure of the inverted pyramid also serves as a method for breaking writer's block. The article, conceived, researched, and sourced, sits out there in the ether. Now it needs to be written.

Wanda Smith, 16 years old, lay in her hospital bed, waiting for her second knee surgery in as many months. A salutary attempt, and it includes a person, which is very important. Starting an article with a tear jerker, however, i.e. little Wanda, is hackneyed and unimaginative.

Dr. Ilene Veritas researches the problems facing pediatric orthopedic patients with a vigor sustained by few of her colleagues. No. Yawn. No.

As obesity gains a foothold among children, more and more of them are experiencing fractures which can lead to life-long problems with walking and the activities of daily living.

Obese children are more prone to a type of injury called a slipped epiphyseal plate, in which a child's weight causes the growth plate above the femoral neck to shear, requiring surgery.

There are kids out there who are going to be crippled because we don't pay enough attention to their weight," said Dr. Ilene Veritas, chair of orthopedic surgery at North Sound General Hospital. "This problem is not going to go away.

Wanda Smith, 16 years old, lies in her hospital bed, waiting for her second hip surgery in as many months.

See how that works? The lede. The nut. Turns out a great place for your best quote is right after the nut. Followed by some color. Practically writes itself. Don't forget to write in active tense.

A word about balance. Balance in reporting is critical, and every reporter needs to consider whether a given article represents a fair take on the issue at hand. If an opposing viewpoint is necessary, he or she needs to seek out that viewpoint and give it fair play, even if it is unpopular. At the same time, some viewpoints are more important than others and some are frankly ridiculous, requiring no forum.

A word about editing. When a treasured article passes from the hands of its doting reporter it will usually be turned over to a voracious, graceless, and ham-fisted individual called an editor. Often, this person will be the one who gave the green light for the article to proceed in the first place. Often, this person will hold the key to obtaining permission for pursuing further articles for the same media outlet. They will then, without asking for consent, proceed to rewrite the entire piece, including that cherished lede. There are two basic ways to respond to this indignity: (1) negotiate, understanding that time is a wasting and your options are limited. (2) Refuse publication of this travesty, with the understanding that your work is too important to be ignored.

The types of objectives I've outlined here are no less applicable for certain types of specialty writing. This holds true whether writing for peers in medicine or for the general public. The essentials of writing involve preparedness, accurate sourcing and context, and willingness to revise and rewrite.

There are professional reporters who do nothing but cover medical conferences, writing not for newspapers or consumer websites, but for trade publications or organizations providing Pharma competition research briefs. There are other venues, but the principles are the same. What is it that really makes this idea interesting right now? How is it immediately relevant to people and what are the implications for the future? How do I structure it so that people can get the information they need, quickly?

Conclusions

There are some great writers in the field of medical writing and reporting. Atul Gawande wrote the recent and widely read essay, "Letting Go" published in the New Yorker. Malcolm Gladwell writes about curiously off-beat topics that often have bearing on medicine. There are others, but the key is to become familiar with many medical writers and along the way, consider how they write. How do they put the bricks and mortar together?

Anyone starting out as a reporter will need a copy of The Associated Press Stylebook.

Your local or regional daily newspaper will have most of its medical news articles (those not taken from a bureau such as the Associated Press) written by one or two reporters. Take note of their byline and the topics they select. Read their stories.

The Centers for Disease Control and Prevention publishes the Morbidity and Mortality Weekly Report and will deliver it to your e-mail online. Most state health departments publish a monthly newsletter tracking health trends in their state.

Local and regional medical societies and specialty societies all produce newsletters and have websites. They are hungry for copy. If they don't have an outlet, it is well past time, and an excellent opportunity.

Chapter 26
A Different Angle: Physician and Architect

Ingrid Ganske

> **Key Points**
> - There is increasing need for medical expertise within architecture, especially looking at the relationship between design and health outcomes, increasing financial constraints, and technological advances.
> - Design considerations in healthcare include operational efficiency, patient safety, environmental issues, disaster planning, pandemic preparedness, and physiologic experience.
> - Architectural education can be informal or require a formal degree, depending on your role and degree of involvement with design.

There has been a relationship between medicine and architecture since ancient times. The care of the ill has taken place in a variety of settings, which have been recognized as a factor in the healing process (Currie JC. The fourth factor: a historical perspective on architecture and medicine. The American Institute of Architects: Washington, DC; 2007).

Introduction

Architecture is full of curves. From lofty domes, to elegantly flying buttresses, spiral staircases, and parabolic bridges, architectural curves provide intrigue and a sense of aesthetic completion. The same is often true of a career path. A medical career

I. Ganske, MD, MPA (✉)
Department of Plastic and Reconstructive Surgery, Massachusetts General Hospital,
Boston, MA 02114, USA
e-mail: iganske@partners.org

R.D. Urman and J.M. Ehrenfeld (eds.), *Physicians' Pathways to Non-Traditional Careers and Leadership Opportunities*, DOI 10.1007/978-1-4614-0551-1_26,
© Springer Science+Business Media, LLC 2012

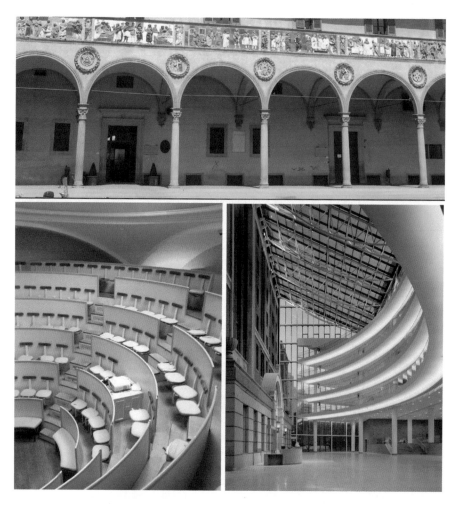

Fig. 26.1 *Top*: Loggia of Ospedale del Ceppo, a medieval hospital in Pistoia, Italy, with a frieze portraying works of mercy. (Wjarek, 2011. Used under license from http://shutterstock.com/). *Left*: Tiered seating in the Ether Dome at Massachusetts General Hospital, Boston, designed by Charles Bulfinch, served as the hospital's operating roomfrom 1821 to 1867 and was the site of the first public demonstration of inhaled ether. (Photo by Dr. Ingrid Ganske). *Right*: Bellevue Hospital Ambulatory Care Pavilion, New York City, by Pei Cobb Freed, 2005, incorporates a historic building by McKim, Mead and White as the public entrance to a facility strategically divided into public, service, and clinical zones (© Paul Warchol Photography, Inc.)

that starts off linearly may take unexpected turns, leading to delightful discoveries. This section will describe some of the unique career twists available for those who have an artistic inclination, an aptitude for spatial conceptualization, or a concern for how the built environment affects our patients and our practice (Fig. 26.1)

Many doctors appreciate architecture – we pause our rushed steps in a well-proportioned courtyard, notice a telescoping sequence of doors down a long corridor,

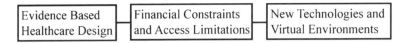

| Evidence Based | Financial Constraints | New Technologies and |
| Healthcare Design | and Access Limitations | Virtual Environments |

Fig. 26.2 Ways physicians can participate in the design process

or comment on a patient's view out their window – but few have taken extracurricular roles in this field and even fewer have made the full-time professional leap to architecture. In light of the rare examples of physician involvement in healthcare architecture, this section will offer a précis on some healthcare design issues, with the goal of inspiring new investigation into the timeless relationship between space and healing.

For those who find this field compelling, the primary challenge lies in carving a niche for yourself within the two relatively separate fields. However, there is increasing need for medical expertise within architecture, and many potential ways to get involved. We are entering a new era for healthcare architecture. First, the field of evidence-based medicine is beginning to examine the relationship between design and health outcomes in order to deliberately employ design strategies that will decrease the spread of nosocomial infections, reduce duration of hospital stays, and increase patient satisfaction. Second, increasing financial constraints are driving a demand for efficiently tailored clinical spaces. And third, technology is opening possibilities of entirely new virtual healthcare spaces; patients can now teleconference, email, or even visit their doctors by video from home. Architects need healthcare providers' input about what entails ideal clinical spaces, what the evolving patients needs and demands are, and the benefits and limitations of new technologies in care giving. There are a number of roles that physicians can play in this dialogue. Some suggestions of ways to participate and to gain additional background in this field are outlined in Fig. 26.2.

What Do Healthcare Architects and Designers Do?

First, what is healthcare architecture? In one sense, healthcare architecture is the design of the actual buildings in which care is provided to the ill. However, health is impacted by our spatial environments at many scales – interior spaces, building structures, surrounding landscapes, and city designs. In each case there are a number of considerations that go into creating healthcare structures and "healthy" environments.

When designing structures and interiors, healthcare architects take into account operational functions of many types, outlined in Table 26.1. Equally concerning are the physiological and psychological effects of the hospital experience. Lighting, color, and nature create ambience that impacts both the patients' and physicians' moods. The acoustic environment affects patients' sleep cycles and the staff's ability to effectively communicate with each other. Small design details can play an

Table 26.1 Summary of design considerations in the healthcare setting

Design considerations for healthcare	Examples
Operational efficiency	Connectivity of different departments, workflow patterns
Patient safety	Preventing falls
Environmental issues	HVAC and airflows, waste disposal
Disaster planning	Arranging alternate routes, structural integrity
Pandemic preparedness	Negative pressure systems, quarantine spaces
Physiologic experience	Lighting, acoustics, colors

important role in individual patient comfort, for instance having private rooms and convenient places for patients to store their belongings, or even choosing the art on their walls from a rotating collection. Children's hospitals, in particular, are canvases for incorporating interactive sound displays, hopscotch hallways, or virtual reality educational games to provide fun, learning, and development throughout hospitalization.

Beyond the design of clinical space, there are also health matters in landscape design and urban planning. Availability of recreational spaces for exercise, safe streets to promote walking instead of driving, vegetation to counteract the effects of air pollution, and availability of shelter for the underprivileged – all these elements impact our patients' health and safety. Physicians may be the first to identify adverse effects of the built environment and, by advocating for community action, they already bridge the fields of health and architecture. There is also a growing body of preventive medicine research examining the effects of particular infrastructure interventions, such as improving mass transit options, on reducing the population burden of obesity and comorbid diseases.

Those, then, are just a sampling of the pertinent design issues in healthcare. Most professionals involved in these building projects are full-time architects or engineers, some with special training or many years experience specifically in healthcare. What these designers *do* on a daily basis evolves as a particular project progresses through various stages of design, drafting, engineering, contracting, and construction.

From conception to completion, building a clinic or hospital takes three to five, or often even more, years – a very different scale than a clinic visit, hospitalization, or surgery. The initial planning stages for an architectural project usually involve a client, such as a hospital board, meeting with a number of design firms who bid on the project. Sometimes they hold a design competition, in which interested firms submit renderings and scale models of a proposal for the job. Once a firm is selected, the board or founder will work closely with the firm to set expectations and parameters for the structures – how many beds the facility needs, what services it will provide, and a budget. The design phase is a collaborative process with architects and structural engineers, requiring numerous mock-ups and routine meetings. As the design goes through several iterations and occasional dramatic alterations, there are tight deadlines, late nights, and lots of coffee. There is a public perception of architects as having glamorous lives and creative autonomy. The reality is that day in and day out, the work is primarily office-based, and individual architects spend most of their time at computers using CAD or similar software. For every artistic idea and creative solution, there is much more time spent carefully drafting every single detail.

Roles for Physicians in Architecture and Design

There are a variety of opportunities for physicians in architecture, short of a full-fledged career change. Most of these are not well-documented and require investigation and initiative on an individual basis. The opportunities that arise for bridging the fields of architecture and medicine will largely be of your own making.

First are consulting type roles. Speak with your hospital administration or facilities committee about the opportunity for physician input into the design of a new wing of the hospital. Different doors may open for physicians of different specialties; the infectious disease doctor has valuable input for the engineering of HVAC and airflow systems to prevent contaminations, radiologists may have ideas about how to integrate their services within other departments to improve clinical communication and efficiency, and an emergency medicine physician may have innovative ideas for mobile care facilities in the case of natural disasters and emergencies. Consulting positions range from helping a specific hospital board, to working on retainer with an architecture firm, or being employed by a management-consulting firm with a division for health systems and structures (see Chap. 10, for more general information).

Second, architectural interventions may be able to improve patient care and population health outcomes. More research is needed, and there is no shortage of questions to examine. For instance, what can the built environment offer to prevent chronic health problems that result from pollution, inactivity, or inaccessibility? Or, on an experiential level, how can spaces improve patient satisfaction, provide camaraderie, and overall efficiency of services? Both architects and physicians are studying these relationships. Look for partnerships with the architectural department in your local University.

In a third category are public health, advocacy, or international health roles. It may be possible to work with the local or statewide department of public health or urban planning to bring a healthcare perspective to city-sized plans. Volunteering with human rights organizations could allow you to advocate for human shelter and access for the disabled members of society. And, in an international setting, the opportunities are even broader, since many physicians setting up care facilities in resource poor areas often have to design and build the very structures in which they can serve.

Finally, the same artistic and structural fascination that may spark one's interest in architecture could be equally applicable to smaller scale designs – for medical devices, orthopedic implants, or prosthetics.

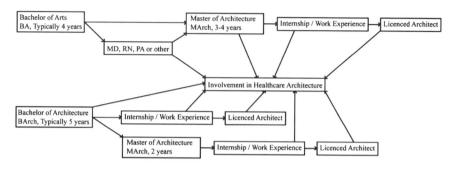

Fig. 26.3 Pathways to a career in architecture

An Architectural Education

Formal Vs. Informal Education

What type of training you might need depends on how sharp of a bend you imagine in your medical career. Are you a physician looking to fully switch careers and become an architect of clinical buildings, or possibly an urban planner promoting public health through clean cities? Or, do you see yourself having a full-time (or at least part-time) medical or surgical practice, while being able to participate in dialogues about the most efficient design of new operating room space, conducting research on the relationship between healthcare spaces and healthcare outcomes. For the former, an architectural degree is necessary; for the latter, however, there are many ways you can gain valuable experience and make forays into the field, without boxing up your stethoscope or loupes (Fig. 26.3).

Formal Education

Becoming a fully licensed architect requires a combination of degree program and internship, much like becoming a physician. An undergraduate Bachelor of Architecture typically takes 5 years to complete, requiring a thesis and internship. Alternatively, an undergraduate Bachelor of Arts with major in Architecture or any alternative area of study could be followed by a 3–4-year Master of Architecture degree. Both degree paths open similar doors. And in either case, architectural degree candidates are expected to take courses in art history, design, computer rendering, physical sciences, and theory as well as courses focusing on engineering and construction. In addition to a degree from an accredited program, architects must complete an internship of typically three years and pass the Architect Registration Examination (ARE).

Unlike pursuing a dual degree in law, business, or public health, for which there are many joint-degree programs, there currently are no schools that offer a combined

Table 26.2 Selected architecture schools with healthcare design programs

Clemson University	M.Arch with concentration in Architecture + Health
Texas A&M	M.Arch with Certificate in Health Systems Design
University of Kansas	M.Arch in the area of health and wellness
University of Illinois-Chicago	Master of Science in Architecture in Health Design
University of Nebraska-Lincoln	Program in Healthcare Design

medical and architectural degree. However, some architecture schools offer programs in healthcare design (see Table 26.2). Most architectural programs require full-time course work, however there are some that offer night time classes so that it is possible to earn a degree while working full (or nearly full) time.

The decision to pursue a formal education is thus a lengthy commitment. It requires either taking a full break from clinical practice and medical studies or possibly taking a scaled-back clinical or research position, in order to be able to fully participate and complete the architectural coursework at the same time.

Informal Experience

Alternatively, there are many ways to gain useful architectural knowledge and skills without getting any additional degrees or licenses. If you have no intention of being able hang out your own shingle as an autonomous architect, you can buff your architectural knowledge and skills in a piecemeal fashion.

One option is taking architecture courses outside of a formal degree program. Many architectural degree programs offer reduced registration prices for community members to take courses without receiving academic credit. Signing up to audit a class on healthcare interiors, the history of hospital architecture, or free hand drawing can provide exposure to the field with a limited time commitment. Additionally, art museums often offer classes or workshops in art and architecture appreciation.

Similarly, professional architecture associations hold meetings and lectures focusing on various topics, including healthcare design. These are typically open to people from any profession. The American Institute of Architecture has a specific subdivision dedicated to healthcare architecture – the Academy of Architecture for Health, which, among other activities, hosts an annual meeting and provides online seminars in the field.

Seek out mentors in both the architectural and medical fields, as it may be hard to find other individuals who straddle both these fields. Contact a local architecture firm that has experience designing healthcare facilities, consider doing a summer internship with the local or state department of urban planning department or simply ask for a tour of your hospital's infrastructure from the building and engineering staff. There are many potential points of entry – the key is to take the initiative and be creative. Your unique perspective as a physician with exposure to and interest in design is valuable and will likely be welcomed.

As a Physician, How Do I Benefit From Incorporating an Interest in Architecture into My Career?

First, as described above, architecture and design affects our patients in innumerable ways. As physicians, it behooves us to continually seek ways to improve patient care and patient outcomes. As we strive to provide constantly better care, innovations in the built environment are an underexamined opportunity for such improvements. Thinking about the spaces in which we work and patients heal may make us better care-givers.

Second, pursuing opportunities in architecture and design may provide unique exposure to hospital administrators and managers. Design and architectural decisions are significant, even monumental, ones. Such decisions require weighing not only health and design issues, but also business, financial, and legal considerations. Participating in the design process may provide exposure to those involved in these aspects of hospital management and administration, potentially advancing or providing unexpected opportunities in similar administrative roles.

Finally, if you are reading this, chances are you have a creative urge, a keen sense of design, and an interest in merging the aesthetic and the functional. Whether dipping a toe in the water – by attending a seminar, providing input into the design of a new medical facility or just thinking about your built environment – or diving in to pursue a full architectural degree, exploring ways to bridge the fields of medicine and architecture may provide an outlet for your creative urges and improve your career and personal satisfaction.

Additional Practical Resources/Websites

Architecture Degree Programs

See the National Architectural Accrediting Board for a full list of programs. http://www.naab.org/architecture_programs/.

Programs that Specifically Offer Graduate Programs in Healthcare Design

Clemson University: Master of Architecture with concentration in Architecture + Health. www.clemson.edu/caah/architecture/1.3.4.php.
Texas A&M: Master of architecture with certificate in health systems design. http://archone.tamu.edu/laup/Programs/Certificates.html.
University of Kansas: Master of Architecture in the area of health and wellness. http://www.saud.ku.edu/architecture/degrees/grad.
University of Illinois-Chicago: Master of Science in Architecture in Health Design. http://www.arch.uic.edu/healthdesign/index.php.
University of Nebraska-Lincoln College of Architecture: Program in healthcare design. http://architecture.unl.edu/programs/research/HDR.shtml.

Programs that Offer Architectural Degrees Through Evening and OnLine Courses

Carnegie Mellon School of Architecture http://www.cmu.edu/architecture.
Boston Architectural College http://www.the-bac.edu.

Professional Organizations

American Institute of Architects (AIA) http://www.aia.org.
Academy of Architecture for Health (within AIA) http://network.aia.org/AIA/Academyof
    ArchitectureforHealth.
American Society of Landscape Architects (ASLA) http://www.asla.org/healthcare.
American College of Healthcare Architects (ACHA) http://www.healtharchitects.org.
American Academy of Healthcare Interior Designers (AAHID) http://www.aahid.org.

Websites, Journals, and Additional Reading

General Information on Architecture School. http://www.architectureschools.com.
Healthcare design magazine. http://www.healthcaredesignmagazine.com.
Healthcare building ideas. http://www.healthcarebuildingideas.com.
Berry LL, et al. The business case for better buildings. Frontiers of Health Services Management.
    2004.
Ulrich R, et al. The role of the physical environment in the hospital of the twenty-first century: a
    once-in-a-lifetime opportunity. Report to the Centre for Health Design. September 2004.
Finch P. Doctors' orders: healthcare architecture, too often a functionalist response to short-term
    budgeting, should increasingly be based on wealth of evidence about how patients respond to
    different physical environments. The Architectural Review. May 2005.
Currie JC. The fourth factor: a historical perspective on architecture and medicine. Washington,
    DC: The American Institute of Architects; 2007.

Chapter 27
Enriching Your Career Through the Arts

Mary E. Thorndike

Key Points

- One can use the arts as a source of personal sustenance and renewal, a means of medical education, professional development and community-building, a research topic, or a healing modality with patients.
- The arts can also be a powerful source of professional development and renewal for medical professionals at all career stages, and can also serve a community-building purpose.
- There are multiple ways that creative arts can be used directly with patients with an explicit goal of healing.

While medicine is to be your vocation or calling, see to it that you have also an avocation – some intellectual pastime which may serve to keep you in touch with the world of art, of science, or of letters. Begin at once the cultivation of some interest other than the purely professional … No matter what it is, have an outside hobby. For the hard-working medical student it is easier perhaps to keep up an interest in literature. Let each subject in your year's work have a corresponding outside author. When tired of anatomy refresh your minds with Oliver Wendell Holmes; after a worrying subject in physiology, turn to the great idealists, to Shelley or to Keats, for consolation; when chemistry distresses your soul, seek peace in the great pacifier, Shakespeare; ten minutes with Montaigne will lighten the burden (Osler [1]).

M.E. Thorndike, MD, MPA (✉)
Division of General Medicine

Harvard Medical School, Department of Medicine,
Brigham and Women's Hospital, MA 02130, USA
e-mail: mthorndike@partners.org

R.D. Urman and J.M. Ehrenfeld (eds.), *Physicians' Pathways to Non-Traditional Careers and Leadership Opportunities*, DOI 10.1007/978-1-4614-0551-1_27,
© Springer Science+Business Media, LLC 2012

Introduction

The goal of this chapter is to discuss some of the myriad ways in which you can link an interest in creative arts with medical practice. Many physicians have training or interest in music, visual art, theater, dance, or writing – and there are a multitude of ways that you can continue these interests in your work as a physician. You can use the arts as a source of personal sustenance and renewal, a means of medical education, professional development and community-building, a research topic, or a healing modality with patients. The following examples highlight ways in which physicians do all of these things, which I hope will inspire you to find ways to link your interest in the arts with your training and practice.

Personal Arts Practice

The simplest and most fundamental way to use the arts to enrich your work as a physician is simply to continue your own personal arts practice. Countless physicians paint, write, play music, dance, act, and sing, and find this to be a rich source of meaning, emotional expression, and personal renewal that resonates deeply with their work. Medical practice is emotionally and interpersonally intense, and all physicians need to find ways to process these emotions either directly or indirectly. For some people this need is met through physical activity, spiritual practice, or talking with friends and family. However, involvement with the arts either as a direct participant or as a consumer is also a deeply satisfying and effective mode of self-care. And it is not necessary to actually practice an art form yourself – reading, looking at artwork, listening to music, or attending performances are things that are available to everyone and can give deeper meaning to both your personal and professional lives.

Arts in Medical Education

Over the last several decades, there has been tremendous expansion in the use of arts in medical education. A 2002 survey of US medical schools by Rodenhauser et al. found that more than half of all US medical school incorporated arts into the curriculum in some way [2]. In general, arts in medical education tend to serve one of two broad purposes: helping students master the basic material and clinical skills; or serving to inspire students to reflect on the humanistic side of medicine, with the goal of becoming more compassionate physicians. The medical humanities movement most often reflects this latter goal, using literature and other art forms to teach reflection and humanistic values. There is a strong medical humanities community in medical education, and many medical schools have departments or institutes of medicine and humanities, or student-published medical humanities journals, or a series of required or elective medical humanities classes. This is probably the most common goal of using arts in medical education.

However, there are also a number of innovative programs that use creative arts to directly teach clinical skills or even preclinical basic science. At the University of British Columbia Medical School, first-year medical and dental students taking their Cardiovascular Physiology block are invited to participate in a photography contest as part of their coursework. Individual students or tutorial groups can submit images of original photography (and in more recent years, video and mixed media works) that represent or interpret in some way the physiologic concepts they are studying. Students submit more than 200 entries per year to this "Heartfelt Images" contest. In an article describing the contest and showcasing several remarkable images, course director Dr. Carol-Ann Courneya points out that student images tend to fall into one of three categories: Using an image to demonstrate a clear understanding of a complex concept; using beautiful imagery to capture a physical quality of the heart; and making new connections by capturing an existing image unrelated to the heart with fresh eyes that connect it to a cardiovascular concept. For instance, a student chose to illustrate atrial fibrillation, in which the atrium is often described as resembling "a bag of worms" with an image of gummy worms in a plastic bag, formed into the shape of a heart.

At Harvard Medical School, first-year students take an elective course called *Training the Eye* which aims to teach the clinical skill of close and accurate observation as part of physical diagnosis through a course that takes place in an art museum. Students attend sessions that teach specific visual observation techniques at Boston's Museum of Fine Arts, and then learn to apply these skills to observation of real patients in the hospital. The course is co-taught by physicians and art educators. Students might learn about texture and patterns by first looking at works by Jackson Pollack and a thirteen-century Iranian sculpture, then hear a lecture on "Texture and Pattern Recognition in Dermatologic Diagnosis," and then observe several patients with various skin conditions to practice what they have learned [3]. A study associated with the course found that students who took this course later scored higher on a test of visual skills, compared with control students who volunteered for the course but were not selected by lottery to enroll [3].

At Albert Einstein College of Medicine, students follow the methodology of Renaissance artists and use drawing as a way of learning anatomy. In a session known as "Da Vinci Night," anatomy professor Dr. Todd R. Olson and portrait artist Andrew Lattimore lead students in drawing not from life but from death, using the cadavers of the anatomy lab as models. In an article about the program (http://www.einstein.yu.edu/home/fullstory.asp?id=512), first-year student Daniel Schaerer noted "The incredible complexity of the hand was somewhat astonishing. We study the anatomy in detail and I can name most of the bones, joints and ligaments that I tried to draw, but actually translating those into lines, curves and shadows made me appreciate the awe-inspiring intricacy of it all." Educational theorists might argue that it also helps them understand the three-dimensional relationships among those bones, joints, and ligaments in a way that is more powerful and enduring than simply studying them from a book.

The above examples use art to help students enrich their mastery and understanding of the material they are studying; many other examples of art in medical education are more broadly focused on humanistic goals of fostering reflection, compassion for patients, and self-knowledge and self-care as physicians. In another example involving an anatomy course that has a somewhat different goal, first-year students at the University of Massachusetts Medical School from 1989 through 2002 were greeted with an assignment before they even arrived at school that asked them to use their creativity as part of preparing for the anatomy lab. In an exercise developed by Dr. Sandra Bertman and Dr. Sandy Marks, students received a packet over the summer with a blank sheet of paper and an attached memo reading: "In the space below, [1] please devise an image of any sort relating to your thoughts or feelings as you anticipate the experience of image dissections [2]. On the attached page, we would appreciate an explanation of your drawing or image [3]. Please mail your image and commentary to Dr. Bertman or Dr. Marks as soon as possible." The students' images were then incorporated (anonymously) into a slide show that they watched before their first session in the anatomy lab. Themes that tended to arise in the students' art included feelings about death and dying, students' fears about feeling repelled or incompetent in the face of dissection, questions about the life led by the cadavers prior to death, and reflections on the common humanity of cadaver and student [4].

At Brigham and Women's Hospital, Dr. Mariah Quinn takes groups of interns to Boston's Museum of Fine Arts for an evening experience that centers around reflection and discussion of art. Looking at selected works of art, the interns reflect on their work and on their patients, and end up discussing themes that range from frustration and distress with the intensity of the intern experience, to deep expressions of grief about patients who have died, to empathy for patients and family members. Dr. Quinn describes one of the works of art and the groups' typical experience as follows:

> We view together a haunting Etruscan Sarcophagus with a relief image of a married couple that is both intimate and somehow strikingly modern in its sensibilities. After a brief introduction to the object by one of the art educators, the interns are invited to express what comes to mind when looking at the object – either concrete observations or responses. Following a period of looking together, we are seated in the gallery and, cued by the questions, "How does this piece relate to the experiences you've had in caring for dying patients?" [5].

A sample of comments from interns who have participated in the program reflect the depth of meaning that is typically experienced:

> … A humanizing experience. I used a part of my brain that has not been used recently. So much of my time is spent dealing with lab values and medical notes. Now I got to think creatively for the first time in awhile….

> … found the experience to be moving – emotionally, spiritually, and physicially – was unprepared for how much I longed for this kind of time away from the hospital

> … I thought our conversation about death in front of the Etruscan Sarcophagus was very meaningful. The piece generated a lot of conversation about issues which are both important and not often talked about in the hospital … [5].

Arts and Professional Development

The arts can also be a powerful source of professional development and renewal for medical professionals at all stages of training. One well-known example is the "Literature and Medicine" program originally developed by the Maine Humanities

Council in 1997 and since disseminated to over 25 states (http://www.mainehumanities. org/programs/litandmed/). The program is a hospital-based humanities reading and discussion program that brings together doctors, nurses, administrators, and allied health professionals in their own workplace for monthly discussion based on assigned reading. Readings can include both fiction and nonfiction works that are chosen to stimulate identification, reflection, or controversy in thinking about the work of caring for patients. For instance, a group might read selections including *The Diving Bell and the Butterfly*, a memoir about living with locked-in syndrome by Jean-Dominique Bauby; a selection of poetry from *Between the Heart Beats: Poetry and Prose by Nurses*, edited by Cortney Davis and Judy Schaefer; the play *Wit* by Margaret Edson, which portrays a woman dying in the hospital of advanced ovarian cancer; and the short story "People Like That Are the Only People Here" by Lorrie Moore, which is about a mother's experience of her young son's diagnosis and treatment for childhood cancer.

The sessions are typically led by a humanities scholar in conjunction with a liaison from the hospital staff. The sessions not only stimulate reflection about patient care, but also lead to revelations about the different perspectives each profession brings to this work, and to increased mutual respect among group participants. Program participants also tend to report increased sensitivity to social and cultural factors in patients' experience of illness, a deeper understanding of the importance of communication with patients and their families [6].

In my own work as Medical Director of the Integrated Teaching Unit (ITU) at Brigham and Women's Hospital, I have the privilege of bringing teams of medical professionals to the Harvard Art Museum twice a month for an evening of reflection and multidisciplinary teambuilding, co-led by the museum's director of education, Ray Williams. A typical group consists of five or six physicians, two medical students, several nurses, a physical therapist, a social worker, and a pharmacist – all of whom are assigned to care for the patients on a particular floor of the hospital. We spend the evening having dinner together, then participating in series of structured discussions about works of art: working together to find the meaning or story behind a particular painting; sharing our emotional reactions to a series of works; or looking to see what a particular work of art says about our work caring for patients.

It is notable that while research has shown the importance of teamwork in healthcare, and that failures in teamwork can be a source of medical errors [7], physicians and allied health professionals are often ill-prepared to work together. Medical professionals are largely trained in completely separate systems (schools of medicine, nursing, pharmacy, physical therapy, and social work), and actually operate within the hospital in separate clinical and administrative units. Even when caring for the very same patients, medical professionals remain "siloed" within their individual disciplines without necessarily even knowing each other's names beyond seeing each others' illegible signatures in the chart.

An important goal of the ITU is to have a fully integrated multidisciplinary team that works together to provide excellent care to all patients and their families. Our experiences at the Harvard Art Museum have been a critical part of building this team. My primary goal for the teambuilding experience is to remove team members from the highly structured, hierarchical world of the hospital and to put them in a setting where everyone has equal access to meaning, everyone can speak with authority and authenticity, and everyone's point of view is valued and needed. When we struggle together to build a theory about the meaning of a work of art, a student nurse and a senior physician-scientist can both contribute insights of substantial depth and meaning.

I also aim to give the group a chance to reflect about their work, and to learn from each other about areas of overlap and difference in how the different disciplines approach clinical care. Standing in front of a statue, a physical therapist can tell a story about her work that makes a medical student see his work with patients in a new way.

The museum experience also serves as a chance for each group to learn something about themselves as a team – patterns of communication, humor, areas of tension, ability to tolerate disagreement, and ability to build on each others' ideas. When the group faces an interpretive challenge, building theories about the meaning of a particular work, many of these features of the group are revealed. When we invite participants to reflect on their group's process, and when we offer observations at the end of the evening about how a particular group worked together, this models a reflective practice that they are encouraged to continue in the hospital.

Finally, I aim to give team members a chance to reflect on the deepest and most mysterious aspects of the life-and-death work they do, and to share those moments with each other in a way that transcends the boundaries of disciplines or hierarchies of training. Works of art facilitate this deeper communion with the questions that run through medical practice – how do we understand suffering? What does it mean to be human? How do we care compassionately for others and yet maintain our own sense of self? Some of our most powerful moments in the museum have involved moments of recognition of these themes in the art we are looking at together, woven through with stories and memories about our work in the hospital.

When the teams return to the hospital after sharing this experience, there is a new sense of connection, of knowing each other in a way that transcends the superficial. People who would have passed each other without noticing 3 days before now stop and talk about their shared patients: "What do you think about Mr. B? This is what I've noticed – how have things gone during your time with him?" "I'm worried about …." "I'm wondering whether you have any experience with …." "Let's meet as a group with Mrs. M and her family and …. " We have other important and necessary structures in place to support teamwork: structured multidisciplinary rounds, sign-out systems, orientations for new team members, and a discharge planning checklist. However, I believe that the connections built at the museum are the transformative elements that truly make the team a team.

Using Creative Arts with Patients

There are multiple ways that creative arts can be used directly with patients with an explicit goal of healing. Art therapy, dance therapy, drama therapy, writing therapy, and music therapy are all established practices with governing bodies and certification for practitioners. There is also an integrated field known as expressive arts therapy in which practitioners move among various disciplines while working with patients. These therapies are usually directed at mental health and social functioning, but some practitioners work with patients with physical illness as well. The goal of these therapies is to use the process of creative expression to allow patients to connect with and express emotions that are difficult to access directly or to express in ordinary conversation. In general, physicians have not been directly involved in these fields and are often ignorant about their benefits. However, physicians are becoming increasingly interested in the potential of creative arts and are forming more collaborative relationships both with expressive arts practitioners and with artists interested in health and illness through organizations like the Society for Arts in Healthcare and the Foundation for Art and Healing.

Rafael Campo is a physician and poet who has written extensively about his overlapping work in the worlds of medicine and literature, and in particular about his use of poetry in his work with patients [8]. Dr. Campo may include poems in his packets of patient handouts given at the end of a visit, or sometimes reads poetry with patients during a visit. He has written movingly about how this stepping back from the concrete details of health and illness and into the emotional, symbolic realm of poetry can open new understanding on the part of both doctor and patient, or bring about transformation in the therapeutic relationship. He also invites patients to write about themselves and their experience with illness, and to share that writing with him at the next visit. Dr. Campo has also led writing groups for patients with particular illnesses, such as HIV, cancer, and depression. He notes that the process of writing about illness gives people a sense of "authorship" over their illness and its meaning, which can be a powerfully healing adjunct to traditional medical therapies [9].

As the director of the Katherine Swan Ginsburg Humanism in Medicine Program at Beth Israel Deaconess Medical Center and Harvard Medical School, Dr. Campo runs a wide variety of medical humanities programs including an annual Medical Humanities Week that features multiple lectures, and events, and which showcases the artistic talent of the hospital's housestaff through an art exhibition and music performance. Dr. Campo has also developed a "Poetry on Rounds" curriculum that encourages medical teams to incorporate poetry reading into their daily clinical discussions.

Another example of an innovative attempt to blend a commitment to the arts with medical practice is Dr. Sam Willis, a family practice physician in Minneapolis, Minnesota. After an experience working to display the work of local artists at the hospital where he worked, Dr. Willis had the idea of opening a medical practice that would provide healthcare for artists and other creative people who might not have health insurance or access to traditional sources of healthcare. He designed a practice that used an innovative economic model but also incorporated an art gallery as an active part of the practice space. Dr. Willis curates or co-curates exhibits in the gallery space and uses this space as an event space for the arts community as well [10].

In an interview, Dr. Willis describes moments when the presence of the art in the office opened or facilitated a conversation with a patient that might not have happened otherwise. For instance, one patient was feeling frustrated over conflicting advice about his wife's recently diagnosed diabetes: it seemed the dietician, the endocrinologist, and the primary care doctor were all saying different things. Dr. Willis started talking with the patient about a mural in his office which looked different depending on where the viewer stood in looking at it: it was possible to see one thing close up; something different from a few steps back; and something still different from 10 ft. back. This led to a discussion of how each professional dealing with the diabetes has a different point of view depending on their particular expertise – and on ways for the patient and his wife to integrate these points of view to a "big picture" that works for them [11].

Research in Arts and Medicine

Some physicians have combined their interests in the creative arts with their research interests, with fascinating results. Dr. Claudius Conrad at Massachusetts General Hospital is both a surgeon and a musician, and has conducted studies on how listening to music affects both critically ill patients in the intensive care unit and surgeons in the operating room. A classically trained pianist who also holds a doctorate in music philosophy, Dr. Conrad published a study in which he showed that patients in the surgical intensive care unit who were fitted with headphones and then exposed to Mozart piano sonatas had lower blood pressure and heart rates, lower levels of epinephrine and Il-6 which are associated with stress response, and needed less sedating medication than patients who wore headphones but didn't hear any music. This study also broke new ground in showing that the patients listening to Mozart also had 50% increased levels of growth hormone in their blood, an unexpected finding with potential to lead to new insights about how patients respond to the stress of surgery and critical illness [12].

Dr. Conrad has also studied the effects of music on performance by his fellow surgeons. In a novel experiment published in *Surgical Endoscopy*, he showed that expert surgeons performed on a laparoscopic simulator with greater accuracy when listening to Mozart than when working under silent conditions or listening to an obnoxious blend of German folk music in one ear and death metal in the other ear [13].

Arts, Medicine, and Community

The arts can also serve a community-building purpose among physicians, as generations of medical students who have taken part in medical student shows can attest. Some medical communities have formal arts groups that perform together. Boston's Longwood Symphony Orchestra draws its musicians from local hospitals and Harvard Medical School, and performs four concerts per year which also serve as fundraisers for medically related causes.

At Columbia University College of Physicians and Surgeons, for more than 40 years medical students have run a highly successful theater company, the Bard Hall Players, which produces three full productions per year. The company produces a musical in the fall, a classic work (often Shakespeare) in the winter, and a contemporary piece in the spring. The productions each involve approximately 40 students, both as cast and members of the production team; some students have extensive, even professional theater backgrounds and others have never participated in theater before. Although there is no explicit attempt to link play choices or the process of producing a play to medical themes, those who participate often feel that they gain skills that are useful in their ongoing medical training [14]. For instance, there is some similarity in the teamwork involved in putting on a show and the teamwork involved in working on the wards in inpatient medicine. Also, acting is fundamentally about empathy – putting oneself into the character of another person – which is an invaluable skill in medicine.

The arts can also be used for health education and to foster social change. On a large scale, organizations like Act Up! or breast cancer advocacy groups have used art and graphic design very effectively to focus attention on activist goals. Although physicians have usually been outsiders to these efforts led by patient activists, there can be a role for collaboration by physician-artists or physicians interested in working jointly with patients and arts communities.

Conclusion

If you love the arts, I hope this chapter has assured you that there are many ways to continue your commitment to the arts and actually use it to enhance your medical career. Although there may be moments in your career when you feel too busy to continue your involvement in the arts, be sure that you never lose track of what you love, and look to find ways to integrate it in your work. Even the busiest intern can read a poem in the morning before pre-rounding, or listen to a beloved sonata while driving home late at night. Look for ways to bring your interest in the arts into the medical arena: find others who share your passion and form a group to read, write, play music, visit museums, or draw together. Think about your patients – is there a way to deepen your connection with them through sharing a favorite art form? Think about your colleagues and your community of practice – how can you find sustenance, connection, and renewal through the arts? I hope that the many examples in this chapter will inspire you to remember that the arts and humanities can be integrated into every aspect of medical practice – from personal practice to medical education, to professional development, to work with patients, to research, and to community-building and social change. The practice of medicine will deeply engage both your mind and your emotions – and staying connected to arts and humanities can deepen this experience in every possible way.

References

1. Osler W. Aequanimitas, with addresses to medical students, nurses, and practitioners of medicine. Philadephia, PA: Blakiston; 1904. p. 213.
2. Rodenhauser P, Strickland MA, Gambala CT. Arts-related activities across US medical schools: a follow-up study. Teach Learn Med. 2004;16(3):233–9.
3. Naghshineh S, Hafler JP, Millier AR, Blanco MA, Lipsitz SR, Drbroff RP, et al. Formal art observation training improves medical students' visual diagnostic skills. J Gen Intern Med. 2008;23(7):991–7.
4. Bertman SL. One breath apart: facing dissection. Ward Street Studio: Newton, MA; 2007.
5. Quinn M. Personal Communication, Oct 11, 2010.
6. Bonebakker V. Literature & medicine: humanities at the heart of health care: a hospital-based reading and discussion program developed by the Maine Humanities Council. Acad Med. 2003;78(10):961–7.
7. Risser DT et al. The potential for improved teamwork to reduce medical errors in the emergency department. Ann Emerg Med. 1999;34:373–83.
8. Campo R. The healing art. New York, NY: Norton; 2003.
9. Campo R. Personal Communication, Sept 13, 2010.
10. Kiser K. Face-to-Face: The artist as physician. Minnesota Medicine, July 2010: Minneapolis, MN; 2010.
11. Willis S. Personal communication, Sept 17, 2010.
12. Conrad C et al. Overture for growth hormone, requiem for interleukin-6? J Crit Care Med. 2007;35(12):2709–13.
13. Conrad C et al. The effect of defined auditory conditions versus mental loading on the laparascopic motor skills performance of experts. Surg Endosc. 2010;24(6):1347–52.
14. Weinstock M. Personal communication, Sept 14, 2010.

Resources

Society for the Arts in Healthcare http://www.thesah.org/template/index.cfm.
Foundation for Art and Healing. www.artsandhealing.org.
New York University School of Medicine Medical Humanities Website. http://medhum.med.nyu.edu/
New York University School of Medicine Literature, Arts and Medicine Database. http://litmed.med.nyu.edu/Main?action=new.
The Center for Literature, Medicine and Biomedical Humanities at Hiram College. http://www.hiram.edu/excellence/litmed.html.
Kent State University Press: Literature and Medicine series. http://upress.kent.edu/series/index.htm.

Part VII
Patient Safety, Ethics, and Additional Career Pathways

Chapter 28
Patient Safety

Alexander F. Arriaga

Key Points

- Errors in medical care leading to patient injury and/or death are common in today's healthcare system, and there is a growing "patient safety movement" across various disciplines to reduce preventable patient harm.
- There are tangible ways for busy clinicians to get the knowledge base and skills needed to participate in high-level patient safety efforts.
- There is a demand for clinicians who have a desire to be involved with patient safety. Such involvement can range from adding additional elements to one's medical profession to transitioning toward a full-time career in the field.

Introduction

Recently, my 86-year-old grandmother was getting up from her couch to turn off the television when, after two steps forward, she felt a bone in her leg suddenly snap. She immediately fell to the ground. With the help of my mother, who happened to be there, she was rushed to the nearest hospital where she received emergency surgery to repair her femur. X-rays showed it had been fractured in three different places. While her surgeon (the attending in charge) was not sure after diagnostic testing what caused her fracture, he discontinued one of her medications and informed her to stop taking it, as there were some reports linking this drug to her type of injury. On the day she was discharged from the hospital, my mother reviewed

A.F. Arriaga, MD, MPH (✉)
Department of Health Policy and Management, Harvard School of Public Health,
Brigham and Women's Hospital, Boston, MA 02215, USA
e-mail: aarriaga@hsph.harvard.edu

R.D. Urman and J.M. Ehrenfeld (eds.), *Physicians' Pathways to Non-Traditional Careers and Leadership Opportunities*, DOI 10.1007/978-1-4614-0551-1_28,
© Springer Science+Business Media, LLC 2012

the discharge plan with the resident, and they confirmed the plan to stop taking the drug in question until the matter was reviewed during a future outpatient visit. The next day, I received a phone call from my mother. The rehabilitation center she had been transferred to placed the drug in question on my grandmother's active medication list, and nearly administered it, due to a miscommunication regarding the medication list as written on her transfer orders.

Errors in medicine are unfortunately much more common than the nonmedical public knows or that clinicians would like to accept. In 1999 the Institute of Medicine (IOM) released an influential report titled *To err is human: building a safer health system*, where the authors reported that medical errors caused up to 98,000 deaths per year (the equivalent of a jumbo jet a day). In 2006, *Time* magazine published an article "Q: What scares doctors? A: Being the patient," where they reviewed several landmark articles on medical errors, including a 2003 study by the Rand corporation indicating that hospitalized adults in the United States received, on average, only 54.9% of recommended care for their conditions. In a 2002 survey conducted by the Harvard School of Public Health, over one third of doctors reported errors in their own or a family member's medical care. Medical error continues to be a hot button issue to this day. In the November 2010 issues of the New England Journal of Medicine, there was a published case report of an orthopedic surgeon who mistakenly performed the wrong operation on one of his patients, and a separate study of over 2,000 random admissions from 2002 to 2007, where the trends that the investigators observed suggested that there was still a need for widespread improvement in rates of patient harm from medical care.

Fortunately, there has been growing interest over the past several decades toward improving patient safety. In the 1970s and 1980s, Jeffery Cooper, Ellison C. Pierce, Daniel Raemer, and other leaders in the field of anesthesiology launched a series of studies and efforts that revolutionized the ability for patients to safely receive anesthetic care. Their works moved forth the notion that a comprehensive view of the causes of medical complications involves not only patient factors (such as patient age and disease status), but also human factors (such as fatigue, poor communication, inadequate supervision) and equipment/system design. In 1990, the cognitive psychologist James Reason published the book *Human Error*, which captured the attention of both the medical and nonmedical communities in his description of the frailty of the human mind in high-risk systems. His model on the dynamics of accident causation, known by many as the "Swiss Cheese" model (Fig. 28.1), has been widely cited and illustrates the notion that patient harm often stems from the occurrence of many failures that go through the holes of a complex system. In parallel to these works, there have also been landmark studies such as the California Medical Association Medical Insurance Feasibility Study and the Harvard Medical Practice Study. These studies quantified, on a large scale, the preventable adverse event rates in American hospitals. Their review of tens of thousands of medical records brought to light that negligence in patient management contributes to an alarmingly high rate of in-hospital adverse events (27.6% of over a 1,000 adverse events observed in the Harvard Medical Practice Study were attributed to negligence). These works set the foundation and background for future intervention efforts, including computerized provider order entry systems and evidence-based pathways of care.

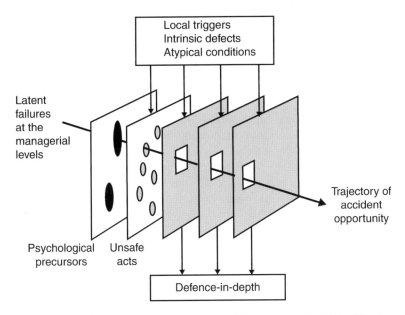

Fig. 28.1 The dynamics of accident causation (Reason J. Human error. Cambridge, UK: Copyright © 1990 Cambridge University Press. Reprinted with the permission of Cambridge University Press.)

Over the past 20 years, there have also been individual physicians who have pioneered additional patient safety efforts. The surgeon and writer Dr. Atul Gawande has published a series of articles, books, and studies that have both influenced health policy and have improved patient safety at an international level. The anesthesiologist Dr. Angela Bader has led several efforts and investigations targeted at ensuring patients are in an optimal medical condition to safely undergo an operation. The internist Dr. David Bates has played a pivotal role in using information technology to reduce drug-related and other medical errors. The surgical oncologist Dr. Caprice Greenberg has led several recent efforts involving the use of advanced technology (such as natural language processing and multistream synchronized audiovisual recording) to make surgical care safer. Dr. William Berry, formerly a full-time operating cardiac surgeon, transitioned to a career in patient safety at the turn of the millennium. Since then, he has become an established leader in the science of implementing patient safety efforts at a population level.

In addition to the Institute of Medicine, there are now numerous organizations actively committed to improving patient safety. Dr. Fred Shapiro, an anesthesiologist who had a strong desire to address the exponential growth of surgical procedures in the office-based setting (i.e., outside a hospital or ambulatory surgical center), founded the Institute for Safety in Office-Based Surgery. At a broader level in the field of medicine, we now have the Institute for Healthcare Improvement (IHI), the National Patient Safety Foundation, the Agency for Healthcare Research and Quality, the World Alliance for Patient Safety, and patient safety groups in practically all healthcare specialties.

These efforts toward patient safety have also been paralleled by successes and lessons learned from other fields. Other high-reliance industries, such as aviation, nuclear power, and the military have long embraced the notion of safe processes. Many of their accepted practices, such as using safety checklists, having dedicated safety officers on staff, and having guidelines for critical-event provider communication, have made their way into the healthcare field. There are now companies, such as Roth Cognitive Engineering, where eminent cognitive psychologists (experienced in intelligence analysis, military command and control, and railroad operations) provide consultation to healthcare institutions on how to make their systems safer. The business sector has also embraced the importance of patient safety. Inspired by the *To Err Is Human* report, a group of large employers launched the Leapfrog group, an organization that allowed these employers to leverage their health insurance purchasing power to encourage efforts to reduce medical mistakes. The organization is now a consortium of purchasers that provide health insurance for over 37 million Americans across the United States, with sponsorship from both profit and nonprofit organizations. In all, these efforts from various medical and nonmedical disciplines have been coined by many as the "patient safety movement," a movement that continues to gain momentum.

Why Pursue Patient Safety?

At a fundamental level, the reason to pursue patient safety is obvious. Healthcare practitioners are trained to provide optimal care for their patients and to first do no harm. We are all a patient at some point, and it is not difficult to see the tangible benefit of avoiding adverse events in medical care.

There are important decisions related to patient safety that are actively being made that impact everyday clinical care. In 2010, significant changes were made to regulations that govern resident duty hours, which require individual healthcare professionals and hospital leadership to alter their approach to resident training, use of physician assistants and nurse practitioners, and overall resource allocation. The American Recovery and Reinvestment Act of 2009 contained legislation that prioritized the promotion of electronic medical records and the creation of a national health information system that can be used across organizations. Leaders of the Agency for Healthcare Research and Quality (a division of the United States Department of Health and Human Services) and the RAND corporation (a nonprofit institution devoted to improving policy and decision-making through research and analysis) have set frameworks for effective patient safety systems (Fig. 28.2). The Joint Commission, an independent, not-for-profit organization that accredits and certifies over 18,000 US healthcare organizations and programs, contains numerous patient-safety-related criteria for accreditation, including their National Patient Safety Goals (which have included goals such as preventing wrong-site surgery,

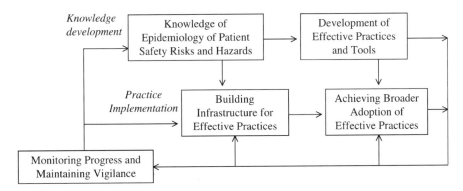

Fig. 28.2 The components of an effective patient safety system (Reprinted from Farley DO. Battles J. Evaluation of the AHRQ Patient Safety Initiative: Framework and Approach. Health Services Research 2009;44(2):628–45, Part II. With permission from John Wiley & Sons, Inc.)

medication errors, and communication breakdowns between caregivers) that were first put into effect in 2003. Healthcare providers involved in patient safety are at the forefront of making these decisions and implementing improvement efforts.

How Can I Benefit from Involvement in Patient Safety?

As a result of the widespread attention associated with the patient safety movement, there is a demand for professionals who are familiar with the salient issues in patient safety and have insight on how to improve care. With all the organizations mentioned above (and the many more in existence), there are opportunities at every level to play a role in patient safety. Policymakers regularly call upon patient safety experts for testimonials in congressional hearings and to inform their decision making. There are millions of dollars in grant funding that healthcare providers are eligible to apply for if they have an idea on how to make care safer. Many hospital systems have dedicated patient safety teams that interact directly with the hospital and organizational leadership. By devoting a portion of your time to patient safety efforts, you can be involved with an effort that is inherently rewarding, and one that can provide the opportunity to be involved with hospital leadership, healthcare administration, and breakthrough research.

How Can I Benefit My Patients?

In addition to improving the quality of patient care and fostering a healthcare system that minimizes medical error, you can use your knowledge of patient safety to empower your patients to play a role in improving their own care. There is an expanding body of research that supports the notion that medical errors are less likely in a system where patients are informed and involved. Many populations of patients can better their care by simple measures such as having an updated and complete medication list on their person, as well as encouraging their providers to adhere to proper hand hygiene. The World Health Organization has its own initiative titled Patients for Patient Safety, which is led by patients and emphasizes the role that patients and consumers have in improving their healthcare quality and safety. A recent review article in *Mayo Clinic Proceedings* (referenced below under "landmark works") contains a suggested research agenda and a proposed model for such patient participation.

What Kind of Education and Background Is Needed?

There are many ways to get involved in the field of patient safety. While an advanced degree is not necessary, a master of public health or public policy degree are some avenues to gaining the literature base, research skills, and/or policy analysis skills essential to developing and implementing improvement efforts. If a full degree is not practical at the stage of your career, there are several institutions that offer summer programs designed for practicing clinicians interested in clinical effectiveness (e.g., The Harvard School of Public Health offers such a program annually). As previously mentioned, many hospital organizations have dedicated patient safety teams that likely would benefit from the clinical expertise you can bring to their efforts. The Joint Commission and other regulatory bodies issue and regularly update patient-safety mandates for hospitals and healthcare organizations. If you are knowledgeable in this area, or even have the desire to help fulfill such mandates, then reaching out to your department chair or practice leader may be an accessible starting point.

If you are at a loss for ideas, one suggestion would be to look at your day-to-day practice and brainstorm for problems you foresee being the potential cause of preventable patient harm. Review the literature to assess what the known incidence of the problem is, and whether any previous efforts have had success. You will then want some structured way of measuring this problem for your population of interest, whether it is to just characterize the phenomena or design an intervention to improve care. To quote Dr. Gawande:

> *Count something.* Regardless of what one ultimately does in medicine – or outside of medicine, for that matter.... You don't need a research grant. The only requirement is that what you count should be interesting to you.[1]

The IHI website contains a handful of free general tools you may be able to use to structure and track your project (http://www.ihi.org/ihi/workspace). Depending on the scope of your idea, you may want to consult with a biostatistician and

---

[1] Gawande A. Better: a surgeon's note on performance. New York: Metropolitan Books; 2007.

epidemiologist to review the design of your initiative. You should also consult your organization's Institutional Review Board (IRB) to obtain approval for or exemption from regulations surrounding quality improvement and research efforts in healthcare.

To help you get started, here is an annotated listing of some of the landmark works in the field of patient safety. It is not intended to be comprehensive, as it would not be feasible to do so in a chapter of this scope. Some are fast reads, and all are engaging and full of ideas and/or calls to action. Whatever your path for involvement in patient safety may be, you will be exploring an active field that offers the potential to see the practical and immediate impact of your work. There is a demand for motivated clinicians with interests ranging from adding a component to one's medical profession to transitioning to a full-time career in improving patient safety.

Annotated Selection of Landmark Works in the Field of Patient Safety

Leape LL. Error in medicine. J Am Med Assoc. 1994; 272(23):1851–57. [A landmark review article in patient safety, this publication provides an overview of the causes of errors in healthcare, and draws from lessons learned from literature on human cognition and other high-risk fields outside of medicine. It also provides suggestions on how to create safer healthcare systems].

Pierce EC. The 34th Rovenstine Lecture: 40 years behind the mask – safety revisited. Anesthesiology. 1996;84:965–75. [An excellent review of the history of patient safety in anesthesia, a field that has made substantial progress over the past decades in reducing adverse events].

Cooper JB, Newbower RS, Long CD, et al. Preventable anesthesia mishaps: a study of human factors. Anesthesiology. 1978;49:399–406. [A transformational publication in the study of errors in the provision of anesthetic care. The authors used a critical incident analysis approach to understand the distribution and etiologies of adverse events in anesthesia].

Vincent, C. Patient safety. London: Elseiver; 2010. [A succinct and easy read written by an international expert in the field of patient safety. A great source of information for any healthcare professional].

Kohn LT, Corrigan JM, Donaldson MS, editors. To err is human: building a safer health system. Washington, DC: National Academy Press; 1999. [This influential and shaping report, which is available for free at http://www.iom.edu/Reports/1999/To-Err-is-Human-Building-A-Safer-Health-System.aspx, provides a comprehensive summary of types and etiologies of errors in medicine, as well as calls to action and suggestions for improvement].

Brennan TA, Leape LL, Laird NM, et al. Incidence of adverse events and negligence in hospitalized patients: results from the Harvard Medical Practice Study I. N Engl J Med. 1991;324:370–6.

Leape LL, Brennan TA, Laird N, et al. The nature of adverse events in hospitalized patients: results of the Harvard Medical Practice Study II. N Eng J Med. 1991;324:377–84. [This two-part series in the New Engl J Med. describes the Harvard Medical Practice Study, a key set of investigations into the incidence and nature of adverse events in hospitalized patients].

Bates DW, Cullen DJ, Laird NM, et al. Incidence of adverse drug events and potential adverse drug events. Implications for prevention. ADE Prevention Study Group. J Am Med Assoc. 1995;274(1):29–34. [This study investigates the incidence and preventability of adverse drug events, one of the most common causes of errors in healthcare. These investigators/study group have also authored several subsequent key studies on this topic].

Gawande A. Complications: a surgeon's note on an imperfect science. New York: Picador; 2002.

Gawande A. Better: a surgeon's note on performance. New York: Metropolitan Books; 2007.

Gwande A. The Checklist Manifesto: How to get things right. New York: Metropolitan Books; 2009. [This trilogy of books by surgeon and writer Dr. Atul Gawande tells the story of many of the successes and pitfalls in medicine, including an account of some notable initiatives in patient safety. An entertaining and informative read].

Haynes AB, Weiser TG, Berry WR, et al. A surgical safety checklist to reduce morbidity and mortality in a global population. N Engl J Med 2009;360:491–9. [International patient safety effort to implement a surgical safety checklist to reduce morbidity and mortality in a global population. The Safe Surgery Saves Lives checklist is currently used in thousands of hospitals around the world].

Jha AK, DesRoches CM, Campbell EG, et al. Use of electronic health records in U.S. hospitals. N Engl J Med 2009;348:651–6. [This recent study reviews the adoption of electronic health records by United States hospitals, a widely discussed topic, particularly with regards to health policy and national funding. It was preceded by a similar study, also published in the New Engl J Med, addressing the ambulatory care sector].

Longtin Y, Sax H, Leape LL, et al. Patient participation: current knowledge and applicability to patient safety. Mayo Clin Proc. 2010;85:53–62. [A recent publication, this article reviews the current literature on patient participation to improve patient safety, and includes (1) specific suggestions for the role of patients to prevent medical errors, (2) a proposed model for patient involvement to improve patient safety, and (3) a research agenda for future work].

Additional Practical Resources/Websites

Joint Commission: http://www.jointcommission.org/

The Joint Commission National Patient Safety Goals: http://www.jointcommission.org/patient-safety/nationalpatientsafetygoals/, http://psnet.ahrq.gov/resource.aspx?resourceID=2230.

Institute of Medicine: http://www.iom.edu/

World Health Organization, World Alliance for Patient Safety: http://www.who.int/patientsafety/en/

Patients for Patient Safety: http://www.who.int/patientsafety/patients_for_patient/en/

Institute for Healthcare Improvement: http://www.ihi.org/ihi

Patient Safety page: http://www.ihi.org/IHI/Topics/PatientSafety/

Interactive Tools and Improvement Tracker: http://www.ihi.org/ihi/workspace.

National Patient Safety Foundation. http://www.npsf.org/

Agency for Healthcare Research and Quality (AHRQ): http://www.ahrq.gov/

Institute for Safety in Office-Based Surgery (ISOBS): http://isobsurgery.org/

National Center for Patient Safety: http://www.patientsafety.gov/

Chapter 29
Bioethics

Lisa Soleymani Lehmann

> **Key Points**
>
> - Bioethics provides an opportunity to reflect on the meaning of our actions, how we interact with patients, their family members, what our core values are and what we should do when values conflict.
> - Bioethical deliberations make a real and immediate difference to the lives of patients, to the culture of our healthcare institutions, and to healthcare policies within our society.
> - The analysis of ethical questions is fundamental to the work of bioethics. Students interested in developing an expertise in bioethics should consider some formal training in moral philosophy.

Introduction

I cannot imagine a career in medicine that would be more intellectually stimulating, personally fulfilling and meaningful than being a bioethicist. Ethical issues permeate every field of medicine and ethics is at the core of what we do as physicians. No matter what area of medicine you choose, there will be ethical questions that you will encounter. Whether you treat patients at the beginning of life or the end of life, whether you are a surgeon who operates or an internist who deliberates, whether you help couples create life or put patients to sleep there will be an ethical dimension to your work. The practice of medicine is inextricably bound to considerations of ethics.

L.S. Lehmann, MD, PhD, MSc (✉)
Division of General Medicine, Brigham and Women's Hospital, Harvard Medical School,
1620 Tremont Street, 3rd floor, Room BC3-2G, Boston, MA 02120, USA
e-mail: llehmann1@partners.org

R.D. Urman and J.M. Ehrenfeld (eds.), *Physicians' Pathways to Non-Traditional Careers and Leadership Opportunities*, DOI 10.1007/978-1-4614-0551-1_29, © Springer Science+Business Media, LLC 2012

Bioethics is a multidisciplinary field, which is defined more by the questions it focuses on than a particular method of inquiry. Challenging questions arise from a consideration of the moral dimensions of the practice of medicine, the science of medicine, and the integration of new technology into medicine. These questions can be considered through the lens of many disciplines including philosophy, law, theology, public health and the social sciences. By engaging in a deliberative process that is focused on the normative question of what we ought to do, clinical ethicists try to improve the quality of patient care. We help healthcare providers, patients, and families by uncovering the assumptions behind different positions, evaluating the soundness of arguments, and reflecting on the consequences of different courses of action. Bioethics provides an opportunity to reflect on the meaning of our actions, how we interact with our patients and their family, what our core values are and what we should do when values conflict.

Why Pursue a Particular Interest?

The opportunity to develop an interest in bioethics is a privilege that is likely to enhance your practice of medicine, the experience of your patients and your personal sense of fulfillment. As a bioethicist I am fortunate to constantly confront new and challenging questions, to ponder philosophical conundrums, and to rethink moral assumptions. This intellectual engagement does not however occur in a vacuum. It transpires in the context of real conflicts that are calling for resolution. In clinical bioethics the deliberative process has an immediate practical consequence since a decision needs to be made in order for medical care to proceed. Bioethical deliberations actually make a difference to the lives of patients, to the culture of our healthcare institutions, and to healthcare policies within our society.

The questions that we consider have a profound impact on people's lives. Should we have age limits for the use of in vitro fertilization? Should we lighten the sedation of a patient with a high cervical spine injury who is now quadriplegic in order to ask her if she would like to continue living on a ventilator? How do we elicit a terminally ill patient's preferences for care at the end of life in a way that is empathic and preserves hope? Should we respect a pregnant woman's refusal of a c-section that we believe is necessary to save the life of her fetus? How should we disclose an error to a patient and their family? How should we make decisions for a patient that does not have mental capacity and does not have any family members or close friends? How should we allocate scare resources such as organs for transplantation? Do undocumented immigrants have the same right to nonemergent healthcare as citizens? Who should decide if an extremely premature newborn should be resuscitated? A consideration of these questions shapes the practice of medicine both within our healthcare institutions and as a profession.

As a Physician, How Can I Benefit Personally?

Engagement with the field of bioethics will help facilitate your own moral development. It will give you the opportunity to clarify your own values and beliefs. Do you believe that physicians should provide assistance to patients who are terminally ill and want to die? Is it ok to respect the preferences of parents who do not want their 25-week-old premature infant resuscitated? Are you willing to operate on a Jehovah's Witness who refuses all blood products? How sacred is patient confidentiality? What will you do if you have access to confidential patient information that if shared against a patient's wishes can prevent a life threatening illness in someone else? By considering these questions in advance you will be better prepared to respond to ethical dilemmas when they arise in your practice.

Bioethics will hone your critical reasoning skills. The ability to assess the soundness of arguments and the ability to develop cogent positions on controversial subjects is a fundamental skill of bioethics. Through reading the literature of bioethics and engaging in conversations about what we should do in different circumstances, you will develop your critical thinking skills. This process will also allow you to more effectively convey your perspective on controversial questions to others within the profession.

Bioethics will help make you a more humanistic physician, and thereby enrich your ability to care for patients as persons. The tendency for physicians to focus on treating diseases and a perhaps overly optimistic belief in the benefits of technology may cause us to lose sight of the individual patient who is before us. Bioethics attunes physicians to a humanistic approach to caring for patients. The humanities encourage an exploration of the meaning of illness and suffering and sensitivity to the human experience that is frequently overshadowed by our technological focus. This perspective has the potential to enrich both the experience of physicians and patients.

How Can I Benefit My Patients?

Although I am not aware of any empirical evidence to suggest that physicians who are engaged in ethical reflection and discussions have improved patient outcomes, it is likely that your patients will benefit from your exposure to bioethics. Your attention to the ethical dimensions of the practice of medicine is likely to help you develop a close rapport with your patients. Many ethical issues arise in the daily practice of medicine, and by giving thought to these questions in advance you will be better prepared to care for your patients. You will have considered what to do if you make a serious error and how to share that with your patients. As you are immersed in the day-to-day care of your patients, you will likely be more prepared to step back and consider the goals of care for your elderly patient who may be deteriorating postoperatively. You are likely to develop patient-centered communication skills and hopefully will recognize the importance of advance care planning with your patients. Attention to these questions is likely to have a significant impact on the care you provide to your patients.

Education, Other Background Needed

There are many educational pathways to a career that integrates bioethics and medicine. One of the most interesting aspects of bioethics is the diversity of voices that reflect on challenging bioethial questions. My personal journey has combined training in medicine with philosophy and clinical epidemiology. My background in philosophy has honed my analytic thinking skills that are necessary for illuminating the ethical debates that arise in clinical medicine. Clinical epidemiology has given me the empirical research methods necessary to pursue empirical research questions that have significant implications for the ethical practice of medicine. As a bioethicist at an academic medical center, I split my time between patient care, clinical ethics consultation, bioethics education for medical students and residents, and research in bioethics. This, however, is just one example of how one could develop a career in bioethics.

Many clinicians may be interested in some exposure to bioethics without pursuing a full-blown career as a bioethicist. One way to gain this exposure is through participation in a hospital ethics committee or by shadowing a hospital ethicist. Although there is significant variability in the role and function of ethics committees at different institutions, participation in the discussions of ethics committees is a good starting point for exploring an interest in bioethics. These committees frequently reflect on clinical cases that arise in the hospital, assist with the development of hospital ethics policy, and provide an opportunity for multidisciplinary discussion of ethical questions. Many also provide case consultations, and participating in consults could be a valuable addition to your clinical education.

Students interested in developing an expertise in bioethics should consider some formal training in moral philosophy, as the analysis of ethical questions is fundamental to the work of bioethics. If you want to develop a career that is primarily focused on bioethics, it is crucial that you choose a particular discipline through which you can consider ethical questions, that you obtain formal training in that discipline and seek out mentors and role models who are doing bioethics. This will allow you to bring a unique perspective to bioethical questions and to do this with the rigor of your discipline.

The field of bioethics has evolved so that there now exist educational opportunities to purse graduate work directly in bioethics or to focus on bioethics through graduate programs in philosophy, law, health policy, literature, public health, theology, and the social sciences. Each of these disciplines has made unique contributions to the field of bioethics. Formal training will allow you the time to master the literature of bioethics, engage in conversations that will hone your critical thinking skills, and provide you with a systematic disciplinary framework from which you can consider bioethical questions. Ideally, bioethicists will have a familiarity with all of the multiple disciplines that contribute to the analysis of ethical questions in medicine and will be able to synthesize information from diverse disciplines. More recently, there is a proliferation of medical schools offering Certificates, Masters, and PhD degrees in bioethics and the opportunity to pursue combined MD/PhD or MD/JD programs that focus on bioethics.

Additional Practical Resources/Websites

The American Society of Bioethics and Humanities (ASBH) is the professional organization for bioethicists. Attending their annual meeting is a good place to start exploring the diversity of voices and issues in bioethics. The ASBH *Core Competencies for Healthcare Ethics Consultation* and *Improving Competencies in Clinical Ethics Consultation: An Education Guide* offer guidelines for the knowledge and skills necessary for clinical ethics and may be of particular help to individuals interested in clinical ethics consultation. If you are seeking further education on the ethical dimensions of research, you should consider the educational opportunities offered through Public Responsibility in Medicine and Research (PRIM&R). In addition to the discussion of bioethics questions in medical, legal, and humanities journals, there are journals specifically devoted to bioethics.

Additional Resources

American Society of Bioethics and Humanities. Core competencies for health care ethics consultation and improving competencies in clinical ethics consultation: an education guide. Glenview, IL: ASBH; 2009. http://www.asbh.org/publications/content/edguide.html. Accessed 18 May 2011.

Beauchamp TL, Childress JF. Principles of biomedical ethics. Oxford: Oxford University Press; 2009.

Vaughn L. Bioethics: principles, issues and cases. Oxford: Oxford University Press; 2010.

Chapter 30
Spirituality and Medicine

Mary Kraft

Key Points

- Ways to incorporate notions of spirituality into patient conversations.
- Spirituality can aid in conversations with challenging patients.
- Acknowledging spirituality in ourselves and our patients contributes to our sense of professional satisfaction.

The Physician's Role

Guerir quelquefois	To cure sometimes
Soulage souvent	To help often
Consoler toujours	To comfort always

Attributed to Edward L. Trudeau, M.D., 1848–1915

"There are no atheists in foxholes." World War II aphorism, author unknown

Introduction

Mr. C is a 67-year-old male who came to our preoperative clinic for an evaluation prior to a radical prostatectomy. He was a bit disheveled and spent our interview time refusing to make eye contact and responding to my questions with monosyllables. After explaining

---

M. Kraft, MD, MPA (✉)
Department of Anesthesia, Baystate Medical Center, 759 Chestnut St.,
Springfield, MA 01199, USA
e-mail: mkraft@massmed.org

R.D. Urman and J.M. Ehrenfeld (eds.), *Physicians' Pathways to Non-Traditional Careers and Leadership Opportunities*, DOI 10.1007/978-1-4614-0551-1_30,
© Springer Science+Business Media, LLC 2012

anesthesia to him, I handed him the consent form, which he promptly threw back in my face, muttering, "It doesn't matter what it says here, it's all in G-d's hands now."

What would you do if you were me? Get angry? Ignore the outburst and pursue the task at hand? Or, understanding Trudeau's definition of the physician's role and the idea that there are no atheists in foxholes, explore his outburst?

The goal of this chapter is to demonstrate how one can incorporate notions of spirituality into one's relationships with patients, so both doctor and patient are enriched. I will also set forth some guidelines for talking about religion, per se, and include resources for those interested in delving further into the subject.

Spirituality and Religion

What is spirituality? One definition is "Spirituality is the aspect of humanity that refers to the way individuals seek and express meaning and purpose and the way they experience their connectedness to the moment, to self, to others, to nature, and to the significant or sacred" [1].

Religion is how groups of people come together to express a common notion of spirituality. Not everyone is religious, but everyone has a way of expressing spirituality. If the doctor is curious, the root of the patient's spirituality is easily discovered.

Skeptics often ask if conversations about spirituality or religion are appropriate to medical care. Koenig gives at least five compelling reasons which are listed in Table 30.1 [2].

The patients agree. In a survey of Ohio patients, 83% (of 921 respondents) wanted to discuss spirituality in some form with their doctors [3].

What's In It For Me?

The most common response from medical students and house officers, when encouraged to have a spiritual conversation with their patients is "I haven't got time." My counter to that is that you don't have time NOT to do it.

We give patients spiritual care when we let them know by our questions and responses that we care about what they care about, for example, what gives them meaning in life, or what meaning the illness at hand has for them.

Table 30.1 Reasons to discuss spirituality and religion with patients

Many patients are religious, and religious beliefs help them to cope
Religious beliefs influence medical decisions, especially when patients are seriously ill
Religious beliefs and activities are related to better health and quality of life
Many patients would like physicians to address their spiritual needs
Physicians addressing spiritual needs is not new, but rooted in the long historical relationship between (sic) religion, medicine, and healthcare

Adapted from Koenig [2]. With permission from Templeton Press ©2002

We are taught to ask patients what brought them to us today, the "chief complaint." What happens if, after the patient tells us about his/her right upper quadrant pain, we ask, "what concerns you most about this pain?" Eliciting the patient's "chief *concern*," changes the dynamic from complaint to concern, which is what really matters most to the patient [4]. Thus, if the patient tells you s/he's worried about a liver abscess like Uncle John once had, you can tailor your usual history questions and differential diagnosis explanations in reassuring tones. We get to the patient's fears quickly, and that makes the rest of the interview go much more smoothly. The concern question puts the patient more at ease and gives him/her the understanding that s/he is not just the embodiment of symptoms. By this question, the doctor establishes his/her wish "to comfort always" and perhaps ease the patient out of the foxhole of worry. The patient relaxes, you relax, and each of you leave the encounter satisfied that a moment of healing took place, even if the patient leaves for his MRI with the same pain.

Foxholes

We and our patients often find ourselves knee deep in foxholes in the course of a medical encounter (Fig. 30.1). For us, these foxholes may look like too many patients for the time allotted, patient acuity, fear of missing something, fear of

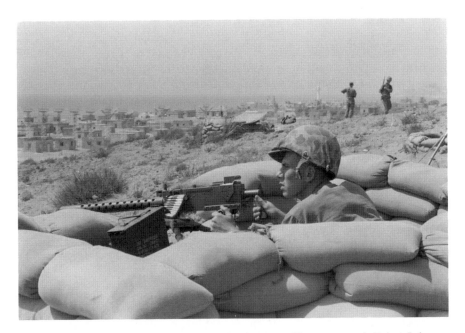

Fig. 30.1 A U.S. Marine sits in a foxhole and points a machine gun towards Beirut, Lebanon. Courtesy of Library of Congress, Prints and Photographs Division, U.S. News & World Report Magazine Collection (LC-U9-1472E-36)

malpractice suits, fear of doing harm, a psychologically complicated patient in the middle of a busy day, and/or a general feeling of frustration at administration and paper work. For our patients, the foxholes look like the doctor's office, the MRI machine, the hospital, and especially the operating room.

Illness interrupts our lives. Stein writes that illness prompts patients to have feelings of betrayal, terror, loss, and loneliness [5]. The North American Nursing Diagnosis Association (NANDA) defines foci of spiritual distress as feelings of uneasiness in the spheres of meaning (the meaning of life, the meaning of the illness), hope, love, trust, and forgiveness [6]. Even though Stein doesn't use the vocabulary of "spirituality" per se, one can easily see the overlap in ideas.

Patients rarely visit the doctor with a story of how they feel betrayed by their bodies, but as they express their concerns, one often finds threads of Frank's illness narratives, which then become huge clues for us in how to enter into the conversation with our patient [7].

The Narratives

The first narrative Frank describes is the "restitution narrative." Its plot has "the basic storyline: 'Yesterday I was healthy, today I'm sick, but tomorrow, I'll be healthy again.'" We like patients who come with this narrative, especially if we can restore health with an antibiotic or a few stitches.

The second narrative, the "chaos narrative," is "the opposite of restitution: its plot imagines life never getting better." We have all encountered patients whose life has been turned so completely upside down by their illnesses or their anxiety about their illnesses, that it takes a long time (and is sometimes nearly impossible) for them to give us a direct answer to a direct question. (e.g., Is the pain sharp or dull? Does anything make it better or worse?) "Chaos," writes Frank, "feeds on the sense that *no one* is in control. People living these stories regularly accuse medicine of seeking to maintain its pretense of control – its restitution narrative – at the expense of denying the suffering of what it cannot treat .... The challenge of encountering the chaos narrative is how not steer the storyteller away from her feelings .... The challenge is to *hear*."

"Quest stories," Frank's third narrative, "meet suffering head on; they accept illness and seek to *use* it." These are the stories we hear from our cancer patients, or from patients who have gone through a life-changing illness. Patients expressing themselves in this narrative often use the metaphor of illness as a journey, and the many memoirs written about illness are written from this perspective. We often find these stories uplifting, even if they are tales of suffering, because the "storyteller's responsibility is to witness the memory of what happened, and to set this memory right by providing a better example for others to follow."

Space for the Stories

If one accepts the premise that listening to patients' stories is important to both the patient's and physician's well being, the next question is where to make the space in the time allotted. Metaphorically, this space is in the hyphen of the doctor–patient relationship. Carson writes, "The hyphen simultaneously signifies separation and synergy, disjunction and conjunction. It calls attention to the distance between parties to the clinical encounter. And then, in the blink of an eye, it is a bridge across the divide" [8]. It is in that very precious moment of silence and rest between the out breath and the in breath. It is in the pauses we sometimes need to force ourselves to take in our often rapid barrage of questions.

What is essential to creating the hyphen? Surely we all intend to do our best, to pay attention to the patient, but often we are distracted by knowing that there are 20 more patients in the office, that we have to pick up the car before the repair shop closes, that we have a lecture to give at 5 p.m., etc. Patients are very keen on intuiting these distractions and will not be forthcoming in their stories when they perceive our distractedness.

To achieve a meeting of doctor and patient on the hyphen, we must be in a state of quiet readiness. A list of tips for obtaining this state is listed in Table 30.2.

Perhaps you will comment that this is easier said than done, and I would agree. Preparing ourselves to do work in this way requires introspection and a willingness to let go of some of our ego (e.g., "I may have gone to medical school but I don't always know best"). This preparation can be accomplished over time with meditation, repetitive physical activity, or eliciting what Benson calls "the relaxation response" [9]. When we can create a space of quiet and stillness within us, we can create that space for our patients, and in a few moments of silence, trust is built and healing happens.

In preparing for this state of quiet readiness, Feldstein teaches about taking a few moments to stop and prepare our "attention" and "intention" before entering the room. In preparing one's attention, stop and take a full and complete breath, letting go of preoccupations. Or, while standing at the sink, hand washing can be transformed from infection control to spiritual preparation – feeling one's feet well grounded, bringing awareness to the breath, and imagining the water washing away distractions. Then, while focused, we take a moment to say to ourselves our intention as we enter the room. For example – to meet my patient in their world as it is for them and accompany them from there; or whatever time I have may I be fully present; what matters most for them is what matters for me [10].

Table 30.2 Tips for achieving quiet readiness

Take a moment to take a breath
Focus on the intention to provide the best care possible
Remember that a moment or two of silence with the patient may produce great insights into the patient's world of health and illness

While conversing with our patients, our silence allows our curiosity to flourish, and we become ready to engage in deep listening with our patients. We can attend not only to their words, but to the spaces between their words and their body language. In this way, we can see the uniqueness of each individual and each clinical situation, greet each day fresh and new, and avert professional burnout.

When we take seriously the goals of medicine to relieve often and comfort always, we are freed up to listen without having to fix or problem solve everything we hear. Listening and being-with *is* doing something and can be powerfully healing.

When we sit on the hyphen, we free ourselves to ask hard questions and broach subjects that are difficult. The story of Mr. C. whom you met at the beginning of this chapter, illustrates how this can all work out as a win-win situation for both patient and doctor.

During our interview, I speculated that Mr. C. was either very worried or very depressed, and my attempts at "breaking the ice" were hugely unsuccessful. It was difficult to "like" this man who spoke in monosyllables and refused to make eye contact. In the moment in which he threw the consent form at me and said "It doesn't matter what it says here, it's all in G-d's hands now," I understood that he was hugely worried about the outcome of his anesthesia. Then, very calmly, I said, "Mr. C. are you trying to tell me you're afraid of dying during this anesthetic?" The clouds dramatically broke! He made eye contact. I did a brief spiritual history (details on "how to" to follow), and he left my office with a lot of eye contact, a warm handshake, and a grateful "thank you."

There is nothing high tech about this kind of healing. Shafir, in *The Zen of Listening* talks about "getting into the movie" of the patient [11]. In the next section, I will address some of how to do this.

Spiritual Caring and History Taking

Frank Ostaseski, founder of the Zen Hospice Project in San Francisco, has lectured about the following five points in the spiritual care for the dying. In the years since I first heard him speak, I have found them to be invaluable in the care of the living.

1. "Bring your whole self to the bedside." As noted earlier, it is important to free your mind of everyday clutter when doing this work. One may not be successful 100% of the time, but with practice, the success rate grows, as does your patients' and your satisfaction with the conversations.
2. "Accept everything, reject nothing." Sometimes the "red herring" that the patient throws into the conversation is a key to something pressing on his/her mind. For example, I once asked a 39-year-old woman if there was a possibility she could be pregnant. She answered, "I suppose I might if I were still with a man." I let the remark go for the moment and circled back to it later. She almost immediately then told me a story of abuse, both from her father and former husband, and that she had then fallen into a relationship with a woman that was a good relationship.

I asked her if she were happy now, she said yes, end of conversation. Two days later, she told everyone in the operating room that I was the best doctor to ever come down the pike. All I had done was listen.

3. "Seize the opportunity." Both the stories of Mr. C. and the woman above illustrate the importance of asking a question from curiosity (not from the textbook).
4. "Find a place of rest in the middle of things." Patients will tell you their stories only if you are quiet long enough for them to get a word in edgewise. If you are having difficulty with an issue, pause and reflect. When I am moved to do this, I often share my pause with the patients, experiences which have produced a few tears across the hyphen and have been some of the most enriching of my professional life. For example, one day a mother, her 25-year-old daughter with a rare genetic disease, and the daughter's caretaker came into my office. The daughter was about to have major scoliosis surgery to make it easier for her to sit in her wheel chair. The chart was replete with DNR orders, so I had to discuss the matter, but watching the triad was reminiscent of paintings of Sts. Elizabeth and Mary and the Baby Jesus, and I was having difficulty composing myself enough to talk about the DNR. Finally I plunged in, introducing the topic by saying that I was having a great deal of difficulty in doing so. The patient's mother and I shed a few tears, and the mother told me that she was glad that the doctor taking care of her daughter was "human."
5. "Intimacy of not knowing." One never truly knows what another person is thinking. In a moment of shared silence, a bond of intimacy over this very topic is created [12].

As for spiritual history taking, there are many question sets available, and I would encourage those interested in studying these in detail to read Chapter 7, "Resources on Spirituality and Health," in Koenig's book. For the purposes of this chapter, I will present two of my favorites, "FICA" and "HOPE."

The FICA Spiritual Assessment Tool was developed by Christina Puchalski, MD, FACP, founder and executive director, The George Washington Institute for Spirituality and Health at George Washington University Medical Center.

F-faith	What is your faith tradition?
I-important	How important is your faith to you?
C-church	What is your church or community of faith?
A-apply/address	How do your religious and spiritual beliefs apply to your health? How might we address your spiritual needs? [13]

When I use this tool set, I often ease into it in the interview by following my questions on family with community. For example, "Who is your family? Who will take care of you and your family during your recuperation? Do you belong to a larger community? Is it a faith community?" The other questions flow quite naturally from the answers to these questions.

Drs. Gowri Anandarajah and Ellen Hight, from the Brown University Department of Family Medicine, published the HOPE Questionnaire in 2001 [14], as outlined below.

Hope: Sources of hope, meaning, comfort, love, and connection

> What sustains you and keeps you going?
> What are your sources of hope, strength, comfort, and peace?
> What do you hold onto during difficult times?

Organized religion: Are you part of a religious or spiritual community? Does it help you? How?

> What aspects of your religion are helpful and not so helpful to you?

Personal spirituality and practices: Do you have any personal spiritual beliefs that are independent of organized religion?

> What aspects of your spirituality or spiritual practices do you find most helpful to you personally?

> Effects on medical care and End of life issues?

Has being sick affected your ability to do things that usually help you spiritually?
As a doctor, is there anything that I can do to help you access the resources that usually help you?
Are there any specific practices or restrictions I should know about in providing your medical care?

Beyond the Comfort Zone

Sometimes in the course of asking these questions, you may be confronted with two types of responses that make you uncomfortable. The first is the patient who asks you to pray with him/her. The second is the patient who makes you his/her spiritual confidante, disclosing spiritual or religious issues that are clearly beyond the scope of medical practice. Often patients are comforted by having a witness to their prayers. It doesn't matter whether or not you are of the same or similar religious tradition as they are, it matters that you care enough about them to just be present or hold their hands while they pray. Sometimes I ask patients if they are prayerful and would like to offer a prayer and tell them that I will give them space and witness to do that. Sometimes they respond by asking me to offer a prayer, and what works best here is a simple petition that the Divine guides the hands and hearts of all of those taking care of the patient and bring the patient swift comfort and healing.

As an example of a disclosure beyond the scope of medical practice, there was a 70-year-old woman who came into our preoperative clinic before undergoing a hysterectomy for an early stage endometrial cancer. She seemed quite anxious, and as I asked some questions, it became quite apparent that she was still feeling guilty over a decision she had made 20 years previously, i.e., encouraging her daughter to discontinue life support on the daughter's anencephalic baby.

While physicians are quite accustomed to hearing confessions, we are not trained or ordained to give absolution. My response to the patient above was to refer her to her pastor for further discussion on the topic. My response to a patient who does not have a relationship with clergy but clearly has a pressing issue is to refer the patient to a hospital chaplain. Hospital chaplains are well trained (see section below) to handle such issues and can be enormously helpful in helping a medical team deal with a "difficult" patient, a "difficult" family, interteam issues about particular patients, and for debriefing after a traumatic medical event.

Avenues of Exploration

If this chapter has piqued your curiosity or whetted your appetite for learning more about the relationship between spirituality, religion, and medicine, I suggest you explore some of the resources listed at the end of this chapter. Medical schools that are a subset of larger universities often offer dual degree programs with their divinity schools. Clinical pastoral education (the formal chaplaincy training program that prepare clergy to be certified as chaplains) has, over the last 12 years opened portions of this training to medical care providers at both the Massachusetts General Hospital (MGH) and Yale-New Haven Medical Center through generous grants from the Kenneth B. Schwartz Center (http://www.theschwartzcenter.org/programs/cpe.html), so that medical providers and clergy can learn from each other how to better care for the whole patient. As the first physician "graduate" of the program at MGH, I not only learned how to better care for patients and myself, but also many interpersonal techniques that have stood me in good stead with my patients and colleagues.

References

1. Puchalski C et al. Improving the quality of spiritual care as a dimension of palliative care: the report of the consensus conference. J Palliat Med. 2009;12(10):885–904.
2. Koenig H. Spirituality in patient care. Philadelphia: Templeton Foundation Press; 2002.
3. McCord G et al. Discussing spirituality with patients: a rational and ethical approach. Ann Fam Med. 2004;2:356–61.
4. Feldstein, B. As taught in spirituality and meaning in medicine, Stanford University School of Medicine, personal communication.
5. Stein M. The lonely patient. New York: HarperCollins; 2007.
6. Thiel, MM. Personal communication, adapted from NANDA-I, Nursing Diagnosis: Definitions and Classifications, NANDA International; 2007–2008.
7. Frank A. The wounded storyteller. Chicago: The University of Chicago Press; 1995.
8. Carson R. The hyphenated space: liminality in the doctor-patient relationship. In: Charon R, Montello M, editors. Stories matter. New York: Routledge; 2002. Chapter 18.
9. Benson H. Timeless healing. New York: Fireside; 1996.
10. Feldstein B et al. The role of clergy and chaplains in healthcare. In: Serlin I et al., editors. Whole person healthcare, volume two: psychology, spirituality and health. Santa Barbara: Praeger; 2007. Chapter 7.

11. Shafir R. The zen of listening. Wheaton: Quest Books; 2003.
12. Ostaseski, F. lecture notes.
13. Puchalski CM, Romer AL. Taking a spiritual history allows clinicians to understand patients more fully. J Palliat Med. 2000;3:129–37.
14. Anandarajah G, Hight E. Spirituality ad medical practice: Using the HOPE questions as a practical tool for spiritual assessment. Am Fam Physician. 2001;63(1):81–8.

Resources

Divinity schools. Many universities have Divinity Schools associated with them. Students interested in pursuing their individual religions in-depth might explore the possibility of taking courses or obtaining a dual degree.

Chaplaincy education. Professional chaplains have advanced degrees or ordination in their respective religions. However, due to the interfaith nature of their work, they also obtain additional training in Clinical Pastoral Education Programs. For more information on these programs, Please see this web site: http://www.acpe.edu/. It is the site for the Association for Clinical Pastoral Education and offers a plethora of useful information.

Chapter 31
Complementary and Alternative Medicine

Darshan Mehta

Key Points

- Complementary and alternative medicine (CAM) is used by a significant proportion of people in the United States.
- Many CAM practices are being integrated into conventional care.
- There are increasing number of opportunities for medical trainees and practicing physicians to pursue clinical and research training in CAM.

Introduction

The healthcare practices of people in the United States include the allopathic model of illness and treatment. However, they also include traditions that have evolved throughout history and culture. Given the diverse backgrounds of the people living in the United States, along with the variations of explanatory models of wellness, illness, and symptom management, many individuals seek multiple modalities as a part of their self-care as well as treatment. Some individuals may also choose to employ certain modalities in place of established standards of care. Given the increasing popularity of complementary and alternative medicine (CAM), it is becoming more imperative for physicians and physicians-in-training to be better versed in understanding patient choice and preference in their treatment.

D. Mehta, MD, MPH (✉)
Benson-Henry Institute for Mind Body Medicine, Massachusetts General Hospital,
151 Merrimac Street4th Floor, Boston, MA 02130, USA
e-mail: dmehta@partners.org

R.D. Urman and J.M. Ehrenfeld (eds.), *Physicians' Pathways to Non-Traditional Careers and Leadership Opportunities*, DOI 10.1007/978-1-4614-0551-1_31,
© Springer Science+Business Media, LLC 2012

What Is Complementary and Alternative Medicine?

According to the National Center for Complementary and Alternative Medicine (NCCAM) at the National Institutes of Health (NIH), CAM is a group of diverse medical and healthcare systems, practices, and products that are not generally considered part of conventional medicine. As broadly defined by NCCAM, there are four main domains of CAM use: mind-body medicine; biologically based therapies; manipulative and body-based practices; and energy therapies. Mind-body medicine focuses on the interactions among the brain, mind, body, and behavior, and how these approaches affect physical functioning and promote health. Examples include meditation, yoga, and tai chi. Biologically-based practices include herbal and dietary supplements. Manipulative and body-based practices focus primarily on the structures and systems of the body, including the bones and joints, soft tissues, and circulatory and lymphatic systems. This includes techniques such as massage therapy and spinal manipulation. Energy medicine includes practices such as Reiki therapy and magnet therapy; these techniques are based on theories of energy field manipulation. Finally, there are broad systems of medicine, such as Ayurvedic medicine and traditional Chinese medicine, which have evolved over periods of time and employ multiple modalities toward treatment and health. While CAM has historically been used to refer to these modalities, many individuals and institutions are utilizing the term integrative medicine to best reflect the nature of interactions between multiple modalities – allopathic and nonallopathic.

How Prevalent Is Complementary and Alternative Medicine?

According to a nationwide government survey released in December 2008, approximately 38% of U.S. adults aged 18 years and over and approximately 12% of children use some form of CAM (Fig. 31.1). As mentioned in this report, it was estimated that U.S. adults spent $33.9 billion out-of-pocket on visits to CAM practitioners and purchases of CAM products, classes, and materials. There is some scientific evidence around the efficacy of some CAM modalities; however, for many modalities, there are still many questions with regard to the safety and efficacy of these CAM modalities in the treatment of medical conditions. In addition, understanding the use of CAM is an important aspect of delivering patient-centered care. Healthcare providers need to be able to ask individuals about their use of CAM. It may not be sufficient to ask about CAM use as simply a treatment of illness; rather, it may also need to be queried in the context of well-being and promotion of care.

Fig. 31.1 Complementary and Alternative Medicine Use by U.S. Adults and Children (Adapted from Barnes PM, Bloom B, Nahin R. Complementary and alternative medicine use among adults and children: United States, 2007. CDC Natl Health Stat Report. 2008;10(12):1–23. http://nccam.nih.gov/news/camstats/2007/graphics.htm with permission from National Center for Complementary and Alternative Medicine, NIH, DHHS)

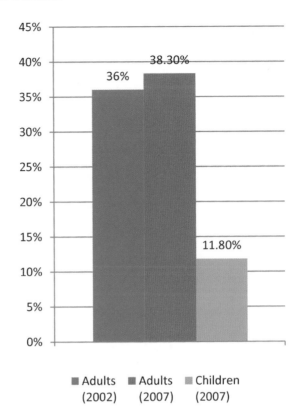

Incorporating Complementary and Alternative Medicine into Your Practice

There are increasing numbers of opportunities for medical students, residents, fellows, and practicing physicians to further their knowledge and practice in integrative medicine. In 2000, the Consortium of Academic Health Centers for Integrative Medicine (www.imconsortium.org) was established to advance the principles and practices of integrative healthcare within academic institutions. Presently, the consortium consists of 46 academic medical centers (Table 31.1). In order for an institution to be part of the consortium, it must have an established program in Integrative Medicine that includes ongoing work in research, education, and/or clinical activity. In addition, the institution must have evidence through senior leadership of its commitment to the field of integrative medicine. These institutions are quite diverse in their offerings, as some may have research and educational opportunities, while other institutions may have evidence of all three activities. Nonetheless, the Consortium is able to identify key individuals who are committed to furthering this field at their respective institutions.

Table 31.1 Academic health centers with complementary and integrative medicine programs

United States

Arizona	*Massachusetts*	*Pennsylvania*
University of Arizona	Boston University School of Medicine	Thomas Jefferson University
California	Harvard Medical School	University of Pennsylvania
Stanford University	University of Massachusetts Medical School	University of Pittsburgh
University of California, Irvine	*Michigan*	*Tennessee*
University of California, Los Angeles	University of Michigan	Vanderbilt University
University of California, San Diego	*Minnesota*	*Texas*
University of California, San Francisco	Mayo Clinic	University of Texas Medical Branch
Colorado	University of Minnesota	*Vermont*
University of Colorado at Denver School of Medicine	*New Jersey*	University of Vermont College of Medicine
Connecticut	University of Medicine and Dentistry of New Jersey	*Washington*
University of Connecticut Health Center	*New Mexico*	University of Washington
Yale University	University of New Mexico	*Washington, DC*
Hawaii	*New York*	George Washington University
University of Hawaii-Manoa	Albert Einstein College of Medicine of Yeshiva University	Georgetown University School of Medicine
Illinois	Columbia University	*Wisconsin*
Northwestern University Feinberg School of Medicine	*North Carolina*	University of Wisconsin-Madison
University of Chicago Pritzker School of Medicine	Duke University	**Canada**
University of Illinois at Chicago School of Medicine	University of North Carolina at Chapel Hill	*Alberta*
Kansas	Wake Forest University School of Medicine	University of Alberta
University of Kansas	*Ohio*	University of Calgary
Maryland	The Ohio State University	*Ontario*
Johns Hopkins University	University of Cincinnati College of Medicine	McMaster University
School of Medicine	*Oregon*	*Quebec*
University of Maryland	Oregon Health and Science University	Laval University

Adapted from Consortium of Academic Health Centers for Integrative Medicine. Member Institutions. http://www.imconsortium.org/about/members/home.html

There are also an increasing number of opportunities for medical trainees to pursue research within CAM. There are federally funded opportunities that allow individuals to further research training in the study of CAM. For example, Harvard Medical School offers a 3-year postdoctoral fellowship that prepares physicians to be academic faculty, with content and research expertise in CAM. Through this program, individuals also acquire an MPH or MS degree at the Harvard School of Public Health. In addition, individuals are prepared to become independent investigators through the development and analysis of original investigations. For many federally funded programs, individuals are invited to apply upon completion of a residency. For medical students and residents who are interested in research, these endeavors require more creativity. That is, it is important to identify mentors and/or centers that have independent funding. As an example, there are NCCAM research centers that may have budgeted positions for medical students and residents.

Over the past decade, many opportunities have evolved for medical practitioners to advance their clinical skills in CAM. For medical students and residents, there are different types of opportunities. As an example, for those individuals who are interested in an immersion program, the University of Arizona offers both an online experience as well as elective rotations. In addition, for those physicians who desire an in-depth experience, there is a 2-year distance fellowship that comprises of online training alongside residential experiences. There are multiple opportunities at academic medical centers to have clinical training in particular modalities. For example, UCLA, Stanford and Harvard medical schools offer intensive courses for physicians to be trained in medical acupuncture. There are ample courses that provide continuing medical education for physicians who are interested in learning updates and/or overviews of CAM modalities. Finally, the American Board of Integrative Holistic Medicine (www.integrativeholisticdoctors.org) offers a nonaccredited certification within this field.

Conclusions

As future physicians think about their medical careers, CAM practices are becoming a part of the standard clinical environment. While concierge medicine and medical spa practices often offer CAM services as part of individualized care, CAM services are increasingly being offered in multiple settings. Given the rising costs of healthcare, many healthcare leaders are looking at CAM services as a means to providing cost-effective care. A recent Institute of Medicine summit brought together thought leaders in integrative medicine to see how these modalities could be incorporated as the United States undergoes a transformation of healthcare delivery.

In summary, CAM use is quite prevalent, and there are many opportunities for physicians and physicians-in-training to avail themselves. The body of literature of scientific research continues to expand with regard to safety and efficacy. As physician awareness and comfort around CAM increases, this will assist them in providing patient-centered care, as they help their patients navigate through the multitude of choices that exist within the healthcare system.

Additional Resources

Barnes PM, Bloom B, Nahin R. Complementary and alternative medicine use among adults and children: United States, 2007. CDC Natl Health Stat Report. 2008;10(12):1–23.

IOM (Institute of Medicine). Integrative medicine and the health of the public: a summary of the February 2009 summit. Washington: The National Academies Press; 2009.

National Center for Complementary and Alternative Medicine. www.nccam.nih.gov.

Consortium of Academic Health Centers for Integrative Medicine. www.imconsortium.org.

American Board of Integrative Holistic Medicine. www.integrativeholisticdoctors.org.

Chapter 32
Volunteering in Your Community: Think Globally, Act Locally

Jean Hess

Key Points

- Choose a community volunteer experience that best suits your desire to help individuals or organizations, your professional goals, and your current skills and knowledge.
- There are many potential benefits of volunteering in your community, including gaining cross-cultural skills, finding inspiration and personal satisfaction, learning about diverse groups of people, improving your medical skills and knowledge, helping decide about future goals or career plans.
- An individual in any stage of his or her career can find opportunities to volunteer. Opportunities for involvement range from small local organizations to established large national and international organizations.

Introduction

The goal of this chapter is to help you translate passion into action, whether you are a premedical or medical student, resident, practicing or retired physician, or whether you are in an academic or nonacademic setting. It will help you consider *what you want to do, where and why you want to do it,* and provide some *resources* to help you make it happen. Act now: the sky is the limit!

Volunteering is experiencing a growth spurt, brought on in part by a new wave of support and legislation. In 2008, 61.8 million Americans volunteered, contributing

J. Hess, MS (✉)
Harvard Medical School, Boston, MA 02115, USA
e-mail: jean_hess@hms.harvard.edu

R.D. Urman and J.M. Ehrenfeld (eds.), *Physicians' Pathways to Non-Traditional Careers and Leadership Opportunities*, DOI 10.1007/978-1-4614-0551-1_32,
© Springer Science+Business Media, LLC 2012

GETTING STARTED	
WHAT MOTIVATES YOU:	**CONSIDER:**
Singular issue or event	Geography/Location
Nature of the project	Transportation Needed
Benefits to agency	Time you have available
Benefits to you	Skills
Learning new skills	Is training available?
A particular person/people	Available staff
Giving back	Mentoring
Working with a specific population	Clear goals for the project
Being able to use/improve language skills	Time that projects takes place
Meeting new people	Values of agency concordant with your own
Career development	Are volunteers recognized?
Learning about self and others	
Being able to act on firmly held beliefs	

Fig. 32.1 Considerations for choosing a volunteer activity

eight billion hours of volunteer service worth $162 billion [1]. Campus Compact, a national coalition of academic institutions that focuses on campus-based civic engagement, service and service-learning, reported in 2008 that 31% of college students in their member institutions were involved in these activities, from K-12 education, alleviating poverty, hunger, and homelessness, to tutoring, voter registration, and much more. In April 2009, President Obama signed landmark national service legislation in the form of the Edward M. Kennedy Serve America Act, greatly expanding the services and resources of the Corporation for National and Community Service. Clearly, huge numbers of people are volunteering!

Volunteering means providing support to individuals, groups, organizations, or institutions without pay. There are countless types of volunteer opportunities and different ways to talk about service. Community service is often associated with social justice issues in that it focuses on underserved and underresourced populations; health and medical volunteering tend to focus on these populations as well, especially for people interested in issues of health disparities. But opportunities abound in *all* kinds of organizations, whether they are in healthcare, education, the Girl Scouts, state and local government agencies, your local YMCA, local charities, or large foundations (See the Resources section for a wide array of organizations and use the suggested databases to help you get started). The most important thing is finding an organization that is a good fit for you and your skills, and an agency or issue that you find inspiring and are passionate about. Sometimes, people are just waiting to be asked. A list of key points to consider when choosing a volunteer opportunity is listed in Fig. 32.1.

Many different forms of assistance can be provided. When people speak about volunteering, they are usually referring to some kind of community service work that targets those most in need. Within the context of academic institutions and on university campuses, community service has been primarily co-curricular (not for credit), even though learning often takes place. For over a decade, service-learning classes have been springing up all over the country. Service-learning is a pedagogy or teaching strategy where community service is integrated into the classroom as part of a course. It typically includes service, didactic learning and reflection. The learning in service-learning is more intentional than it is when someone is solely doing a community service project. The two words are often combined ("community service-learning") or used interchangeably, but experts in the field agree that there is a distinction between the two. For the purposes of this chapter, volunteering will be the word most often used to connote working in underserved communities. References to community service and service-learning will be identified primarily in the "On Campus" section.

This chapter takes a look at some of the reasons why people volunteer and the benefits gained. It gives advice about how and where to find volunteer opportunities, whether you are a pre-medical or medical student, resident or practicing physician/faculty. Finally, it provides resources for people interested in looking for volunteer opportunities, with a focus on health-related activities.

Benefits of Volunteering

There is nothing quite as satisfying as feeling like you've made a difference – this is perhaps the overarching reason why people decide to go into medicine. You can make an impact in many, many ways: on individual lives, on a program or agency, on a particular issue, through direct service or advocacy, and even on yourself.

Recent studies on health gains from volunteering demonstrate that benefits are not only limited to the beneficiaries of services. In fact, people who provide support through volunteering often have more gains in health than those who are receiving services: studies on the relationship between health benefits and volunteering show that those who do the volunteering accrue more health benefits than those who are receiving the services [2].

There are many other benefits of volunteering and a summary is provided in Table 32.1.

Table 32.1 Benefits of volunteering

- Being part of a community
- Participating in new activities
- Gaining specific skills
- Increasing self-confidence
- Learning about diverse groups of people
- Gaining cross cultural skills
- Helping decide about future goals or career plans
- Gaining a sense of achievement
- Living longer
- Finding inspiration and personal satisfaction
- Stepping outside your comfort zone
- Having fun

How to Find Volunteer Opportunities on Campus

Community service and service-learning have spread exponentially across the spectrum of education institutions in the last decade, from K-12, to undergraduate colleges and universities, to graduate school programs such as medical schools. Typically, students who wish to attend medical school have engaged in some sort of service; it is seen as a requirement for admission. Following are some general ways to find volunteer opportunities for premedical and medical students.

Student volunteers have myriad choices in accessing community service resources. They include student service and interest groups that include service in their mission; offices of community affairs or service; service-learning classes; faculty mentors involved in service activities; databases of service opportunities; and various scholarships and awards pertaining to service.

Service-Learning Classes: An attempt to better organize and codify the various meanings and goals of community service and service-learning has led to a variety of strategies to achieve the goal of commitment to service; service-learning is perhaps the premier pedagogy. Undergraduate students are probably most familiar with service-learning, but it has recently made many gains in graduate school settings. The Liaison Committee on Medical Education (LCME) created a requirement in 2007 regarding service-learning as a standard for medical schools: "Standards for Accreditation of Medical Education Programs Leading to the MD degree: IS-14-A: Medical schools should make available sufficient opportunities for medical students to participate in service-learning activities, and should encourage and support student participation" [3]. In addition, the American Medical Association (AMA) passed a resolution in 2004 that supports the concept of service-learning as a key part of medical school and residency curricula and promotes the kind of experiences that include collaborations with a community partner/agency to improve the health of communities.

Dedicated Campus Centers: In addition to service-learning courses, there are a plethora of community service offices on most undergraduate and graduate school campuses. Campus Compact reports in the 2008 Membership Survey of its 1,190 institutions that 94% have at least one office or center devoted to community service and/or service-learning [4]. When looking for these offices, undergraduates, medical students, residents, and faculty should look for offices for community service or service-learning, and/or departments or centers that articulate values such as community-campus partnerships and outreach. Established with a variety of different missions, the overall goal of these offices is to link people with volunteer activities. Many of these opportunities can be found through a "community" link on a school website's homepage. There are many health-related and student organizations which focus on volunteering. Several of these organizations are listed in Table 32.2 and more detailed information is contained in the Resources section.

A popular way for students to volunteer is in medical clinics, some of them student-run. Over 100 student-run clinics exist across the country and can often be found through medical school websites if they have a community service section.

Table 32.2 Health-related student organizations with a volunteer focus

- The American Medical Association (AMA) has a student section with a plethora of information on grants, fellowships, internships, international health experiences, ways to get involved in advocacy projects, and more. Resources are also available to residents and physicians
- The Student National Medical Association (SNMA) is a national organization (with school and regional chapters and conferences) that vigorously includes community service in its mission
- The American Medical Student Association (AMSA) has many action committees and interest groups
- The American Association of Medical Colleges (AAMC) sponsors the annual Medicine in the Community Award, a generous grant program for student-led community service projects

Medical clinics, immunization clinics, health promotion activities, student/faculty collaboratives, mobile health clinics, and student-run health clinics provide volunteering opportunities for everyone from undergraduates to medical students, to residents and practicing physicians. Clinics serve as training grounds for students and a place for doctors to "give back" in the form of direct services to community members and teaching students a variety of skills. Most clinics work with underserved populations in under-resourced, usually urban, areas and often have the dual mission of training future healthcare providers while providing a variety of direct services to needy clients, usually for free.

There is currently a renewed focus on finding more systematic ways to educate students in democratic values and citizenship, how to create mutually beneficial community–campus partnerships, and the promotion of all kinds of volunteering, advocacy, and civic engagement programs. Community–Campus Partnerships for Health (CCPH), a nonprofit agency founded in 1997, brings together myriad strategies for addressing these issues. Other organizations exist on the local, state, national, and international levels (see the Corporation for National and Community Service and Campus Compact in the Resources section), and community-based scholarship, especially through community-based participatory research, is gaining more recognition both nationally and internationally.

For Residents and Practicing Physicians

Service-learning is one way that residents and faculty can engage with communities. Many academic institutions now offer service-learning courses and some include service-learning and community-based research in their tenure and promotion processes. In addition, some residency programs are offering service-learning types of programs in community-oriented primary care where residents are required, as part of a course, to develop sustainable projects and partnerships with community sites. Residents interested in community-oriented primary care and family medicine will usually find community service and engagement an integral part of their residency programs. Physicians in academic settings benefit from the recent changes in the promotion and tenure process that recognize community-based work and research.

Clinical Translation and Science Awards (CTSAs), funded by the National Institutes of Health, now exist at 46 institutions in 26 states. One of the goals of the CTSAs is to improve the health of communities by engaging community partners in order that research can move quickly into clinical practice. Many sites maintain internal databases that provide a way to search for faculty with similar interests.

CCPH works with faculty to increase recognition for community work. They clearly articulate the relationship between goals such as eliminating health disparities and how they are tied to community-based teaching, research, and service. Their work includes the recent establishment of a free, online website that helps community-engaged scholars publish and distribute peer-reviewed, health-related scholarship that are in forms other than journal articles (such as curricula, videos, policy reports, and resource guides). See http://www.ces4health.info/. Community partners and academic peers both review everything submitted to CES4Health.

On the CCPH general website (see Resources) viewers can read about the "Faculty for the Engaged Campus," view resources (such as the "Community-Engaged Scholarship Toolkit"), find a database of faculty mentors, and join a discussion group for other faculty interested in community-engaged scholarship. An extensive variety of other resources are available.

Residents and practicing physicians can obviously find many volunteering opportunities on their own; service does not necessarily have to be part of courses or research. If you are affiliated with an academic institution, chances are that some of the resources that are available to students are also open to residents and faculty. These include the means to find opportunities through internal databases and assistance from staff at campus offices that work to match people with needs at community sites.

Since residents and physicians do not have access to other student resources, an easy place to start looking is with larger, well-known organizations (the reader can find volunteering opportunities at many of the agency suggestions in the Resources section of this chapter). Most national organizations have local chapters that are easily accessed from the main homepage of their websites. Easily finding the website for a national organization through a search engine on the internet (for instance, organizations such as the American Red Cross, the American Cancer Society, and Habitat for Humanity) will provide easy navigation to a local chapter in your state where volunteer opportunities will be prominently featured. Examples of the kinds of opportunities available at these agencies include administrative support, serving on boards of directors, and working on specific projects that pertain to the particular organization. You can pursue activities that run the gamut from disaster relief, to health and safety issues, to running support groups or teaching in an after-school program, to planning and implementing a fundraising event, to working on just about anything that helps fulfill the mission of an organization. Smaller, local grassroots organizations are sometimes harder to find but can be just as rewarding. Oftentimes you can find these organizations advertising for both paid jobs and volunteer opportunities on the databases in the Resources section. Many smaller nonprofit agencies utilize idealist.org to publicize openings.

Hopefully this short chapter has convinced you that anyone who is interested in volunteering can find an excess of opportunities. All you really need to do is find something you feel passionate about – then hopefully you can translate that passion into action. Talk to anyone you know who has volunteered, especially at establishing community relationships over time, and you'll be sure to find a satisfied and inspiring individual. Your colleagues are often the best place to start.

References

1. Key Findings from the "Listening Post Project," a national survey of Nonprofit Organizations done in partnership with the Corporation for National and Community Service. July 2009. www.VolunteeringInAmerica.gov. Accessed May 2010.
2. Corporation for National and Community Service, Office of Research Policy and Development. The health benefits of volunteering: a review of recent research. Washington, DC: CNCS; 2007.
3. Liaison Committee on Medical Education. Functions and Structure of a Medical School: Standards for Accreditation of Medical Education Programs Leading to the M.D. Degree. June 2008. http://www.lcme.org/functions2008jun.pdf. Accessed 4 June 2010.
4. Campus Compact. 2008 Service statistics: highlights and trends of campus compact's annual membership survey. Boston: Campus Compact; 2009.

Examples of Resources

National Organizations:

http://www.ama-assn.org/: The American Medical Association website provides ways for students, residents, and physicians to become involved in particular issues.

http://www.nationalservice.gov/: The Corporation for National and Community Service is a federal agency that oversees Senior Corps and AmeriCorps and a variety of special initiatives. Their website provides ample information about volunteering and offers a wide range of links from funding information to other service-related topics. It also includes the Learn and Serve America Program that provides grants to schools, higher education institutions, and community-based organizations that engage students, their teachers and others in service to meet community needs.

http://www.compact.org/: A national collaboration of over 1,000 colleges and universities located in 35 states that focuses on service, service-learning, and civic engagement in higher education. The Campus Compact VISTA program joins the missions of Campus Compact and AmeriCorps*VISTA through projects that build community–campus partnerships to fight poverty.

http://depts.washington.edu/ccph/index.html – Community–Campus Partnerships for Health is a nonprofit agency that works to promote health by linking academic institutions and communities. They maintain an extensive website, online newsletter, on-line discussion groups and provide access to a broad range of resources for students, faculty and staff.

http://www.servicelearning.org/resources-parents-how-get-your-child-started-service-learning#where: The National Service-learning Clearinghouse supports schools (higher education and K-12),

community-based agencies, and tribal programs to strengthen local communities through service-learning projects. It provides information on syllabi, jobs, publications, and volunteer opportunities.
National health-related organizations with state chapters: American Heart Association, American Red Cross, American Lung Association, etc.

Fellowships, Grants, and Awards

http://www.schweitzerfellowship.org: The Albert Schweitzer Fellowship is a national program that provides stipends to students in the health professions who seek to "turn idealism into action," with an emphasis on creating leaders in service for a lifetime. It has sites in Boston, Baltimore, the Bay area, Chicago, Houston, greater Philadelphia, Los Angeles, New Hampshire/Vermont, New Orleans, North Carolina, and Pittsburgh. Their website has a listing of possible volunteering sites in each city.
http://www.aamc.org/about/awards/cfc/start.htm – The American Association of Medical Colleges (AAMC) Medicine in Community Grant Program provides funds for student-led community programs.
http://www.aauw.org/learn/fellows_directory/community.cfm: The American Association of University Women (AAUW) provides Community Action Grant Awards to female students providing service in community sites.
http://www.usg.edu/carteraward/: The Jimmy and Roslyn Carter Partnership Award. This award honors a recipient where the partnership program addresses critical areas of public need undertaken by a college or university in partnership with a community group.
http://www.atpm.org/pasp/index.html: The Paul E. Ambrose Scholars Program (given annually through the Association for Prevention Teaching and Research) is a Washington, D.C.-based program that familiarizes health professions students with influential public health professionals and prepares them to become leaders in public health through advocacy and service.
http://www.compact.org/initiatives/campus-compact-awardsprograms/: Variety of awards such as the Frank Newman Leadership Award which recognizes students with financial need and civic leadership potential and provides financial support and mentorship to help them achieve academic and civic goals. The Thomas Erlich Civically Engaged Faculty Award recognizes one faculty member each year for exemplary engaged scholarship and enhancing higher education's contributions to the public good. Student Leaders in Service is an AmeriCorps Education Award Only program, which engages college students as part-time AmeriCorps members.
http://www.neche.org. The Ernest A. Lynton Award for Faculty Professional Service and Academic Outreach: An annual scholarship to a faculty member who connects his or her experience and scholarship to community outreach.
http://nhsc.hrsa.gov/: National Health Service Corps (NHSC) scholarship and loan repayment programs. Scholars must serve one year for each year they receive a scholarship (minimum two years) and work in a health professional shortage area in a primary care field. NHSC also recruits primary care clinicians who are dedicated to providing care in NHSC-approved sites for underserved people.

Where to Find More Information and Local Opportunities

Your colleagues.
Hospital-based Community Benefits and Community Outreach Offices.
State and city affiliates/chapters of national organizations.
United Way affiliates.

Campus Compact state offices.

Community Health Centers and statewide associations of health centers (For instance, http://www. massleague.org has information on sites, careers, loan repayment and more).

Schools: pre-school, K-12, charter and pilot schools, community colleges, colleges and universities, graduate programs.

Faith-based, arts and cultural, and neighborhood organizations.

YM/YWCAs.

Mentoring, tutoring, and after school programs.

Large agencies such as the Red Cross, American Lung Association, American Diabetes Association, American Cancer Society, American Heart Association, and other disease-specific programs and events.

Local public health departments or state departments of health in your city; health education and public health programs.

Healthcare policy and advocacy organizations on the local, state, and national level.

Adult Education, GED and ESOL (English for Speakers of Other Languages) classes, health literacy organizations or projects, libraries.

Population specific agencies such as those that work with immigrants and refugees, teens, English-language learners, specific races and ethnicities, women, at-risk youth and others.

Economic and neighborhood development organizations.

Health-related (broadly defined) agencies such as Habitat for Humanity, healthcare organizations and shelters for the homeless, literacy agencies, programs in sexual health for teenagers, rape crisis centers and domestic violence shelters, elderly organizations, sports-related organizations, housing, food and nutrition, and more.

Sample Volunteer Databases

Volunteer Solutions is a program of the United Way that matches individuals to volunteer opportunities in the community. They are at http://volunteer.united-e-way.org/.

Volunteer Match has opportunities around Boston and the entire country. They can be found at http://www.volunteermatch.org/; http://idealist.org/ has opportunities locally and internationally; http://servenet.org/ is an extensive site with information about volunteering locally and nationally. It has information on how to get involved, how to help nonprofits and other volunteer resources.

Find a way to be a mentor through the National Mentoring Partnership (and their state affiliates) at http://www.mentoring.org. http://www.dosomething.org helps you find information by cause, zip code, length of time, etc. (youth-focused action site).

Part VIII
Real-Life Stories

Chapter 33
Leaders in the Successful Pursuit of Nontraditional Careers in Medicine

Christopher W. Baugh, Mark A. Bloomberg, Spencer Borden, Maria Young Chandler, Joseph S. Fastow, Jonathan P. Gertler, Richard Kalish, Lisa Bard Levine, N. Stephen Ober, and Peter L. Slavin

Key Points

- Alternative careers for physicians are very diverse. No two are exactly the same.
- There are numerous reasons why physicians seek alternative career tracks.
- The opportunities for physicians outside clinical medicine are great.
- Those considering alternative careers should network with those physicians who have made the leap. Their stories are invaluable.

C.W. Baugh, MD, MBA
Department of Emergency Medicine, Brigham and Women's Hospital,
Harvard Medical School, Boston, MA, USA

M.A. Bloomberg, MD, MBA
HealthNEXT, Sudbury, MA, USA

S. Borden, IV, MD, MBA, FACR, FAAP, FACPE
Concord, MA, USA

M.Y. Chandler, MD, MBA
University of California, Irvine, USA

The Children's Clinic, Long Beach, CA, USA

Association of MD/MBA Programs, Inc., Sunset Beach, CA, USA

J.S. Fastow, MD, MPH, FACEP
Physician Management, Ltd., Bethesda, MD, USA

J.P. Gertler, MD, MPH, FACEP
Back Bay Life Science Advisors, Boston, MA, USA
e-mail: jgertler@BBLSA.com

R.D. Urman and J.M. Ehrenfeld (eds.), *Physicians' Pathways to Non-Traditional Careers and Leadership Opportunities*, DOI 10.1007/978-1-4614-0551-1_33,
© Springer Science+Business Media, LLC 2012

Introduction

Throughout this book we have provided detailed information on alternative career paths for physicians. This chapter pulls this information together into a series of personal case studies of real world physicians who have successfully made the transition from full-time clinician to leadership positions in their chosen fields. We've attempted to capture diverse career options in fields such as finance, consulting, healthcare administration, academia, and entrepreneurship to name just a few. Each contributor provides a candid profile of their personal background and insight into their career decision-making process. The "stories" are all different, but certain common themes emerge. One consistent observation is the immense satisfaction each contributor has with his/her chosen career. Another theme is the continued strong bond and identification with clinical medicine. As the director of an MD/MBA dual degree program and a mentor to numerous physicians seeking alternative careers, I am consistently asked the same questions, "How do I make the correct career decision and what are my options." I hope this chapter sheds some light on these important and fundamental questions.

Christopher W. Baugh, MD, MBA

Dr. Christopher W. Baugh is an Emergency Physician at Brigham and Women's Hospital (BWH) in Boston (Fig. 33.1). In 2009, Dr. Baugh graduated from the Harvard-Affiliated Emergency Medicine Residency and joined the Brigham faculty as Director of the Emergency Department (ED) Observation Unit – a closed ten-bed unit within the ED where patients can spend up to an additional 24 hours undergoing additional treatment and evaluation after their initial ED evaluation. Shortly after taking on this role, Dr. Baugh began to lead the clinical planning for a new urgent care center in Foxborough, MA, which he currently directs since its launch in September of 2010. Dr. Baugh received his BA degree from Johns Hopkins University and MD and MBA degrees from the University of Pennsylvania.

R. Kalish, MD, MS, MPH
Boston Medical Center HealthNet Plan and Boston HealthNet, Department of Medicine, Boston Medical Center, Boston, MA, USA

L.B. Levine, MD, MBA
Navigant Consulting, Inc., Needham, MA, USA

N.S. Ober, MD, MBA (✉)
Business Incubation, Boston University Technology Development, MD/MBA Dual Degree Program, Boston University School of Medicine, Boston, MA, USA
e-mail: sober@bu.edu

P.L. Slavin, MD
Department of Administration, Massachusetts General Hospital, Boston, MA, USA

Fig. 33.1 Christopher W. Baugh, MD, MBA. Medical Director, Brigham and Women's ED Observation Unit. Medical Director, Brigham and Women's Urgent Care Center. Clinical Instructor, Harvard Medical School

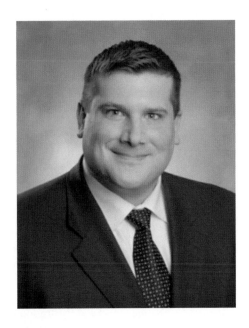

Career Roadmap

- BA Johns Hopkins University
- MD University of Pennsylvania
- MBA Wharton Business School
- Emergency Medicine Residency, Harvard-Affiliated Emergency Medicine Residency
- Clinical Instructor in Medicine, Brigham and Women's Hospital
- Medical Director, BWH ED Observation Unit
- Medical Director, BWH Urgent Care Center at Foxborough

Personal History

I was born and raised in Marin County, California and attended St. Ignatius College Preparatory in San Francisco. My father was a small business owner and was the owner/operator of a Shell gas station while my mother worked various jobs before finding her niche as a real estate agent. I certainly was not exposed to the practice of healthcare growing up, so it's no surprise that I arrived at my chosen career path a little late. In my childhood I was very focused on being the model student-athlete but I had no concrete vision of my eventual career path. I fell in love with the sport of football and my criteria for college were the following: (1) East Coast location (I wanted the experience of being on my own), (2) strong academic environment that wouldn't limit my options for whatever I wanted to do after college, and (3) a realistic opportunity to play football for all 4 years of college. I found all of these traits at Johns Hopkins, a Baltimore school known for rigorous academics and a Division III football program that promised copious time on the field. Whenever someone hears that I went to Hopkins for college, they assume that I was set on becoming a physician all my life, but to be honest, I didn't decide on medicine until at least 2 years after heading to Baltimore. Once there, I thrived on the competition both on the field and in the classroom. Hopkins' notoriously difficult premed curriculum was yet another challenge that I took on and I was thrilled to see that I could excel there – don't get me wrong, Organic Chemistry (aka "Orgo") freshman year kicked my butt and gave me serious pause about continuing down that path, but I pushed forward. I spent time shadowing on a kidney transplant ward and in the operating room at the University of California at San Francisco during my winter break that first year and I continued to take courses in Economics at Hopkins – the other area of study that I connected with in those early days. My main take away from that experience was that doctors were very frustrated with the administrative aspects of medicine, but still loved taking care of patients. This was in the winter of 1996 – the peak of the managed care wave, and doctors were certainly feeling it. This sense of helplessness and frustration really stuck with me and drove me to try to understand why the healthcare system operates the way it does. When deciding how my life would incorporate science and economics, I considered several career visions. I thought about bench top research, life as a PhD student, postdoc, and perhaps one day as part of a biotech start-up company. I spent 3 years doing bench-top research, supported by grants from Pfizer Pharmaceuticals and the Howard Hughes Medical Institute over my summer breaks. In the end, I felt that I needed the human connection of caring for patients to be a central aspect of my work, so medical school was in my future. I ended up with a minor in Economics and major in Biology, which was a nice combination to help me think about the business and science of healthcare, or at least know which questions to ask when given the opportunity. My undergraduate experience ended on a high note, as I was awarded Phi Beta Kappa and All-American honors for football.

Because I had settled on medical school relatively late (beginning of junior year), I felt unprepared to take the MCAT at the usual time – in the spring of that year. As a result, I pushed it off until August of my fourth year. While the extra time was very useful in allowing me to prep for the test, it also put me behind in applying for medical school in that immediate application cycle. I also had a sense that once I started medical school, my life would inevitably lead to one responsibility after another with no real time off. As a result, I decided that it would be an ideal time to spend a year out of school between college and medical school. I moved in with my girl-friend and we found an apartment in Northern Virginia. I took a position at the Princeton Review in Washington, DC and got my first taste of office work. After about 6 months of a brutal commute (I had enough time to read everything Kurt Vonnegut had ever written on the DC Metro) and waiting for the clock to strike 5 p.m. every day, I decided life was too short so I quit and started working as a sub-stitute teacher in the local school system. I quickly found regular work at South

Lakes High School as a tenth grade Geometry teacher and very much enjoyed the combination of short days and teaching. During this year I thought hard about which medical school made the most sense for my interests – I wanted a very good school that would prepare me well for whichever residency I wanted but also one with both access to and support for coursework around the business of healthcare. In college, I had always envisioned going back home to UCSF, but life took me in a different direction. That girlfriend I moved in with became a fiancée, and with her family on the East Coast and the relative lack of business school access at UCSF, the University of Pennsylvania emerged as the ideal school for me.

I had also assumed that I was going to be an Orthopedic Surgeon prior to medical school – I still loved football and I was trying to think of a specialty that would keep me close to the game. However, I soon realized a few important lessons early in medical school (1) while spending time in the operating room was interesting to me, I could imagine being happy in a specialty that did not involve operating, (2) the job of an NFL team Orthopedist was not quite as glamorous as I had imagined, (3) the life of a surgeon is very hard on family (and I planned on starting one in residency), and (4) it would be very difficult to pursue significant administrative interests and work less than full time as a surgeon. As I was realizing all of this I discovered Emergency Medicine. From the start I was hooked – in contrast to the days when I was staring at the clock for my day to end, I would see hours fly by in the rush of a shift in the ED. I loved meeting people and getting the first shot at figuring out what was wrong. I loved being there for patients when they had nowhere else to go or no one else to care for them. Even the business of Emergency Medicine was inherently interesting to me – the logistics of running a busy ED was like a case study in operations. All the while I was discovering my interest in Emergency Medicine, I was continuing along the path toward broadening my understanding of the healthcare system. I took an internship as GlaxoSmithKline during the summer break between first and second years of medical school and applied to the Wharton MBA program at Penn.

> *"The MBA buys some degree of access and credibility, but the knowledge and experience gained through the education are what really opens doors and allow me to exceed expectations in my administrative roles."*

I thought hard about the timing of the MBA. I knew that I wanted the content and experience of the MBA but I was worried that I hadn't done enough at that point in my life to get the most out of the coursework. Also, I knew that a residency would follow, likely delaying most meaningful use of my MBA toolkit while also causing decay of one of the most useful perks of a top-tier MBA – my network. However, in retrospect I am grateful that I decided to move forward with the combined degree at that time. An MBA is a huge investment, both in terms of time and money. It is not a trivial thing to go back to school for 2 years after being in the workforce for some time. People often get locked into jobs and commitments, such as a mortgage and family, which are often enough to deter seeking this experience in mid-career, especially for a physician. As a result, many physicians seek executive MBAs and other part-time degrees. While these can also be valuable, I feel very fortunate to have a full-time Wharton MBA in my background, and I have no doubt that it has already benefited my career trajectory immensely. The MBA buys some degree of access and credibility, but the knowledge and experience gained through the education are what really opens doors and allows me to exceed expectations in my administrative roles.

At the end of my time at Penn I had an amazing experience with management consulting that almost derailed my future as a clinician. Spending a summer in the New Jersey office of McKinsey & Company was a revelation – I had never before been surrounded by so many smart, hardworking individuals in my life. The culture of under-promising and over-delivering, constant performance feedback and innovative thinking was intoxicating. I came surprisingly close to accepting a full-time offer to join them after graduation, but that desire for a connection with patients that originally drove me to pursue medical school was just too strong, so after graduating from Penn with Alpha Omega Alpha honors and an MD/MBA degree, I headed off to Boston for an Emergency Medicine residency at Brigham and Women's and Massachusetts General Hospitals.

My 4 years of residency was a blur – my wife and I had two children and I became an Emergency Physician. I tried very hard to maintain my B-school skill set and ended up publishing a paper looking at ED Observation patients through the lens of an options analysis. This was exactly what I was looking for – a direct application of tools from the business world in a healthcare environment. I finished residency in 2009 and stayed on the faculty at Brigham and Women's Hospital. There is tremendous synergy between my clinical practice and administrative roles in a large academic hospital environment. Drawbacks include overcoming resistance to change and navigating a very political workplace. My wife and I bought our first house last year in Wellesley, MA and we are very happy being quite busy working hard and raising our family. In terms of the long-term future from here, I like seeing patients too much to leave the practice of medicine, so working administratively in an academic medical center is a really nice fit with me for the foreseeable future.

Lessons Learned

- Don't spend the time and money for business school "just because it's there"; same goes for MD degree
- Physicians with MBA training tend to think about problems in a different way than others
- Never underestimate the power of networking
- Having an MBA on your resume may help you land an interview (with the right audience), but it's up to you to exhibit and communicate the MBA skill set
- You have to start making decisions that close opportunities and paths at some point in order to progress further down another

Mark A. Bloomberg, MD, MBA, FACPE

Dr. Mark A. Bloomberg is the Chief Medical Officer of HealthNEXT, a new company that works with self-funded employers to create a culture of health within their workplaces (Fig. 33.2). The chronology that has led him to this role is outlined above. In a career that began with the solo practice of general internal medicine, he found himself immersed health plan medical management when his local hospital medical staff asked him to lead a newly formed IPA. This led to his leaving practice to assume a major role with first a major regional health maintenance organization (Tufts) and years later with a major national preferred provider organization (PHCS). Following these positions, he created his own consultant practice focused on healthcare quality improvement. He increased his teaching commitments to include roles at Tufts University School of Medicine and Harvard School of Public Health. As a consequence of his consulting efforts, he was asked to lend his expertise first to a start-up company focused on electronic medical records and most recently to a new company which assists major employers in creating a culture of health within their locations with the intention of shaping a healthier workforce as a way to improve productivity and reduce healthcare expenditures.

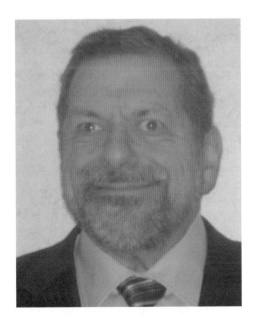

Fig. 33.2 Mark A. Bloomberg, MD, MBA, FACPE. Chief Medical Officer, HealthNEXT

Career Roadmap

- BA Boston University, 1970
- MD College of Medicine and Dentistry of New Jersey – Rutgers Medical School, 1974
- Internal Medicine Residency, Saint Elizabeth's Hospital of Boston, 1974–1977
- MBA Northeastern University, Boston, MA, 1990
- Private Practice, General Internal Medicine, Waltham, MA, 1977–1988
- Medical Director, West Suburban Health Plan, Waltham, MA, 1982–1987
- Corporate Medical Director, Tufts Associated Health Plans, Waltham, MA, 1987–1995
- Chief Medical Officer, Private Healthcare Systems, Inc. (PHCS), Waltham, MA, 1995–1998
- Associate Clinical Professor of Medicine, Tufts University School of Medicine, Boston, MA, 1988 – present
- Senior Physician Surveyor, National Committee for Quality Assurance, 1991 – present
- President and Consultant, The Bloomberg Healthcare Group, 1998 – present
- Adjunct Lecturer in Health Policy and Management, Harvard School of Public Health, 2004 – present
- Chief Medical Officer, WiFiMed, Inc., 2004–2009
- Chief Medical Officer, HealthNEXT, LLC, 2010 – present

Personal History

I was raised in Trenton, New Jersey and followed my sister to Boston University for my undergraduate training. I was focused on medicine and after receiving my BA in Biology returned to New Jersey and enjoyed the in-state tuition at Rutgers Medical School. My wife and I wanted to settle in New England and so I obtained my Internal Medicine training at Saint Elizabeth's Medical Center in Boston. Following my residency I started a solo practice in Waltham, a small city 10 miles west of Boston. The practice grew rapidly and as a member of the medical staff of Waltham Hospital was asked to chair the Quality Assurance/Utilization Management Committee. I found this responsibility to be challenging and rewarding, allowing me to work with my clinical peers to promote better medical decision-making. When the medical staff created an IPA to affiliate with Blue Cross Blue Shield of Massachusetts and accept HMO patients, I was asked to be the part-time medical director because of my QA/UM experience. Over the next 5 years the IPA grew rapidly and the increased work load (what had begun as a 5 h/week job had become 20 h/week) was creating a strain on my medical practice.

I was all set to step down from my role as IPA medical director and devote all of my time to medical practice when Tufts Associated Health Plan, a growing HMO in the Boston area, asked me to become their first full-time medical director. In what was probably the most difficult decision in my life, I decided to leave medical practice and take the position at Tufts. Once there, I was part of an eight person senior management team that guided the health plan through a period of rapid growth and program development. The HMO grew from 40,000 to 500,000 members during my tenure and I was responsible for developing the quality improvement program, including the effort to achieve National Committee for Quality Assurance (NCQA) accreditation. To assist in this goal I became an NCQA physician surveyor and began to survey HMOs across the country, an activity I continue to this day, 20 years later.

My success at Tufts led to my being recruited as the Chief Medical Officer (CMO) of Private Healthcare Systems, a national preferred provider organization with six-million enrollees where I was effectively the Chief Operating Officer of a $50 million business unit with 300 employees performing telephonic utilization management across the country. While there I spent 3 years fulfilling that role and found myself gradually coming to the conclusion that I was not enjoying the responsibility for overseeing a large national operation and was actually doing an inadequate job leading my portion of the company. This convinced me to leave PHCS and I formed my own business providing both teaching and consulting in the area of healthcare quality improvement. I began teaching a course each at Tufts University School of Medicine and Harvard School of Public Health and continued my work with NCQA. I also developed a course on managed care for the American College of Physician Executives, an organization I had been a member of since 1984. While filling a variety of consulting roles, I was asked to assist in the development of a new tablet-based electronic medical record and served as the CMO of WiFiMed which I supported for 5 years until it was merged into another company. Most recently I was asked to serve as CMO for HealthNEXT which assists large self-funded employers create a culture of health within their plants so as to increase worker productivity and reduce overall healthcare costs.

Along this 33-year journey, I have been the fortunate recipient of much mentoring and assistance from a wide variety of peers, supervisors, and business colleagues. It has been my experience that everyone with whom I came in contact had valuable lessons to teach me, if only I would be open to listening and learning. I have also found that it is very important to listen to that inner voice that informs you if you are enjoying the position you are in and the roles you are expected to play. Self-awareness, self-confidence, and strong personal values are the keys to professional success.

Lessons Learned

- Always treat others with the same courtesy and respect you expect of them
- Focus on what you can do for others and they will focus on what they can do for you

- Never allow yourself to be talked into taking actions you feel violate your personal values – you will always regret them
- Never stay in a position you are not enjoying – life is too short and your best career interests will not be fulfilled
- Look for opportunities to be mentored and pay that forward by mentoring others
- Never burn bridges or make enemies – you will inevitably meet them again
- Always network with as many professional colleagues as possible
- Don't be afraid to take risks – life's best lessons come from failure
- Build upon your clinical training and experience – you will likely become an "interface" professional and will need to translate both medicine and management to others

Spencer Borden, MD, MBA

Spencer Borden, MD, MBA, CPE, FAHCE, FACR, FAAP, FACPE, is Senior Managing Scientist at Exponent, a scientific and engineering consulting company, where he heads a new consulting practice in the pharmaceutical, biotech, and medical device sectors (Fig. 33.3). Exponent has over 600 consultants (over one half with doctorates) in over 90 scientific disciplines. Dr Borden was formerly director of employer outcomes research at Johnson and Johnson Healthcare Systems, Inc. J & J Healthcare Systems is a division of J & J that supports the 250 independent operating companies under the J & J umbrella. Borden develops workplace-based dem-

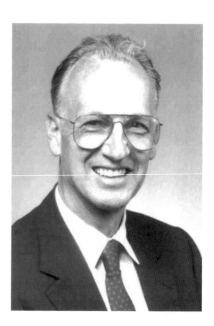

Fig. 33.3 Spencer Borden, MD, MBA. Senior Managing Scientist. Exponent, Inc.

onstration projects to show the value of J & J products and services for the employer market sector. Borden ran his own independent consulting company, Integrity Consulting, LLC, for 10 years and consulted with large employers, business coalitions on health, 13 major pharmaceutical firms, and three major biotechnology companies in areas of human capital management and health and productivity management. Previously, he was medical director at Aetna Life Insurance Company, MediQual Systems, Inc., and Value Health Sciences. He was Senior Medical Consultant for Watson Wyatt Worldwide, an employee benefit consulting company. He also spent 20 years in academic pediatric radiology, chairing the pediatric radiology departments at Massachusetts General Hospital and Children's Hospital of Philadelphia.

Career Roadmap

- Harvard College
- Dartmouth Medical School
- Harvard Medical School
- Boston Children's Hospital
- Massachusetts General Hospital
- US Air Force
- Children's Hospital of Philadelphia
- Wharton School, University of Pennsylvania
- Aetna Life Insurance Company
- MediQual Systems, Inc.
- Wyatt and Company
- Value Health Sciences
- Integrity Consulting, LLC
- Johnson & Johnson Healthcare Systems
- Exponent, Inc.

Personal History

I enrolled at Harvard College, wanting to be a physical anthropologist (archeologist). But the anthropology department was very weak in physical sciences, so I transferred my major to biology. I took a minor in fine arts. After college, I took organic chemistry in the summer semester, having avoided it all my undergraduate years. Married, I got a job in the Radiology Department of the Peter Bent Brigham Hospital in Boston, working under E. James Potchen, MD, then a resident in Radiology. Jim and I helped start the Nuclear Medicine Department at the Brigham. Jim later became Chair of Radiology at Michigan State University.

At the recommendation of Francis D. Moore, MD, the Surgeon-in-Chief at the Brigham, I submitted 15 applications to the most prestigious medical schools in the country. I got 13 rejections rather quickly. Finally, I was admitted to the College of Physicians and Surgeons at Columbia University, and sent them my $200 deposit. The prospect of living on 168th Street in New York City with my wife and 6-month-old daughter was not appealing to me. I had not yet heard back from Dartmouth Medical School, so I went to Hanover, and hung around the Medical School, talking to whoever would listen to me. Finally, they accepted me and I told Columbia to keep my $200, as I was going to Dartmouth. My wife, daughter, and I moved to a condo in Wilder, Vermont. Dartmouth was a 2 year school, majoring in laboratory medical sciences. It was a great class of 50 students, including about one half being women. My wife bore us a son at Dartmouth, and I transferred to Harvard Medical School for my third and fourth years of Medical School. At Harvard, I became acquainted with N. Thorne Griscom, MD, and E.B. D. Neuhauser, MD, the Chair of Radiology and Boston Children's Hospital. Both became role models for me and I selected Pediatric Radiology as my career choice.

I was selected for a Pediatric Internship by the Internship Match at Boston Children's Hospital. It was 1 year of 36 h on, and 12 h off, for a yearly stipend of $1,200. It was a huge amount of work, but I learned a lot and was very satisfied with my progress. I learned that I had no limits on the amount of work I could accomplish and that my first clinical instincts were almost always correct. My second daughter was born then.

After Children's, I moved to the Diagnostic Radiology residency at Massachusetts General Hospital, under the direction of Lawrence Robbins, MD, the Department Chairman. My interest in Pediatric Radiology became widely known, and I had many months of rotating through that section during the 3 years of residency. I started the Pediatric Radiology Teaching Collection, adding 5,000 cases there. I was named Teacher of the Year in the Department.

I took a year-long Chief Residency in Pediatric Radiology under Dr. Neuhauser at Children's, which was terrific fun and very stimulating. My timing was fortunate, as Dr. Neuhauser retired shortly thereafter.

Participating in the Berry Plan of the Armed Services, I had selected Radiology as my specialty and received a 4 year deferral to complete my Radiology training. So, I entered the US Air Force as a Major and was stationed at Malcolm Grow USAF Hospital in Washington, DC, as a staff member in the Radiology Department. The clinical workload was not challenging; I read 5 years of the Radiology, Pediatric, and Orthopedics journals literature. I saw the Saturday Night Massacre and the End of the Vietnam War during my 2 years there.

I returned to Mass General Hospital at Chief of Pediatric Radiology and grew the Pediatric Radiology Section in staff, cases, and Teaching Collection cases. I was Director of the Pediatric Radiology Section for 3 years.

I was recruited to be Radiologist-in-Chief at Children's Hospital of Philadelphia (CHOP) and Associate Professor of Radiology and Pediatrics at the University of Pennsylvania. The Radiology Department there was without a Chief for 4 years and was in disarray. I formulated a 5 year development project, adding Ultrasound and

Nuclear Medicine, new film viewers, library, and new staff. I completed this plan in 6 years, at a cost of $6 million.

In 1983, hospital admissions and length of stay were declining in all hospitals across the US. The general attribution was due to the implementation of prospective payment (DRGs) by Medicare. I correctly saw this as a power shift from providers (hospitals) to payors (Medicare and insurers). If payors could redefine provider services and recomputed how to pay for them, they have assumed control of the provider space. I saw the next logical target – physicians. In the end, my prediction came true, with the adoption of Resource Based Relative Value Scales for physician compensation. This disempowerment of physicians' trend is continuing up to the present.

Because of these seismic changes, I wanted to get in front of these trends and I enrolled in the Executive MBA program of the Wharton School at the University of Pennsylvania. I loved my classmates (55 of them from all walks of middle management), the curriculum content and the opportunities in the business side of healthcare. At the end of my first year, I notified the Dean of the University of Pennsylvania that I would be departing, after the installation of my successor.

After my successor was installed at CHOP, I took a job at Aetna Life Insurance Company in Hartford, CT. I was asked by Aetna to set up a Medical Technology Assessment Unit, so they could pay for medical and surgical services that were effective, and not pay for those that were not. This was a huge culture challenge for an indemnity insurance carrier, used to paying claims without clinical scrutiny. I proposed a five-person, $5 million per year Tech. Assessment Unit for them, which they turned down. Four years later, they recruited Bill McGivney, MD, from the AMA, to set up this very same unit I had proposed. Being ahead of the curve is as bad as not being on the curve at all.

I was recruited to MediQual Systems, Inc., in Westborough, MA. MediQual made a software program, called MedisGroups, which measured severity-adjusted morbidity and mortality rates of hospital care. It was my introduction to statistical quality control, as compared to inspection quality control at Aetna. The difference was profound. I worked in the Database Services Division and sold the need for MedisGroups at hospitals used by large employers and business coalitions on health, the customers of hospitals. At one time, we had state-wide legislative mandates to install MedisGroups in all the hospitals over 100 beds in Pennsylvania, Iowa, and Colorado. Only Pennsylvania is still using the system, and is still publishing their results through the Pennsylvania Healthcare Cost Containment Council (PHC4).

Through my friend, Jim Braun, I was recruited to be the Senior Medical Consultant at Wyatt and Company, an Employee Benefit Consulting Company. It later merged with Watson Consultants in the UK and finally with Towers Perrin, to become the current Towers Watson. I worked with consultants and actuaries on employee benefit strategies and benefit designs. I learned that my first customers were Wyatt consultants, and that they would introduce me to their clients and consulting projects. This tour of duty grounded me in my consulting career and gave me many of my consulting skills.

I joined Value Health Sciences (VHS) in Santa Monica, CA, as a virtual employee living in Concord, MA. They made software to precertify surgical procedures and to measure the clinical performance of physician groups (the Practice Review System – PRS). Pfizer was a 50% venture funder of these products. Since I was on the East Coast, I became the client lead contact with Pfizer and had ready access to their Headquarters on East 42nd Street in NYC. I worked with their field teams (Tactical Area Customer Units – TACUs), to deploy our software to hospitals, health plans and physician groups. At the same time, I assisted Pfizer in starting up their Employer Unit, to market their products to employers. Pfizer liked my work with them so much that they offered to be my first client, if I were to start my own consulting company. Given that strong stimulus, I did form my own consulting company.

I named my firm Integrity Consulting, LLC., using the name to depict my values. I expanded my work with Pfizer, later engaging 13 other pharmaceutical and biotechnology companies on developing their approach to the Employer Marketplace. I worked closely with John Herrick of Schering-Plough for over 7 years.

I was recruited by Rick Heine of Johnson & Johnson Healthcare Systems, Inc. to join the Employer Team, which was then forming. I was Director of Employer Outcomes Research for the Employer Team. I performed four Outcomes Research studies and helped write a 100 page manual on how to perform an Employer-Based Outcomes Research Study, which was widely circulated in J&J.

An executive recruiter introduced me to Exponent, Inc. Exponent is a scientific consulting company, with over 600 consultants in 90 different disciplines. Over half of the consultants have a doctorate in their specialty. I became their Senior Managing Scientist in the Health Sciences Practice. I marketed their consulting services into the pharmaceutical, biotechnology, and medical device segments, using my extensive contacts there.

I have had many opportunities for personal development and I have seized them. I learned that I am an avid risk-taker. My high school, Milton Academy, did not have a crew team. When I enrolled at Harvard College, my classmate, Nick Bancroft, and I tried out for the crew team. Nick's father and grandfather were each Harvard Crew Captains, so rowing was in his pedigree. No one in my family was an oarsman. So, we both learned how to row in our freshman year, each making the Freshman Team by the time of the Yale Race (which we won). We made the Harvard Varsity Crew in our sophomore, junior and senior years, with Nick in the No. 2 seat and I rowed both No. 5 and 7 on the starboard side. We beat Yale by 7 lengths in our sophomore and senior years, but lost to them by 1/4 length in our junior year. I had grown one inch in college (to 6 ft. 5 in.) and grew 20 lb of muscle to 195 lb. My growth in teamwork and hard work was equally great. Rowing was the high point of my college years.

> *"Clinical work fixes one patient at a time. Medical Management work fixes many patients and the system that serves them."*

One week after the Yale Race in my senior year, I married my sister-in-law. My older sister had married her older brother 8 years earlier. I loved being married, working in a hospital, and having children at an early age. I had three children before the end of my Internship year. My children and my sister's children are all double first-cousins, and share the same four grandparents. Being a spouse, a parent, and a dedicated student in Medical School, Internship and Residency training, was the equal of three full-time jobs. In retrospect, I did the latter two better than the former. I got a divorce after 17 years of marriage.

My colleagues in Academic Pediatric Radiology thought I was crazy to enroll in the Executive MBA Program at the Wharton School of the University of Pennsylvania. My executive, legal, accounting, and management friends thought it was a brilliant move. They were right. I was entirely ready to explore Healthcare Business, after 20 years in Academic Medicine. I never looked back.

I did join and make many contributions to Professional Societies over the years. I was elected to Fellowship Status in the American College of Radiology, the American Academy of Pediatrics, the American College of Healthcare Executives, the American College of Medical Quality and the Center for Health Value Innovation. I achieved Distinguished Fellowship Status at the American College of Physician Executives, and currently serve as a Director on the Board of Directors of the American College of Physician Executives.

Lessons Learned

- Build a large network of business friends. They are your colleagues, your fans, your potential recruits, and people to console you and encourage you. Your friends can be the source of potential new jobs and business challenges. They can share their triumphs and tragedies with you, and rely on your listening and strength.
- Take risks. Accept a new job or project in an area in which you have incomplete knowledge. Smart people can succeed in any location. Eagerness to learn is the prerequisite. Apply your enthusiasm, intellect, and energy, and you will succeed. Search for a mentor. Mentors can teach you, encourage you, show you the potential traps, and serve as a role model for your development.

Maria Young Chandler, MD, MBA

Maria Young Chandler, MD, MBA launched the MD/MBA joint degree program at the University of California, Irvine (UCI) in 1997 enabling medical students to obtain both their business and medical degrees simultaneously (Fig. 33.4). The mission of the program is, *to train a select group of physicians in the aspects of business who will lead our community and the healthcare industry toward a solution to the incredible challenge we are faced with of providing patients with quality care that is financially and ethically responsible.* She believes wholeheartedly that physicians

Fig. 33.4 Maria Young
Chandler, MD, MBA. MD/
MBA Program Director, UC
Irvine. Chief Medical Officer,
The Children's Clinic.
President, Association of
MD/MBA Programs

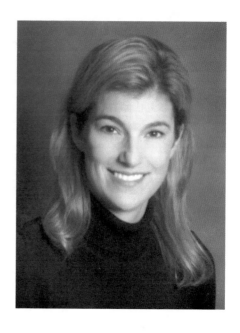

of the future need business skills to be better leaders as well team members. After
obtaining an MBA herself to improve her administrative skills, in 1997 she accepted
the task of establishing a dual degree program at UCI. Many national organizations
were publicizing the leadership roles of physicians and the business skills they
require which aren't offered in traditional medical curriculum. For example, The
Association of American Medical Colleges stated (4/97) that future physicians must
"acquire leadership skills," be able to "analyze financial data," and "negotiate contracts." According to Hospitals & Health Networks (8/97), physicians held leadership positions in more than 50% of the cases in hospitals, managed care settings,
and group practices. Dr. Chandler's larger ambitions led her to establish the
Association of MD/MBA Programs, and spearhead UCI in hosting the first annual
conference in 2003. She has since cohosted every conference at Jefferson, Emory,
Dartmouth, Baylor, Washington, DC, Wright State, and Boston University. This
group has initiated many projects such as tracking the residency choices and career
paths of MD/MBA graduates nationally. Dr. Chandler has also coauthored an article
with Yale colleagues entitled, *MD/MBA Programs in the United States: Evidence of
a Change in Healthcare Leadership* (Academic Medicine 2003). At that time there
were few programs nationally. By 2010 there were over 65 programs at the 130
medical schools. UCI's program continues to be one of the most well established
and largest programs accepting 15% of each entering class. UCI MD/MBA students
are aspiring to fields in healthcare such as policy, administration, academics, information technology, biotechnology, and entrepreneurial adventures. She is one
of only two physicians at UCI who holds dual appointments at both the schools of
Business and Medicine. Dr. Chandler also serves as the Chief Medical Officer of
The Children's Clinic, a six site nonprofit federally qualified health center based at

Long Beach Memorial Medical Center/Miller Children's Hospital in Long Beach and an affiliate teaching institution of UCI. She has been employed there since the completion of her residency in 1992. The Clinic has been in existence for over 70 years and in 2010 provided well over 70,000 patient visits. Dr. Chandler earned her BS and MD degrees as well as completed her pediatric residency training at the University of California, Irvine. She received her MBA degree from Pepperdine University. She is board certified in Pediatrics and is a Fellow of the American Academy of Pediatrics.

Career Roadmap

- BS UCI
- MD UCI
- Pediatric Residency UCI
- MBA Pepperdine University
- MD/MBA Program Director, UCI
- Chief Medical Officer, The Children's Clinic
- President/Founder, Association of MD/MBA Programs

"I slept and dreamt that life was joy. I awoke and saw that life was service. I acted and behold, service was joy
(Rabindranath Tagore (born 1861))."

Personal History

My parents headed west with me when I was 6 months old on route 66 from Kentucky until they reached the beach for my father to be a resident at UCLA. He finished a child psychiatry fellowship at Cedars-Sinai and bestowed on me his love and appreciation for children. I wanted to experience that joy and had decided to become a doctor by the time I was 9 years old. When my grandmother told me that I should "marry a doctor," I said I was going to BE a doctor. She had gone to college, as had her mother in the early 1900s. She had a long career in finance which she shared with me when I stopped to see her every day on my way home from grammar school. My family had moved to Orange County with her and my new brother. I went on to be a cheerleader, Harbor Princess, tennis player, and valedictorian ALWAYS keeping my most important goal in mind, to be a doctor. During my senior year of high school, my father took me to an informational session at UCI. He sat me next to a colleague who I informed of my plan to attend there just before he was introduced as the Dean of the medical school.

I felt fortunate to have Dean Stanley van den Noort, a distinguished neurologist as a role model through my undergrad, medical school, pediatric residency, and faculty member before his final days last year. During my residency, I rotated through an affiliated nonprofit community health center, *The Children's Clinic*, and I knew I had found my new home. I was unaware of these wonderful organizations that serve those in need. I started there directly after residency working 6 days/week, taking night call, and rounding on weekends. I loved teaching residents and medical students; however, I wasn't done searching for new knowledge. When my mom sent me an article entitled, "MDs getting MBAs" after 2 years of work, I knew it was the direction I needed to take. I was fortunate that the Clinic's CEO was a physician with a dual degree and supported my plan to further my education. I enrolled in a night program at Pepperdine University because they would allow me to take 4 years to obtain my MBA degree. I felt it was necessary for me to feel comfortable at the table with business leaders. I used the new information I learned on the job and I quickly realized its value. The teaching style was new to me, a team approach, asking others for input rather than taking tests and giving orders alone. I understood how important the training was in order to develop my own cohesive style. It was a good lesson and early enough in my career to help me be more effective. I found you must know enough about yourself to bring the best out of others and that more minds ARE better than one. Since finishing my MBA, I became Medical Director of the Clinic and eventually Chief Medical Officer. I sent a letter to the medical school Dean at UCI offering my guidance to others contemplating an MBA degree. He sent a letter back asking if I would help realize their dream to start an MD/MBA dual degree program, and we did. I continued to grow the program, coauthored an article, hosted the first annual conference, and founded the national Association of MD/MBA Programs. I reap such reward from mentoring these students on projects which show so much insight so early in their career such as "Optimizing Patient Flow in a Comprehensive Gastroenterology Center: An Efficiency Analysis," and "Assessing the Market and Feasibility of a University Medical Simulation Center" which served as the basis for our new Center which opened earlier this year. I have many to whom I owe thanks. Besides my father always encouraging me to strive for more and my mother being my rock, along the way I encountered important mentors. First is the CEO of the Clinic, Elisa Nicholas, MD, MSPH, who has been a wonderful partner and friend for 20 years with the vision of "growing healthier communities." Second is Dr. Alberto Manetta who had the dream of starting an MD/MBA program. Third is Roger Schenke, founder of the American College of Physician Executives (ACPE), who in the 1970s believed physicians make great leaders. He recognized our Association as an "academic" version of his and was the instigator of our nonprofit incorporation. I feel fortunate to have found a way to affect healthcare on a national level and continued my first passion of caring for children. From the 4 year old who compliments me on my necklace to the teen who offers that she'll put extensions in my hair, to the mother who says she considers me a sister, my heart is full.

Lessons Learned

- Recognize successful partnerships you have and maximize them (*Working Together by* Michael Eisner, past CEO of Disney).
- Read the books your mentors recommend to you. Mine were *True North* by Bill George, past CEO Medtronics and professor Harvard Business School, it helps me remember to be true to myself; and, *Kitchen Table Wisdom* by Dr. Rachel Naomi Remen, it helps me remember to stay true to my patients and have empathy.
- Reach out to those who inspire you and you'll be surprised what you'll get back.
- Be open to learn from others no matter how small the pearl.
- Emulate the traits of those who you admire most.
- Remember that an MD degree doesn't make you good in business or people skills; both take hard work and knowledge.
- Stay humble, "Be happy" (I refer you to the work of Sonja Lyubomirsky, PhD, Stanford University).
- Affect change in as big a way as possible.
- Treat your life as seriously as you would your own company ("We are CEOs of our own companies: Me, Inc," *The Brand Called You*, 1997 by Tom Peters).

Joseph S. Fastow, MD, MPH

Joseph S. Fastow, MD, MPH was born in Philadelphia, Pennsylvania and he received his BA in Biological Sciences from Rutgers University, his MD from Boston University School of Medicine and his MPH from The Johns Hopkins University Bloomberg School of Public Health as a Robert Wood Johnson Foundation Clinical Scholar (Fig. 33.5). Dr. Fastow was one of the first residents in the emergency medicine residency at The Johns Hopkins Hospital. He is board certified in emergency

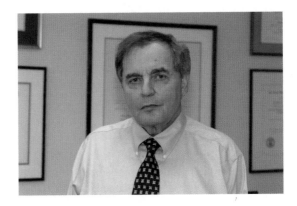

Fig. 33.5 Joseph S. Fastow, MD, MPH. President. Physician Management, Ltd.

medicine and a Fellow in the American College of Emergency Physicians. He founded Physician Management, Ltd. in 1975 and has operated contracts for professional services in emergency medicine, urgent care, internal medicine and pediatric hospitalist, and intensivist and house coverage at more than a quarter of the hospitals in Maryland as well as hospitals in surrounding states.

In addition to his clinical and administrative responsibilities, Dr. Fastow has held many leadership positions during his 35-year professional career. These include Chairman of Council and Chairman of the Executive Committee of the Medical and Chirurgical Faculty of Maryland (Maryland State Medical Society), President of the Maryland Chapter of the American College of Emergency Physicians, President of the Calvert County Medical Society, and Director of Emergency Services at Calvert Memorial Hospital. He has held clinical faculty positions at The Johns Hopkins School of Medicine, Georgetown University School of Medicine, and is currently a Senior Associate in the Department of Health Policy and Management at the Johns Hopkins Bloomberg School of Public Health. Dr. Fastow has had numerous publications in professional journals on topics related to emergency medicine and medical malpractice as well as numerous local and national presentations on medical liability in emergency medicine, the business of medicine from the emergency medicine perspective, and entrepreneurship in medicine.

Career Roadmap

- Rutgers University
- Boston University School of Medicine
- Pennsylvania Hospital
- Bureau of Radiological Health and NIH
- George Washington University Hospital
- Johns Hopkins Hospital
- Johns Hopkins School of Public Health
- Physician Management, Ltd.

Personal History

Growing up in a small town in New Jersey, I was always a science fan and the study of medicine fascinated me. I majored in biology at Rutgers and when it came time to decide on a medical school, I chose Boston University because I wanted a small school and BU was the second smallest medical school in the country.

I was not sure what specialty I wanted to pursue when I graduated, but internal medicine seemed to have the broadest exposure to patient care. I completed a straight medical internship at Pennsylvania Hospital in Philadelphia and spent the following

2 years doing various projects with the Public Health Service at the Bureau of Radiological Health and the NIH in Bethesda, MD. These were critical years for me because they afforded me the opportunity to take stock of my career priorities and goals. In 1972, a cardiologist friend mentioned that his hospital had agreed to fund night and weekend coverage for their CCU because the fulltime cardiologists lived more than 30 min from the hospital. Seeing a business opportunity to provide physician services to hospitals, I began calling cardiology fellows in the Baltimore-Washington metropolitan area. When I had a critical mass, I contacted the hospital and wrote my first contract.

> *"Listening is an art. You learn very little with your mouth open."*

After my internship, I concluded that internal medicine was not for me. I started an anesthesiology residency at George Washington University Hospital, thinking that I wanted to be an intensivist. When an emergency medicine residency was begun at Johns Hopkins Hospital, I applied and began the residency in 1974. I felt that the spontaneity of emergency medicine was a better fit for me than the regimentation required of anesthesia, and the flexibility of shift work allowed me to be a clinician and a contractor of physician services at the same time. I was fortunate to be offered a Robert Wood Johnson Foundation Clinical Scholarship at Hopkins which enabled me to complete an MPH program at the Johns Hopkins School of Public Health. By 1975, my wife, Ellen and I had formed Physician Management to operate hospital physician contracts in Maryland, Virginia and New Jersey. For the past 35 years, Physician Management has operated contracts for the provision of emergency medicine, internal medicine, pediatric, hospitalist, intensivist, and urgent care services. Until very recently, contracting for physician services to hospitals had not changed significantly over the years. You required the ability to recruit quality physicians by specialty, the resources to document, code and bill for large numbers of inpatient encounters and the business acumen to operate efficiently, negotiate effectively, and retain the trust of hospital administrators and your physicians. That has not changed. However, the environment of hospital medicine has changed dramatically with the passage of major healthcare reform legislation. It has focused attention on the deficiencies in the fee-for-service model, especially in hospitals. The bundling of hospital and physician services is on the horizon. In the future we expect more requests from hospitals to locate physician practice leaders and strong clinicians to be hospital employees, and fewer requests to manage entire programs. Hospital-based physicians will view themselves more as part of a hospital team than as independent vendors of services. As with any major change, opportunities will abound to innovate in association with, or within a hospital network. Quality has always been the gold standard between contracting hospitals and hospital-based physicians. Healthcare reform mandates efficiency as well as quality to stem the unsustainable escalation in healthcare cost. It represents the challenge of a lifetime for hospitals and physicians alike.

Lessons Learned

- Listening is an art. You learn very little with your mouth open.
- The most challenging part of any enterprise is managing people. If you have a knack for it, cultivate it. If not, hire someone who does.
- In business, partnership is the equivalent of a marriage. Enter into it only after a sober analysis of advantages and disadvantages. Divorce is disruptive, expensive, and often leads to the demise of the enterprise.
- Being a clinician and an entrepreneur is a balancing act. Choose your specialty with your entrepreneurship in mind. Shift work is preferred because it gives you control of your time.

Jonathan P. Gertler, MD, MBA

Dr. Jonathan P. Gertler is one of two Founding and Senior Partners at Back Bay Life Science Advisors a boutique strategic advisory firm based in Boston serving the United States CANADA and an international clientele (Fig. 33.6). BACK BAY'S services and capabilities range from innovation management and strategies, initial due diligence, market, and opportunity assessment through life cycle management, commercial and technology development strategies including transactional preparation, and corporate and business development growth and transformational. BACK BAY'S capabilities encompass small and large company needs and also serve to help academic and technical institutions optimize strategies for commercialization of promising technologies.

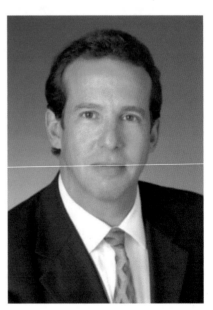

Fig. 33.6 Jonathan P. Gertler, MD, MBA. Senior Partner. Back Bay Life Science Advisors

Prior to founding BBLSA, Dr Gertler served as Senior Partner and Managing Director, Leerink Swann Strategic Advisors where he advised emerging growth and mid- and large cap Pharma, Biotech, and Medical Device companies on similar strategic issues. In addition, since leaving academia in 2001, Dr. Gertler has led several investment banking groups: BioPharma Investment Banking at Leerink Swann and Health Pennsylvania Hospital.

Care Investment Banking at Adams Harkness/Canaccord Adams. He has been responsible for >$4.5 B aggregate consideration in M&A and equity issuances since beginning his investment banking career in 2001.

From 1988–2001, after training at Columbia University (MD), Yale New Haven Hospital (General Surgery) and the Massachusetts General Hospital (Vascular Surgery), Dr Gertler was a practicing academic Vascular Surgeon, first as Chief of Vascular Surgery at SUNY-HSCB in New York from 1988 to 2002 and subsequently at the Massachusetts General Hospital (MGH) from 1992 to 2001. He was Associate Professor of Surgery at Harvard Medical School (HMS) and Codirector of the Vascular Research and Diagnostic Laboratories at the MGH. He has published more than 125 peer reviewed articles, chapters, and abstracts in clinical vascular surgery and endothelial and smooth muscle cell biology and retains an appointment at the Health Science and Technology program as well as the Department of Mechanical Engineering at MIT He has served as an ad-Hoc editor for the Journal of Vascular Surgery, The New England Journal of Medicine, The Journal of Critical Care Medicine, and Surgery among others. From 1986 to 1987, following general surgery training but prior to his vascular fellowship he served as Instructor in Surgery at Yale Medical School and Director of the Surgical Intensive Care Unit at Yale New Haven Hospital.

During the latter stages of his full-time academic career, Dr Gertler was a Venture Partner from 1998 to 2001 for Schroder Ventures, now SV Life Sciences, where he was part of the Medical Device Investment Team with active involvement in five of the Fund's investments. In addition, in 1998 he founded CardioVascular Technologies, an endovascular start-up in the area of embolic entrapment based on one of his inventions. The company was successfully sold in a stock deal to Embolic Protection Inc in 2000 which was subsequently acquired in 2001 by Boston Scientific for $75MM plus an addition undisclosed multiple earn out.

Dr. Gertler is a frequent lecturer and speaker on strategic issues facing life science companies at all stages and continues to publish in this regard.

He currently serves on the external advisory boards of the Petit Institute for Bioengineering at Georgia Tech and Boston University School of Medicine's Dean's Advisory Board.

Dr. Gertler has a BA from Wesleyan University, an MD from Columbia University College of Physicians and Surgeons, and an MBA in Health Policy and Management from Boston University. He is a Fellow of the American College of Surgeons and a member of numerous academic and clinical surgical societies.

Career Roadmap

- Wesleyan University (BA)
- Columbia University (MD)
- Yale New Haven Hospital
- Massachusetts General Hospital
- SUNY-HSCB
- Harvard Medical School
- Boston University School of Management

Personal History

In 2010, A Partner and I started a new strategy consulting firm to finally synthesize what I had learned in my medical and business life. Entrepreneurship is bimodal – young and slightly reckless, full of faith in oneself, and able to withstand the downturn because couch surfing remains a possibility. And then there are those of us who retain that somewhat youthful exuberance but at the same time need to create a unique workplace. I'm there after 20 + years in medicine and 10 in business. My plans had been to be an academic oncologist. Enamored, I thought, of basic research and having been pushed (not so gently) into a medical career by family values and deep expectations, it seemed a logical choice. That changed my first day of clinical clerkships – I was getting surgery out of the way. A NY cop came in shot and dead. I witnessed his resurrection – a female (!) cardiac surgery fellow (this was 1979 – not a lot of them around) cracked his chest, clamped his pulmonary artery, and we ran to the OR, my trembling hands eased into gloves by an old male army nurse who told me to calm down and just help out. I spent the next 3 hours water skiing on the end of an "egg beater" (a lung retractor), while Kathy McNicholas whipped out his lung and anesthesia resuscitated him. He lived. The next day I saw him writhing in bed, swollen, unresponsive, ventilated in the ICU. The next day I saw him sitting up about to extubated. The ICU nurse, in an extraordinary act of kindness, introduced me as "Dr Gertler, one of the doctors who operated on you" He squeezed my hand, looked me in the eye, nodded thank you. And I was gone. Forever hooked. Nothing else I ever wanted to do just surgery.

> *"The privilege in synthesizing the scientific, clinical, cultural, policy and economic underpinnings of life science businesses is the critical contribution of the physician business leader and affords a rare opportunity to have broad impact while still staying close to the intellectual and social attributes that medicine provides."*

I spent the next 3 weeks talking to the (I will leave out his last name but if ever he is reading this and recognizes the story I hope he finds me) about what it was like to die. I learned about how he couldn't go back to police work because he would not have any discipline left in his self protection and would thus be dangerous to the community. (Years later, while on trauma duty as a young assistant professor, another cop told me of a man who had grabbed his gun, pointed it at him and misfired it next to his temple. The cop brought down his nightstick, disarmed, and cuffed the guy and never thought about anything more. Told me that was job, not to get so angry that he kills someone and ruins his own life and others around him. I understood finally what an first mutant meant. Anything more would have ruined more lives). And so I longed to become a surgeon. And I did.

I had the privilege of training at Yale where I learned humanity from the surgical staff, a love of the craft of surgery and the marriage of science to the clinical arts, a love of personal balance, and the continuity of great thoughts in and out of the OR; a deep and still persistent love of helping people through crisis. (See below!) We had world famous writers on our staff (not necessarily the best of the surgeons) and a faculty who loved the venerable institution of Yale for its exposure to all. I left after 6 years as a bundle of academic ambition (a young man's disease as one of my older Yale mentors told me) and then got to go to the than bigger leagues at the MGH for some further training.

And when all was said and done, I went back to NY as Chief of Vascular Surgery at SUNY – Downstate. The belly of the beast if ever there was one. I had cracked my own chests by that time (though the first time I had done so and saved a stabbed young man's life his sister berated me for the lack of peri-crack-chest antibiotics). She was a pharmacist. Let me rephrase. She was an abusive pharmacist. I was a heroic and then deflated third year resident. My Chief Resident, who had come in after the heart was restored, said kindly "I'm so sorry" when he heard that I wasn't treated with adoring appreciation and I quickly had learned that one practices medicine always at risk for being unappreciated but always exposed to some of the greatest events a person can experience.

Downstate was dangerous, gritty, loaded with inequities and poor equipment, and patients in those days died there due to poor care and poor conditions. I would sleep in the hospital by the bedside of my thoracoabdominal aneurysm patients for 2 or 3 days and gradually built a strong service. But when NY was overwhelming and I was tired of the fear and the impossible conditions, the MGH called and I returned.

Over the next 9 years I had a wonderful career. Out publishing, growing in the national societies, and surrounded by bright people and challenges. But also stymied by the hierarchy, stymied by private practice masquerading as academia. One enabling event, years before I ever contemplating leaving medicine, was striking. The NIH had out an RFP for vascular disease center grant – one per institution, salary support, and the chance to move vascular surgery to the next level. We were on the cusp of the endovascular revolution, the biology of vascular disease was emerging at great pace and the MGH was eligible for the award. I worked for months – united neurologists, cardiologists, lipidologists, vascular interventionalists, and, I thought, my colleagues into a web of multidisciplinary excellence – at least on paper. I had been down to the NIH several times to vet the ideas. They loved it I was told.

On a Friday before the Tuesday when the grant was due, – everything written, packaged, and ready to go, my department chairman called to say that a competing grant had surfaced from the Department of Medicine and that since it was only one submission per institution, mine would have to be reviewed against his by the research affairs committee. I was an Assistant Professor, he was a Full Professor. I had spent months with what I thought was full institutional support. I was later told that his was written at the last minute. And I was also told that the institution wasn't ready for a multidisciplinary approach to what had long been a specific silo and specialty dominated disease. Although one day I was assured it would make sense, it just wasn't the time. I brushed it off and went back to work. But I would never accept that or let that happen today.

Needless to say, I lost the review. The other grant went in to the NIH and didn't make it past the first cut. Triaged out, as they say in the parlance of NIH study sections. And I learned something very sad about the world of medicine. The currency differs, but human nature is the same.

I worked happy and interested and motivated. And that never changed or changes.

In 1996/1997, getting close to the stage of chiefship or chairmanship I decided to get an MBA in Health Policy and Management. I figured that any leader in Medicine should be able to go toe to toe with any consultant, any manager, or any guy or gal who spouted discounted cash flows and NPV's as criteria for medical policy decisions. My MBA was discouraged – just do your cases and publish your papers I was told. But I was also stubborn and a surgeon (often wrong, never in doubt) and I completed the MBA with interest in my "spare time". Plus the MGH was crawling with consultants and newly minted administrators replete with clipboards and jargon – some were my fellow MD's, some RN's, and some MBA's. I truly believed then, as I still do, that one deeply steeped in medicine with the operational experience of business can have a huge positive impact on the way all aspects of medicine develop – whether technology innovation or improved access to care.

And then other things began to happen. Carotid angioplasty was becoming a hot topic. It occurred to me that there was no way that balloons should be shoved into the carotid system without the care and precautions we took during carotid endarterectomy. And so, with an MIT colleague, I invented an embolic entrapment device. Made every mistake in the book starting the company – the wrong angel investors, the wrong prototypers, and no regulatory knowledge – you name it. But our IP was robust, and as I was learning a little of the venture game, we managed to get a stake in what turned out to be a highly successful company developing a competitive device by selling our IP to them. We did far worse than we could have and far better than we deserved. But it was a remarkable experience. And for the record, my colleague was and is one of my closest friends. I still have the contract we hand wrote to each other that stated that the minute our economic venture impacted our friendship we would shut it down. And we would have in a heartbeat.

And then a venture group came calling as well. I joined what was then Schroder Ventures as consultant and then a venture partner while still going full bore at the MGH. It was a young group and there was a lot of maneuvering by the younger Partners and Principles and clueless doesn't do justice to my lack of knowledge – not only of the business and venture world but of the way peopled worked and managed their ambitions. It was a fascinating experience, a great trajectory of learning both by example and by involvement and I am forever grateful for that as I am for all that preceded it.

In 2001, my long suffering otolaryngologist wife finally thought to tell me that a ratio of two jobs per child (I have three sons) wasn't a great way to spend our life. I loved surgery, I loved research, I loved teaching, I loved invention, I loved venture finance, and I loved entrepreneurship.

And I love my wife and children. It was time to choose.

I had offers within academia that were extremely compelling. I had offers from venture groups. And I had an offer to become an investment banker and head of medtech banking at a local but nationally positioned firm. What does an investment banker do I asked? My friend who was recruiting me, head of banking at the firm, and an ex surgeon himself replied "I'll teach you." But I have no idea what that means or what to do I replied. I'll teach you, he assured me again and with a very rewarding offer in hand as well as the chance to build knowledge in areas I didn't have – the public markets, M&A, corporate finance – the economic tools of reducing science to practice as well as establishing my own independent judgment and network, I took a leave of absence from Harvard and gave it a shot. I have never looked back

My first 5 years in Investment Banking were a great ride. My firm was nontraditional. I wasn't beholden to sales, trading, and research analysts. Rather I could find the companies I wanted to work with, do my own diligence, and advise them transactionally. I was learning on a colossally steep curve and somehow managing to stay out of trouble. It was venture capital with transactional rather than investment revenue – just a different model. After my first major deal closed for a novel endovascular company I was supporting, a very successful deal, my chairman of banking said to me "it's a good thing you don't know what the **** you are doing because you never if you did, would have taken that chance". I had colleagues with integrity and a love of new technology. And I had an enormously rewarding time getting to know other professionals, learning a whole new field, and being part of an entrepreneurial banking culture. I was rapidly promoted to Managing Director and Head of the Healthcare practice and had wonderful success. I was unfettered in my leadership and recruited a diverse group of intelligent and ethical people. New technology development is also fascinating – and though I believe that access to basic care is unbelievably and probably more important – I was just suited to that side of the equation. And for reasons I will explain, I am forever indebted to biotech as well.

My firm sold after my sixth year there. The buyers were real bankers – tough, venal, corporate guys who instituted review processes, revenue targets, hierarchies, and a love for things in life I didn't really appreciate –hard drinking, taking clients to strip clubs, entertainment over intellect as a way to win business.

I was miserable.

I thought it was the new firm. But 3 years and more leadership investment banking roles in other firms later I realized that investment banking had become a bit of a commodity in general – and that it was taking me far away from the things I loved. Medicine still meant and means the world to me. I care about patient advances. I am a geek for science and thoughtful technology. But by then, as opposed to my old days as an undisciplined and unschooled young actor in the venture game, I realized and practiced the critical aspects of business discipline and knew, that without a reasonable funding, regulatory, and commercial plan, the most valuable invention will die on the vine, choked by the poor planning of the entrepreneur or responsible company rather than fed by the discipline of thoughtful development and business people. Better is the enemy of good.

One of my managing types, whom I like as person but couldn't adhere to as a manager (my fault, not his, I am unmanageable) told me that all one needed to control investment bankers was greed and fear. And although certain things in life make me afraid – my children's and wife's safety, the world deterioration politically – I had spent my days cross clamping falling apart aortas and I didn't think money was the definition of self. So, I asked him, how can you manage me when nothing particularly scares me and I'm not greedy? Needless to say I quit investment banking shortly thereafter.

There was another driver. In 2008, my wife was diagnosed with a bad breast cancer, triple negative, probably lymph node spread. She spent the year in chemotherapy, radiation, and surgery and has fallen into the category of those rare few with triple negative with a complete response and thus a wonderful prognosis. It brought me back to the wonder of medicine and made me ever thankful for those targeted therapeutics and novel chemotherapeutic agents that were funded by my financial world but more importantly developed by my scientific and medical world. I was struggling to be the banker I thought I should be – driven by vision and thought rather than transactional performance metrics.

Not a chance that could work in this day and age.

So within my same firm, I moved to the consulting side. It wasn't intellectually different than what I had always done before I was asked to be a commodity transactionally driven investment banker. But the business model was different. It rewarded me real-time for contributions to a company's growth. It allowed me to have an impact on those companies that were developing technologies of meaning. And I needed a way to support my family while I figured out my path forward.

Suddenly I was spending weeks in-depth on projects working through the intersection between clinical need, scientific merit, regulatory milestones, commercial applicability, adoption hurdles, and funding mechanisms. It was the marriage of everything I had ever studied.

I was thinking again.

I was reducing my experience of the last 12 years to helping companies survive and even thrive and, just like the feeling of a great case completed, I felt that it wasn't fact and execution but judgment and insight that carried the day. I loved it. And then I knew I had to do it in my way with hand chosen people who valued the same things.

For whom reward went well beyond the end of the year bonus and who wanted to pull together to contribute something. I needed to create the right platform.

In May 2010 we launched our new firm. In less than a year we have grown extensively, have numerous fascinating strategic assignments with big and small companies alike and have novel business models that include venture returns on the right companies, transactional interplay and honest, non-transactionally driven, data-dependent analyses. We are working across the value chain of early discovery to life cycle management. Our structure is flat, our profits are shared, we mentor commercial people toward the commercial side of our practice while teaching them the science, and we nurture scientists and consultants to understand the transactional and investment worlds that drive growth of companies. Our dogs come to work, we dress up when we need to and dress down when we can. A Wharton applicant for a job in our firm told me it was the closest thing he's seen to a California start-up except that we were wildly busy and profitable ahead of the game. And I am back to being steeped in science, driven by reality, intellectually honest and intolerant of the wrong ethics in my work place.

Lucky me.

> *"It is the clinical and scientific years beyond the degree itself that enable these insights. Balancing time in grade in medicine against gaining primary business experience is a highly individual choice."*

Lessons Learned

So what lessons can I add? Let me review what the mistakes are that science/medical types make and what mistakes financial types make and hopefully create a series of identified pitfalls. Good judgment comes from experience which comes from bad judgment. So you can be assured that these pearls of wisdom – or are they just shiny fecaliths? – aren't theoretical.

- Doctor negatives
  - Medical omniscience for all technologies doesn't exist
  - Technology savvy does not equal business sense
  - Sesquipedalian pontificators (doctors and others who use big words) aren't necessarily clear thinkers
  - Being expert in one area does not render you the smartest person in the room
  - Don't act like the smartest person in the room
  - There is no substitute for 10,000 hours regardless of whether one is dissecting the aorta or dissecting a business plan
  - Listening is a huge skill
  - Your hierarchical powers disappear at the door of your new office
  - So should your ego

- Healthcare Finance Types negatives

  - Business sense without clear technology or systems understanding puts you at a huge disadvantage in creating asymmetric opportunities
  - The game is not just about returning capital in the absence of clinical utility and quality improvements
  - Capital return doesn't occur in the absence of clinical utility and quality improvements
  - Leveraging other people's skill sets without cross functional learning ultimately hurts your business in the long run.
  - That is, don't pigeonhole clinical/scientists
  - Allowing for failure, allowing for risk, needs to be ingrained in the culture
  - Money is not the only reward people seek
  - Healthcare businesses require measurable outcomes in patient care to be justifiable and sustainable

- Pitfalls for MD's in Business

  - Paying too little attention to the nuts and bolts of finance and execution
  - Depending on siloed intelligence to succeed. Getting one's hands dirty is essential to being central to the deal – any deal
  - Allowing yourself to be pigeonholed into a clinical diligence corner
  - Over-relying on your medical degree as a differentiator of expertise – unless you have truly demonstrated expertise in a way that can match founding clinicians, scientists and CEO's/Board members
  - Not learning how to apply expertise and experience over general principles and fields
  - Over-applying general approaches until one has become completely dedifferentiated
  - Being a smart young person in a hurry (the next 540 pages will cover examples of people from both my academic and business experiences)

- Value of the physician perspective in the commercial world

  - Avoidance of spin
  - Hard data analytics
  - Clear understanding of adoption criteria
  - Clear understanding of physician behavior and institutional barricades
  - Balance between technology fervor and ability to reduce to practice
  - Correlation of these multiple factors into a cogent financial model and valuation metric
  - Correlation of numerous factors into a cohesive and flexible strategic plan
  - Ability to distinguish among biases in KOL and community opinions
  - Ability to discern where self promotion undermines credible opinion
  - Recognition of the different currencies in play among the drivers of life science businesses

- Currencies differ: An issue often misunderstood in managing other physicians (or any others as well)
  - Measurable economic success
  - Career advancement, i.e. new aptitudes, capabilities, progress, respect, and network
  - Contribution back to society
  - Utilization of collective experience
  - Partnerships based on trust
  - Life balance

And lastly, but most importantly, the responsibilities of a physician business leader:

- Patient focus
- Provider focus
- Data focus
- Ethical representation/analysis of company attributes, strategies, and operational goals
- Fluency in business capabilities
- Recognition of limits of direct knowledge of specific clinical fields, business issues associated, and utilization of background to consolidate the best information and practices possible

Richard Kalish MD, MS, MPH

Dr. Richard Kalish is the Medical Director of Boston HealthNet, a network of 15 community health centers, Boston Medical Center and the Boston University School of Medicine, and is a Medical Director of the Boston Medical Center HealthNet Plan, a provider-sponsored Managed Care Plan with 250,000 members throughout Massachusetts (Fig. 33.7). The Plan has members with both Medicaid and

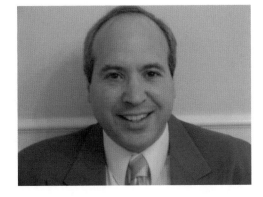

Fig. 33.7 Richard Kalish MD, MS, MPH. Medical Director, Boston HealthNet. Medical Director, Boston Medical Center HealthNet Plan. Assistant Professor of Medicine and Family Medicine, Boston University School of Medicine

Commonwealth Care, an insurance product which came about as a result of the recent healthcare reform in Massachusetts. In both of these roles, Dr. Kalish works with community health centers, hospitals serving the underserved and other safety net providers. The work involves population and disease management models aimed at improving the health of people and communities. The models focus on both chronic diseases and prevention. In addition, he has led practice redesign efforts in the network. Results have included processes to improve access in ambulatory practices and utilizing an electronic medical record for decision support, performance improvement, and to improve communication between healthcare providers.

Dr. Kalish has extensive experience working with public health officials. He worked with Massachusetts DPH officials and others as a member of a steering committee in developing a Strategic Plan for Tobacco Control in Massachusetts in 2006. In a Collaborative effort with DPH and the Massachusetts Association of Health Plans he has been on a Pandemic Flu planning team. At the local level he has worked with the Boston Public Health Commission on multiple prevention and chronic disease control efforts which have involved the Boston community health centers (CHC). At the federal level he has been the lead clinician or Principal Investigator on five Health Resources and Services Administration-funded CHC network grants focusing on coordination of care, capacity building and health information technology. In 2005 he was a civilian volunteer with the Public Health Service in disaster relief efforts in New Orleans after Hurricane Katrina. He has followed up on this commitment with coursework in disaster preparation and mitigation.

As a Board Certified internist, Dr. Kalish has a primary care panel at one of the Boston HealthNet member community health centers, the South Boston Community HealthCenter. He was the Medical Director of this community health center from 1996 to 2001. Dr. Kalish attended Brandeis University where he earned a BA in Economics. He received a Master of Science in Preventive Medicine and attended medical school at Ohio State University. He holds a Master of Public Health in Healthcare Management with an emphasis in Quality of Care and Risk Management from the Harvard School of Public Health. His medical training is in Internal Medicine at Boston City Hospital and he did a General Medicine Fellowship at Beth Israel Hospital in Boston.

Career Roadmap

- BA Brandeis University
- Research Associate, State Street Consultants
- MS Preventive Medicine, Ohio State University
- MD Ohio State University
- MPH Harvard University
- Medicine Residency, Boston City Hospital (merged with Boston University Hospital to form Boston Medical Center)

(continued)

Career Roadmap

- General Internal Medicine Fellowship, Beth Israel Hospital and Harvard Medical School
- Internist, MetroWest Medical Center
- Internist, Mount Auburn Hospital
- Medical Director, South Boston Community Center
- Medical Director, Boston Health Net
- Medical Director, Boston Medical Center HealthNet Plan
- Assistant Professor Medicine and Family Medicine, Boston University School of Medicine

Personal History

Until age 12 I lived in a Boston suburb. My father was a "jack of all trades" for a dress manufacturer for 23 years, never really enjoying any of the work. Dissatisfied with his job, he decided to uproot our family when he bought a small hotel in Miami Beach, a business he knew little about. This was uncharacteristic of him since he is very risk averse. It turned out to be a smart decision because he enjoyed the work. Although my career path has been very different than my father's, it similarly took some unexpected turns that led to a rewarding professional life.

After graduating from Miami Beach Senior High School, I enrolled at Brandeis University where I earned a BA in Economics. To this day, the principles of economic theory, including efficiency and thinking about what goes on at the margin, are those that come most naturally to me.

> **"Try to keep as many doors open as you can."**

On finishing my undergraduate work, I networked with professionals in healthcare and public health. I hoped to land a job in healthcare economics, thinking I could do some good with my interest in the "dismal science" of economics. I began working for a Boston management consulting firm which had federal government health agency contracts. I ended up not working on any of these contracts. I soon realized that this kind of work was not going to be the direction I wanted to take my career. After much soul searching and ongoing discussions with health professionals, I decided I wanted to be a physician with a focus in public health. I then told my employer of this interest and was able to work there part time while I began taking premed classes and exploring the possibility of enrolling in a graduate program in public health. The programs I looked at all indicated I would need to pick an area of concentration. Not knowing the field well enough, I decided to attend a program in Preventive Medicine at Ohio State where I would be able to take the public health core courses without "declaring a major."

I continued my premed coursework in Ohio, and, on after obtaining my Masters degree in Preventive Medicine, I moved to New York where I worked on federal agency contracts focused on collecting data on drug abuse and neonatal herpes. This work brought me in contact with physicians who straddled the fields of medicine and public health, underscoring the idea that there were many opportunities where I could combine my skills and interests. After 2 years of being based in New York City with responsibilities and travel to Boston, Buffalo, and nearby Newark, I returned to Ohio State University for medical school.

When it came time for my residency I wanted to pick a field that would not close any doors in public health and give me unquestioned clinical skills. I also wanted to work in a hospital with an underserved population where my public health interest could be further developed. The Internal Medicine residency program at Boston City Hospital, one of the major Boston University School of Medicine teaching hospitals, fit the bill. Working with physicians who were involved in clinical research led me to enroll in a General Medicine Fellowship at Beth Israel Hospital and Harvard Medical School. The focus of this program was to develop clinical research-ers. At the same time I was able to earn a MPH at Harvard. Now ready to "declare my public health major," I pursued a quality of care and risk management track within a healthcare management concentration. I realized during my fellowship that I did not want to spend most of my career in research, though I did enjoy working on a study describing the cost of major surgery complications. This work combined my interest in economics, quality of care, and clinical medicine.

My first two jobs after my fellowship were as a hospital-employed physician spending 75% of my time doing clinical work with the remainder on helping the hospital and my practice colleagues with performance improvement and other clinical administrative projects. I served on quality and utilization management committees and helped to develop selected clinical guidelines. Capitated Medicare risk contracts were becoming more common. I took on the responsibilities of analyzing the data for my group, trying to find opportunities for both better quality and efficiencies.

My next job as the medical director of the South Boston Community Health Center in 1996 was the first intersection of my interests in clinical medicine, public health, and healthcare management. For the first time I had many people reporting to me. This required me to learn line management on the job. This trial and error experience may not have been ideal, but helped me develop the managerial skills that I use today. I was both exhilarated and exhausted from managing capitated contracts, performance improvement activities, community health programs, and teaching programs for both Boston University medical students and Boston Medical Center residency programs. I also was a part-time primary care provider, a role I maintain at South Boston to this day. A few years into the job at South Boston, Boston HealthNet, the network of 15 community health centers, Boston Medical Center and the Boston University School of Medicine, was growing its clinical inte-gration activities and needed a medical director. I agreed to do this work while maintaining my medical director role at South Boston.

In 2001, the Boston Medical Center HealthNet Plan, a provider-sponsored managed care plan with only Medicaid members at the time was rapidly growing.

I agreed to become a medical director there and decided to give up my medical director role at South Boston while maintaining my clinical practice there as well as the medical directorship of Boston HealthNet.

In 2009, I added another role to my existing responsibilities. I became the Director of Community Engagement for the Boston University Clinical and Translational Science Institute, a NIH funded initiative under the Clinical and Translational Science Awards. The goal is to effectively engage communities and practices in the translational research process. We strive to define research agendas with a voice from the community. I am positioned to match BU researchers with members of the community and community health centers.

These management, academic, and clinical roles require that I work in areas including performance improvement, chronic disease management, care coordination, prevention strategies, community health initiatives, electronic health record implementation and data integration activities, and, of course, cost containment. While the list is demanding, it is validating that I am able to work alongside truly inspiring people trying to improve the lives of disadvantaged people.

Lessons Learned

- Try to keep as many doors open as you can.
- Stay clinically active. It's not just for credibility reasons. It's enjoyable and the perspective is essential.
- You will grow personally and professionally as you speak with others and explore opportunities.
- Constantly develop and cultivate new skills. This is not only valuable, but also fun.
- Career advancement depends on the ability to effectively collaborate.
- Surround yourself with people who challenge and inspire you.
- Pursue your passion. The work may be hard, but it will be more fulfilling. This is truly what matters the most.

Lisa Bard Levine, MD, MBA

Lisa Bard Levine, MD, MBA, is an Associate Director in the Healthcare Practice at Navigant Consulting, Inc. in Needham, MA (Fig. 33.8). She works with leading US healthcare organizations on physician–hospital alignment, performance excellence, and clinical service line development. Her consulting work focuses on financial, operational, and strategic healthcare redesign initiatives that improve quality and safety of patient care. Much of her work recently has been oriented around the Accountable Care Organization (ACO) and the patient-centered medical home model of primary care. Dr. Levine's career has also concentrated on mentoring emerging physician leaders. Prior to her position at Navigant Consulting, Inc., Dr. Levine was a senior consultant at The Bard Group and before that, with the

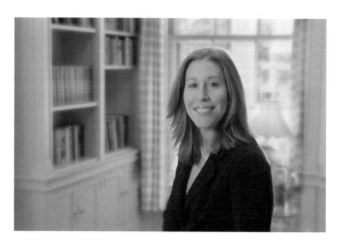

Fig. 33.8 Lisa Bard Levine, MD, MBA. Associate Director. Navigant Consulting, Inc. (formerly The Bard Group)

Mount Sinai Medical School under the Director of Business Strategy, and APM/CSC Healthcare in New York. Dr. Levine graduated from the University of Pennsylvania where she studied healthcare management. She received her MD and MBA from Tufts University and completed her internship at Newton Wellesley Hospital. After initiating her residency at Massachusetts General Hospital, Dr. Levine chose to return to her primary interest in the business and management side of healthcare and returned to her consulting career.

Career Roadmap

- BA cum laude, University of Pennsylvania
- Consultant: APM and CSC Healthcare (NY)
- Consultant: Mount Sinai Medical Center (NY)
- MD, Tufts University School of Medicine
- MBA, Tufts University School of Medicine
- Intern, Newton Wellesley Hospital (MA)
- Resident in Anesthesia and Critical Care, Massachusetts General Hospital (MA)
- Consultant: The Bard Group (MA), now Navigant Consulting, Inc.

Personal History

I knew I would always become a physician. Despite growing up under the mentorship of my father who was a successful primary care physician, physician manager and executive, and later a nationally recognized healthcare consultant and expert, the decisions about my career all came from within. I demonstrated my leadership and management skills early on as the president of my high school graduating class and was recognized as being quite savvy at business. I went to Penn and studied the pre-medical courses… as electives. I wanted to focus my studies outside of science so I tried just about every possible course in college: from sociology to nutrition to economics, Spanish and yes, to costume design (ok, truth: that class somehow fulfilled some requirement needed to graduate. I hope Penn has caught on by now). I spent my free time as the women's ice hockey goalie and captain throughout my 4 years at Penn.

"Know your true north …"

Through coursework and internships, I found that my passion lay at the intersection of the clinical and the business sides of healthcare. I guess that is when I realized that my DNA won, despite trying to fighting it. I was an intern at APM while at Penn (now CSC Healthcare) and worked on a large strategy and operations redesign for a prominent academic medical center. I was put in front of senior leadership very early on: in fact, I can recall one meeting with a Department Head and me alone, and he asked "so what gives you the experience to be telling me this?" and to this day I have no idea how I squeaked out of that meeting, just prior to my senior year in college. But memories of that meeting do bring back some palpitations. After Penn I recognized that there was an in-depth understanding of how healthcare organizations run that I needed to understand before I entered it as a physician. So I returned to APM/CSC Healthcare and worked on the East Coast to help healthcare provider organizations redesign and reorganize how they deliver clinical care, optimize their revenue cycle and develop standardized approaches to patient care.

Ultimately, several of us former consultant colleagues reunited together at the Mount Sinai Medical School and its Faculty Practice as internal consultants. I focused on strategy, revenue enhancement opportunities, and I developed electronic tools for financial reporting and modeling. At this time, I also got the privilege of staffing a large national search for the new chief of cardiovascular surgery at Mount Sinai – I am not sure if Boston has yet forgiven me for recruiting a rising young star from the Brigham and Women's Hospital.

I deferred medical school for a period of time, and realized that after 3 years in operations and strategy of healthcare systems, it was now time to learn how to be a physician and work within this complex system. By this time, I felt prepared and enrolled in an intense MD/MBA program (at the time, this was just about the only integrated program in the country). It was the perfect fit. I vowed that I would never go back to school again after this, unless it was for cooking (ok I have done that now). I was an informed student and carefully explored clinical careers. I analyzed clinical rotations, and took a systems approach to everything. I tended to look at fields of medicine not from the resident's perspective, but from the attendee's perspective – "what would his or her career be like?" I wanted strong clinical training and did an intense transitional internship at Newton Wellesley Hospital (surgery/ICU/medicine), working with amazing physicians. Then I chose to train at

Massachusetts General Hospital in anesthesiology – and I chose that field carefully. Several factors played a role including:

- Where were the people "like me" who understood the business and clinical sides of healthcare and who had experiences and interests in both?
- Where could I find and leverage a strong female mentor who balanced hospital leadership with clinical responsibilities?
- Where could I find a career which would enable me to divide my time and interests between the clinical and business sides of healthcare?
- Where did the physicians seem truly happy?
- Where did the physicians seem to have the ability to balance both a career and a family?
- Where were there significant advances in patient safety?
- Where would I have the time and be able to have an intimate conversation with a patient, comfort them, while managing only their care at the time?
- Where could I feel that at the end of the day I had finished something? I needed some send of instant gratification for patient care and sense of completion.

However rational these elements appear, I soon realized that the decision to pursue whatever clinical field is still for the most part completely uninformed – for it is not until you truly own the patients and are managing their care as a resident and attending do you experience what it is like be a physician. This lesson is difficult for many who like making informed decisions, like just about every medical student I have ever met.

During my internship and the start of my residency I realized a few things:

1. I took my systems perspective everywhere I went and found the urge to uncover why certain systems operated suboptimally; and I wanted to fix them now
2. I found the urge to improve systems of care delivery and couldn't wait, but was not yet in a position to do so
3. I really disliked doing interventional procedures and using needles in any form on patients
4. I missed the business and management side of healthcare

Despite it being a difficult decision, I left clinical medicine. It was the right decision for me and the best decision I ever made. I was worried at what the world around me would say, for clinical medicine is a field in which most people do not leave: I was surprised by the support, encouragement and respect that this "bold" move elicited in people. I could never have anticipated it, but I have been so fulfilled personally, that it confirmed my decision. Coincidentally, the Bard Group was growing, a healthcare consulting strategy firm with niche in marketplace for engaging physicians. The COO hired me as part of the growth strategy and I managed recruiting and grew the firm of healthcare professionals from 10 to 45 in about 2 years. I also developed programs, education, and infrastructure as needed, managed the *Bard Group Weekly Digest,* wrote white papers, and was a physician consultant. It was in December of 2008 that the Bard Group was acquired by Navigant Consulting, Inc. And the rest is history.

One helpful book we often suggest our clients to read is Jim Collins' book *Good to Great*. In his book, Collins tells the story of Isaiah Berlin's essay *The Hedgehog and the Fox*. Berlin had extrapolated from the parable that people are essentially divided into two groups: foxes and hedgehogs. Berlin's premise states that "… foxes are scattered or diffused, moving on many levels…never integrating their thinking into one overall concept or unifying vision. Hedgehogs, on the other hand simplify a complex world into a single organizing idea, a basic principle, or concept that unifies and guides everything." This helped establish what Collins refers to as the "Hedgehog Concept." As defined by Collins "a Hedgehog Concept is a simple, crystalline concept that flows from a deep understanding about the following three circles." There are three intersecting circles: What you are passionate about? What you can be best at? and What drives your economic engine? It is at the intersection of these three circles that I believe you should use to set your own personal compass.

Lessons Learned

- Know your *True North* – know what stirs your passion and what is most important to you and work your life around it to achieve personal peace (family, career achievements, fame, etc)
- Keep an open mind – a straight path is not necessary for success in today's world, and increasingly less common
- Ask lots of questions – about yourself and about the world around you
- Find strong role models – and good peers
- Take risks – and opportunities as they arise
- Read Jim Collins' *Good To Great*
- Remember that Generation Y is vastly different from generations before us: acknowledge this and take advantage of it
- Listen to yourself
- Enjoy what you are doing (or your destination)

N. Stephen Ober, MD, MBA

Dr. N. Stephen Ober is Executive Director of Business Incubation at Boston University (BU), where he assists faculty members commercialize technologies and start new companies (Fig. 33.9). The BU business incubator hosts 13 emerging companies in the Life Science and Engineering industries. In 2008, Dr. Ober became faculty Director for BU's MD/MBA dual degree program. Under Dr. Ober's guidance, the MD/MBA program has grown dramatically and the student run Medicine and Business Association (MBA) boasts over 200 medical student members, making

Fig. 33.9 N. Stephen Ober, MD. Executive Director, Business Incubation. Faculty Director, MD/MBA Dual Degree Program. Boston University

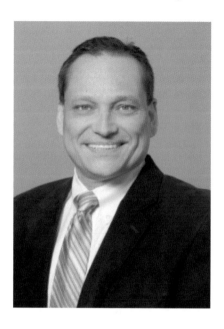

it the largest student organization on campus. Prior to joining BU in 2004, Dr. Ober was cofounder and president of BG Medicine a biotechnology company that developed and applied a unique "systems biology" approach to drug discovery and development. Prior to BG, Dr. Ober was president and chief executive officer of Synergy, a successful health information and data management company. Synergy was founded by Dr. Ober in 1995 and was acquired by ENVOY Corp. in 1998. As part of ENVOY, Synergy developed leading-edge technologies and analytic methods to develop one of the industry's largest and unique healthcare data warehouses based on real-time, patient-level electronic claims data. In March 1999, ENVOY was acquired by Quintiles Transnational, the world's largest Clinical Research Organization (CRO). At Quintiles, Dr. Ober successfully integrated Synergy's data and technology into Quintiles' drug development processes to improve the efficiency of drug clinical trials. Prior to Synergy, Dr. Ober spent 5 years as executive vice president and corporate medical director of Private Healthcare Systems (PHCS), one of the largest national managed care companies in the country. At PHCS (now Multi Plan), Dr. Ober managed product development, quality management, medical management, outcomes management, and headed several strategic systems development initiatives. Dr. Ober received his BA and MD degrees from Boston University, his clinical training in surgery and orthopedic surgery from University of California San Diego, and his MBA from the Harvard Graduate School of Business.

Career Roadmap

- BA Boston University
- MD Boston University
- Orthopedic Surgery Residency, University California San Diego
- MBA Harvard Business School
- Corporate Medical Director, Private Healthcare Systems, Inc.
- Founder and CEO, Synergy Healthcare, Inc.
- President Synergy Division, Quintiles Transnational
- Cofounder and President, BG Medicine
- Consultant, Philips Medical Systems
- Executive Director, New ventures and Business Incubation, Boston University

> *"Never give up in pursuing a career interest, no matter how bleak the prospects may look."*

Personal History

I grew up in a suburb of Boston to a middle-class family. My father had an entrepreneurial spirit and started a trucking company with his brothers when I was quite young. At the age of 3 I was diagnosed with fibrous dysplasia, a rare congenital bone disease effecting my left leg and right arm. I had approximately 13 major orthopedic surgeries and numerous hospitalizations to treat femur fractures and complications by the time I was a college sophomore. These medical experiences early in life had a great negative psychological impact on me at the time; however, I also developed a tremendous interest in medicine – especially orthopedics. In retrospect, I think this fascination with the profession of my treating physician might have been some type of defense mechanism. By focusing on the technical aspects of my care there was less time to dwell on the pain and disappointments I was experiencing. During college I was fortunate enough to be selected for an early acceptance program to BU School of Medicine. While on crutches for much of my medical school years, I managed to fulfill all the requirements and graduate with my class. Upon graduation I was fortunate to be accepted to several orthopedic surgery residency programs. For my general surgery internship I matched at University California San Diego. I was thrilled with my choices and looked forward to 6 years of residency in a specialty which I loved. However, late in my internship year my fibrous dysplasia once again caused me to sustain another severe hip fracture. While undergoing treatment, I built a strong relationship with the orthopedic attending managing my care. In addition to being at the top of his clinical career, he had interests outside medicine and had performed many business pursuits on behalf of the hospital and others. He quickly became my mentor and he spoke a great deal about the realities of life as a surgeon with fibrous dysplasia. In a nutshell, he strongly recommended that I find a different career that would be less physically demanding on my leg and a career where time off for treatment of my condition would be less disruptive than orthopedic surgery. I thought he was crazy. But the more we spoke and the more time I had to reflect on the reality of my situation, the more I came to realize that he was right. So after leaving the residency program, I spent the following year networking with physicians working outside full-time clinical medicine and working with BU professor Dr. Richard "Dick" Egdahl, a surgeon, hospital administrator, and entrepreneur. This year was a turning point in my life. The guidance and mentorship Dr. Egdahl provided me was invaluable as I weighed my career options. Together we started a successful medical software company called Health Payment Review, Inc. (HPR). My main responsibility in the company was sales, marketing, and client support, areas that I immediately enjoyed. The fast pace, long hours and short-term rewards (commissions on signing new customers) reminded me of being a surgical resident. After that year I was determined to utilize my clinical training in a way other than direct patient care. The software developed by HPR was an expert system that used clinical algorithms to appropriately code medical claims for physician reimbursement. As a physician I was very effective at communicating the logic utilized by the system to arrive at an appropriate decision. I learned quickly that my credibility as a clinical "expert" was actually greater outside the medical realm than inside. However, I knew nothing about the world of business. Not being board certified in a clinical specialty also made me feel inadequate as a physician. To address both these issues I decided to go back to the classroom and obtain an MBA. I was fortunate to be accepted to the Harvard Graduate School of Business in 1989 at the age of 30, older than all of my business school peers. Adjusting to the classroom experience and being the oldest in my class section was difficult at first. But with hard work and support from my wife and friends I graduated with my classmates after 2 years of full-time study. For me, attaining the MBA was akin to being board certified in orthopedic surgery. I also learned a great deal during those 2 years about myself as I planned my new career track. I realized early on that I enjoyed being the "boss" and making my own decisions. Combining that with the positive experience at HPR, I knew that the only career for me had to involve starting my own company. Unfortunately, there was one major obstacle that kept me from doing this right after business school – money. Years of living on a house officer's salary and the Harvard tuition had taken its financial toll. I knew my entrepreneurial dreams would have to wait until I had enough capital to pay down my debts and endure the financial risk inherent in starting a new venture. This is where the blend of my clinical expertise and new business credential really paid off. I was quickly offered a position as the executive vice president and corporate medical director of Private Healthcare Systems, one of the largest managed care companies in the country at the time. The six figure salary and the senior role reinforced my belief that I made the right decisions. After 5 years at PHCS I left to finally fulfill the dream of starting my own company. The rest of my story to present involves starting other ventures over the years and eventually ending up working at my alma mater in a position that affords me the opportunity to mentors entrepreneurs and work closely with a variety of start-up companies. I consider myself blessed to have the good fortune of meeting mentor along my journey and receiving sage advice along the way. I love what I do and have no regrets about what I have accomplished. When given lemons I simply made lemonade.

Lessons Learned

- Never give up in pursuing a career interest, no matter how bleak the prospects may look.
- Find and use mentors. They are your greatest asset.
- Network, network, and network. Talk to as many people in the fields that interest you as possible.
- Explore all career alternatives no matter how extreme they may initially feel.
- Enter your new career search with the same focus, dedication, and determination you had when you were a medical student and full-time physician.
- Try to test the new career waters first by doing part-time work in your field of interest before jumping in full time.
- Never forget your clinical roots. You have a truly unique skill set that people recognize. Learn how to leverage this credibility and use it at every step in your journey.

Peter L. Slavin, MD, MBA

Since January 2003, Dr. Peter L. Slavin has served as president of the Massachusetts General Hospital, an institution to which he has dedicated much of his career (Fig. 33.10). Dr. Slavin first joined the hospital staff as a primary care physician in 1987 after completing his residency in internal medicine there. In his first years at the MGH, in addition to practicing and teaching medicine, Dr. Slavin held various management roles, notably developing the hospital's first quality and utilization management program.

In 1994, Dr. Slavin was selected senior vice president and chief medical officer of the MGH, as well as medical director of the Massachusetts General Physicians Organization, the largest multispecialty physician group in the state, 1 year later. During this time, Dr. Slavin – an avid Boston sports fan – also was on the medical staff of the New England Patriots and New England Revolution.

In 1997, Dr. Slavin was recruited to serve as the first president of the newly merged Barnes-Jewish Hospital in St. Louis, Missouri, the largest teaching hospital in the state. Two years later, he returned to Boston and became chief executive officer of the MGPO, as well as chair of the MGPO Board of Trustees. In 2003, he was appointed president of the MGH.

Fig. 33.10 Peter L. Slavin,
MD, MBA. President.
Massachusetts General
Hospital

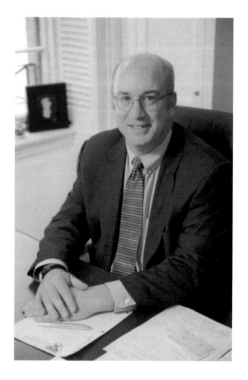

At the MGH, Dr. Slavin has championed transparency and tracking measures of performance to improve care, overseeing the establishment of the Center for Quality and Safety. To ensure that quality care is accessible to all, Dr. Slavin was a strong advocate in creating the Disparities Solutions Center, and has worked to ensure that improving community health is integral to the fabric of the MGH, leading the adoption of a revised hospital mission statement to reflect this commitment in 2007. Dr. Slavin has cultivated a culture of innovation at the MGH, made evident by the recent establishment of an Innovation Support Center and the impressive amount of funding available for research at the hospital. Currently, Dr. Slavin and other hospital leaders are increasing their focus on efforts to improve care while reducing costs.

> *"Never take your eye off the ultimate goal of providing great patient care."*

Dr. Slavin has adeptly guided the MGH as its campus transitions to meet growing demands of patient care and research, supervising the opening of a number of new facilities, including the Lunder Building, a state-of-art patient care facility housing the latest in technology and slated for completion 2011 – the hospital's bicentennial. Dr. Slavin also has helped foster relationships with other institutions, including the Massachusetts Eye and Ear Infirmary, and overseen the integration of Nantucket Cottage Hospital, Martha's Vineyard Hospital and the renowned Benson-Henry Institute for Mind Body Medicine into the MGH family.

As president, Dr. Slavin represents the MGH within a number of organizations and has held leadership positions with the Massachusetts Hospital Association, the Massachusetts Life Sciences Center and the American Association of Medical Colleges. Most recently, in 2010, Dr. Slavin was selected as chair of the administrative board of the AAMC's Council of Teaching Hospitals and Health Systems.

A professor of Healthcare Policy at Harvard Medical School, where he has been a faculty member since 1987, Dr. Slavin speaks widely on the topics of quality and utilization management, the economics of teaching hospitals, and the state of physician practices. In recent years, he has been actively involved in a committee working to design a combined MD/MBA program at Harvard.

Dr. Slavin received his bachelor of arts in biochemistry from Harvard College, his medical degree from HMS, and his master of business administration from Harvard Business School. Early in his career, Dr. Slavin worked in Washington, DC, in the Office of US Representative Ed Markey and the Office of the Director of the National Institutes of Health.

Career Roadmap

- Harvard College
- Harvard Medical School
- Resident in Internal Medicine, MGH
- Staff physician, MGH
- Instructor, HMS
- Harvard Business School
- Senior vice president and chief medical officer, MGH
- Medical director, MGPO
- President, Barnes-Jewish Hospital
- CEO and chair, MGPO
- President, MGH

Personal History

Many physicians have a pivotal moment in their childhood that influenced them to pursue a medical career. For me, that experience came at the age of 5, when I developed a severe case of staphylococcal pneumonia and had to be admitted to the intensive care unit at Boston Children's Hospital.

I was in the ICU for several days, and it wasn't clear that I would survive – but in addition to curing me, the care I received at Children's Hospital truly amazed me. I was mesmerized by the technology my caregivers utilized and inspired by the knowledge and kindness of my physicians, particularly my pediatrician, Albert Frank, MD.

From that time on, I knew I wanted to be a doctor. Growing up in the Boston area, surrounded by nationally acclaimed hospitals and top-notch medical schools, medicine felt like the perfect choice, and I enrolled in Harvard College in 1976 as a biochemistry major. I was not your typical premedical student, though. While I spent a lot of time in the classroom and laboratory, I also was in a number of student organizations focused on political and public policy issues. My family had always been active in local Democratic politics, and early on I was taught the importance of civil involvement and engaging in community issues.

These extracurricular interests eventually led me to volunteer in Massachusetts Democrat Ed Markey's local congressional campaign. He won the election, and I was given the chance to join his staff in Washington, DC, during the summer of 1977. Working with Markey on the issues he addressed as a member of the Health Subcommittee of the Interstate Commerce Committee, I saw how my passion for medicine and politics could intersect.

After graduating from Harvard College, I moved back to DC to be a legislative analyst in the Office of the Director of the National Institutes of Health, learning even more about health policy and the inner workings of Washington. In 1981, I returned to Boston to begin medical school at Harvard.

Among the many specialties I was exposed to at HMS, primary care stood out. I found the science behind primary care to be both broad and challenging. Most important, I cherished the lasting relationships I developed with my patients. I decided to pursue my interest in primary care and applied for a residency in primary care/internal medicine at the MGH, an institution I grew up hearing about. My great-grandfather, an immigrant from Lithuania, had suffered an accident which resulted in a wood chip being embedded in his leg. He developed a severe infection, and for nearly a decade, he and his daughter – my grandmother – traveled weekly to the MGH for care. The care was free, and it kept my great-grandfather alive and well for many years. My grandmother frequently spoke of the MGH and the wonderful care it offered.

As a resident, I found that the MGH lived up to the praise of my grandmother, in addition to exceeding my own expectations. The hospital was vibrant with innovation in research and patient care, and each patient encounter was as educational as it was rewarding. More and more, though, I felt myself drawn to the larger systems at work behind each of my colleague's interactions with patients. I realized that the managers of institutions like the MGH made decisions about healthcare cost, quality, and access on a daily basis, and that these decisions directly and significantly impacted care. Yet I sensed a divide between physicians and managers, and it was apparent to me that someone with a background in both medicine and management might be able to effectively bridge the gap.

Toward the end of my residency, I was fortunate enough to care for an individual who confirmed my theory that medicine and management training might go hand-in-hand: former HBS Dean Lawrence Fouraker. After discussing my career interests and experiences, he encouraged me to attend business school. I was hesitant. I was about to finish my medical training – going back to school seemed counterintuitive. In addition, pursuing both a medical degree and master of business administration was quite unusual at the time.

I eventually decided to follow Dean Fouraker's advice and applied and was accepted into HBS. My education there was as intensive and stimulating as medical school, and had a similar takeaway: I learned how to diagnose an organization's problems and come up with a treatment plan to solve them.

Juggling business school and my career as a physician was as difficult as I expected it to be. I remember one instance at HBS when I was paged during a marketing final and ended up spending much of the exam time on the phone with a patient experiencing chest pain. Fortunately, the patient turned out to be OK, and I passed the exam.

The challenges were as numerous as they were worthwhile. As graduation approached, I was impressed with the number of opportunities available to me. I considered various fields – including nonmedical ones – but finally chose to return to the MGH. There, in addition to practicing and teaching primary care, I took on several key management roles related to healthcare cost and quality, and was proud to develop the hospital's first quality and utilization management program.

Following a change in leadership, in 1994, I was asked to become chief medical officer and senior vice president at the MGH, and in 1995, medical director of the MGPO. I spent several years in these roles, with my most significant management responsibility being to lead an institution-wide effort aimed at redesigning how care is organized and delivered.

In 1997, I was recruited to Barnes-Jewish Hospital in St. Louis, Missouri, where I served as president of the newly merged institution. The experience was amazing, but Boston and the MGH were home, and after 2 years, I returned as chief executive officer and chair of the MGPO. These roles with the MGPO ultimately helped prepare me to take on what has been the most challenging but immensely rewarding position of my career so far: president of the MGH.

Lessons Learned

- Finances are only a means to an end. Never take your eye off the ultimate goal of providing great patient care.
- Hire people who are energetic, talented, and truly believe in sustaining your organization's mission – and then stay out of their way.
- Make career decisions with your head *and* with your heart. Not only will you enjoy what you're doing more, you'll do a better job of it.
- Make sure to maintain a balance between work and personal life. Sometimes this means saying no to professional activities, and that's OK. I view my career as the icing on the cake – time with my wife and two sons is truly the cake.

Index

R.D. Urman and J.M. Ehrenfeld (eds.), *Physicians' Pathways to Non-Traditional
Careers and Leadership Opportunities*, DOI 10.1007/978-1-4614-0551-1,
© Springer Science+Business Media, LLC 2012

Printed by Printforce, the Netherlands